Palliative Psychology

Palliative Psychology

CLINICAL PERSPECTIVES ON AN EMERGING SPECIALTY

E. ALESSANDRA STRADA, PHD, MSCP, CCH, FT, CCFP

Licensed Clinical Psychologist
Palliative Care and Hospice Consultant
Adjunct Faculty, Psychopharmacology Program
Alliant International University, San Francisco
Adjunct Faculty, California Institute of Integral Studies
San Francisco, California

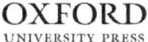

OXFORD
UNIVERSITY PRESS

Oxford University Press is a department of the University of Oxford. It furthers
the University's objective of excellence in research, scholarship, and education
by publishing worldwide. Oxford is a registered trade mark of Oxford University
Press in the UK and certain other countries.

Published in the United States of America by Oxford University Press
198 Madison Avenue, New York, NY 10016, United States of America.

© Oxford University Press 2018

All rights reserved. No part of this publication may be reproduced, stored in
a retrieval system, or transmitted, in any form or by any means, without the
prior permission in writing of Oxford University Press, or as expressly permitted
by law, by license, or under terms agreed with the appropriate reproduction
rights organization. Inquiries concerning reproduction outside the scope of the
above should be sent to the Rights Department, Oxford University Press, at the
address above.

You must not circulate this work in any other form
and you must impose this same condition on any acquirer.

CIP data is on file at the Library of Congress
ISBN 978-0-19-979855-1

This material is not intended to be, and should not be considered, a substitute for medical or other professional
advice. Treatment for the conditions described in this material is highly dependent on the individual
circumstances. And, while this material is designed to offer accurate information with respect to the subject
matter covered and to be current as of the time it was written, research and knowledge about medical and
health issues is constantly evolving and dose schedules for medications are being revised continually, with
new side effects recognized and accounted for regularly. Readers must therefore always check the product
information and clinical procedures with the most up-to-date published product information and data sheets
provided by the manufacturers and the most recent codes of conduct and safety regulation. The publisher
and the authors make no representations or warranties to readers, express or implied, as to the accuracy
or completeness of this material. Without limiting the foregoing, the publisher and the authors make no
representations or warranties as to the accuracy or efficacy of the drug dosages mentioned in the material. The
authors and the publisher do not accept, and expressly disclaim, any responsibility for any liability, loss or risk
that may be claimed or incurred as a consequence of the use and/or application of any of the contents of this
material.

9 8 7 6 5 4 3 2 1

Printed by WebCom, Inc., Canada

Contents

Preface vii
Acknowledgments ix
Introduction to Palliative Psychology xi

1. The First Domain of Palliative Care: Structure and Processes of Care 1

2. The Second Domain of Palliative Care: Physical Aspects of Care 35

3. The Third Domain of Palliative Care: Psychological and Psychiatric Aspects of Care 65

4. The Fourth Domain of Palliative Care: Social Aspects of Care 105

5. The Fifth Domain of Palliative Care: Spiritual, Religious, and Existential Aspects of Care 143

6. The Sixth Domain of Palliative Care: Cultural Aspects of Care 173

7. The Seventh Domain of Palliative Care: Care of the Patient at the End of Life 206

8. The Eighth Domain of Palliative Care: Ethical and Legal Aspects of Care 238

Index 267

Preface

The field of palliative care has grown significantly and has received increasing attention for the great benefits it brings to patients and family caregivers. Health-care professionals who recognize the complex needs created by serious illness are advocating the integration of palliative care close to the time of diagnosis. Old myths about palliative care are being dispelled, and it is now being increasingly offered to patients concurrent with disease-modifying treatment because it provides additional layers of valuable physical, emotional, and spiritual support.

Providing specialist-level and evidence-based psychological assessment and intervention to patients with serious illness and their families can become a critical need. This is especially important when complex clinical circumstances create suffering. While this book is intended to be valuable for different psychosocial professionals, it is written especially for psychologists who are interested in pursuing a career in palliative and hospice care.

I have two goals in writing this book: first, to present several clinical perspectives on the unique and integrated role possible for palliative psychologists on a palliative care and hospice team; and second, to advocate for the formalization of a new specialty, palliative psychology, which defines the roles and competencies of psychologists working in palliative care. Social work and spiritual care have been historically the core psychosocial disciplines. With the necessary training and skills, palliative psychologists should also become fully integrated in the interdisciplinary palliative care team.

My career as a clinical psychologist has focused on palliative care. I have been fortunate to serve as a core member of specialist palliative care teams and to provide care in a variety of inpatient and outpatient settings, including intensive care units, step-down units, oncology floors, chemotherapy and radiation oncology suites, palliative care clinics, and hospice. I have served as a rural community practitioner as well as a program director in an academic setting and multispecialty hospital.

In the different settings, I have found that patients with serious illness and their family caregivers have multiple, complex, and ongoing psychological needs. The specialized assessment and intervention skills of a palliative psychologist can make significant contributions to the relief of suffering. And, by working collaboratively with nurses and physicians, social workers, spiritual care providers, and music and art therapists, palliative psychologists can become valued and relied-upon members of the interdisciplinary palliative care and hospice team.

Acknowledgments

I would like to thank the editorial and production team at Oxford University Press. Their professionalism and support have been critical to the completion of this book.

I could not have written this book or learned anything about palliative care without all the patients and families who have allowed me to bear witness to their unique stories of hope, grief, perseverance, and love. Each story is complex, with deeper layers that often elude our understanding, requiring our full presence with humility and authenticity.

I am also grateful to the mentors and colleagues who have inspired me with their knowledge, talent, wisdom, and intuition. Finally, I would like to thank my very special family for their love and support and their willingness to celebrate every small gift in life, and I give gratitude to my loved ones who are no longer here, but whose presence continues to warm my heart and enrich my life.

Introduction to Palliative Psychology

Developed initially as a medical subspecialty, palliative care in the 21st century has increasingly become an important area also for psychosocial and spiritual care professionals. Specialty trainings and certifications in palliative care are now available not only for physicians but also for nurses, nurse practitioners, social workers, and chaplains. A rapidly growing field, palliative care has become progressively integrated into mainstream care, with 63% of all US hospitals and 85% of medium- to large-sized hospitals reporting the existence of a palliative care team (Voelker, 2011). The significant popularity and growth of palliative care, especially in the outpatient setting, has also evidenced a shortage of palliative care clinicians, which has been estimated between 6,000 and 18,000 (Blackhall et al., 2016). Indeed, as health-care providers, patients and family caregivers become more aware of the potential benefit of palliative care services in serious and advanced illness, as well as end of life, the demand for these services is likely to continue to increase.

The complex needs of increasing numbers of patients living with serious and advanced illness is also a reason for this growth. Most people in developed countries are diagnosed with a serious, chronic, and progressive illness before they die and will live longer with chronic and serious illness due to advancements in medicine. Their disease can last a variable period of time, including many years. The presence of medical and psychiatric comorbidities often adds to the overall burden and distress for each patient.

Living with illness raises numerous physical and psychological challenges for patients and for the family members who care for them. And it impacts every aspect of existence: physical, psychological, social, cultural, spiritual, and existential. Ensuring the best possible quality of life for these patients and their family caregivers has become a mandate for comprehensive and patient-centered health care. It is critically important to address their needs throughout the continuum of care by providing relief not only from pain and other physical symptoms but also from the psychological distress that is associated with the disease process.

Defining Palliative Care

Several definitions of palliative care have been proposed reflecting its comprehensive focus. The World Health Organization (WHO) has championed several global palliative care initiatives, starting in the early 1980s, aimed at improving pain and symptoms management for patients with cancer and HIV/AIDS. It has defined palliative care as "an approach that improves the quality of life of patients and their families facing the problems associated with life-threatening illness, through the prevention and relief of suffering by means of early identification and impeccable assessment and treatment of pain, and other problems, physical, psychosocial, and spiritual" (Sepulveda et al., 2002).

According to the US Department of Health and Human Services Centers for Medicare and Medicare, palliative care means "patient and family-centered care that optimizes quality of life by anticipating, preventing, and treating suffering. Palliative care throughout the continuum of illness involves addressing physical, intellectual, emotional, social, and spiritual needs and to facilitate patient autonomy, access to information, and choice" (Centers for Medicare and Medicaid, 2008). According to the Center to Advance Palliative Care, "The goal is to improve quality of life for both the patient and the family. Palliative care is provided by a team of doctors, nurses and other specialists who work together with a patient's other doctors to provide an extra layer of support. It is appropriate at any age and at any stage in a serious illness and can be provided along with curative treatment" (Center to Advance Palliative Care). Palliative care is also defined as "an interdisciplinary therapeutic model appropriate for all populations with serious or life-threatening illness, the goals of which is to prevent and manage suffering and illness burden for both patient and family from the time of diagnosis onward" (Portenoy, 2014). Furthermore, the *Clinical Practice Guidelines for Quality Palliative Care* (2013) explain that "palliative care is operationalized through effective management of pain and other distressing symptoms, while incorporating psychosocial and spiritual care with constant durations of patient/family needs, preferences, values, beliefs, and culture. Evaluation and treatment should be comprehensive and patient centered with a focus on the central role of the family unit in decision-making. Palliative care affirms life by supporting the patient and family's goals for the future, including their hopes for cure or life prolongation, as well as their hopes for peace and dignity throughout the course of illness, the dying process, and death" (p. 9). While each definition emphasizes different aspects, they all underline the importance of providing expert emotional and psychological assessment and intervention to patients and families across the illness trajectory, from the time of diagnosis to end of life and extending into bereavement.

The rapid growth of palliative care over the last decade and its presence in different settings have highlighted the need to identify specific competencies to ensure clinical excellence. The National Consensus Project brought together major hospice and palliative care organizations and identified eight domains of palliative care and defined clinical practice guidelines (Box I.1). These describe best practices in the different areas of each domain. The latest revision, in 2013, was the result of a collaboration between several organizations: the American Academy of Hospice and Palliative Medicine, the Center to Advance Palliative Care, the Hospice and Palliative Nurses Association, the National Palliative Care Research Center, the National Association of Social Workers, and the National Hospice and Palliative Care Organization.

Palliative care involves both a philosophy and systems of care delivery. The philosophy is grounded in a holistic patient-centered perspective focused on identifying sources of discomfort, distress, and suffering in the patient and the family, and on mitigating

> **Box I.1 Domains of Palliative Care**
>
> 1. Structure and Processes of Care
> 2. Physical Aspects of Care
> 3. Psychological and Psychiatric Aspects of Care
> 4. Social Aspects of Care
> 5. Spiritual, Religious, and Existential Aspects of Care
> 6. Cultural Aspects of Care
> 7. Care of the Patient at the End of Life
> 8. Ethical and Legal Aspects of Care
>
> ---
>
> Adapted and modified from National Consensus Project for Quality Palliative Care. (2013). *Clinical Practice Guidelines for Quality Palliative Care.*

such suffering. Improving quality of life for the patient and the family through continual assessment, identification, and active management of distress represents the essential goal of palliative care, regardless of diagnosis or prognosis. This multifaceted goal is accomplished through a model of care delivery based on careful and ongoing assessment of the multiple and complex needs of the patient and the family that can start at any point during the illness, ideally starting at the time of diagnosis. Palliative care continues during end of life and with expert grief and bereavement support for grieving family members and other caregivers who have been part of the patient's network of support.

Additionally, palliative care does not focus on curing disease; it focuses on allowing the patient to experience the best quality of life possible for as long as possible and supporting the family. "Quality of life" is a complex construct. In this context, it is utilized to indicate the degree to which the patient and the family needs are met in the essential domains of human existence: the physical domain, the social domain, the psychological domain, the spiritual domain, and the cultural domain. Patients and families define for themselves their needs and values as they cope with illness. Palliative care clinicians are committed to recognizing, understanding, and addressing these unique needs, which may continue to evolve in complexity based on the patient's unique circumstances. This includes a commitment to affirming and honoring cultural values and preferences.

Finally, palliative care is best provided within an interdisciplinary model that uses a team of specialists from different disciplines. The interdisciplinary approach is integrative, with the different disciplines working together to address the different needs of the patient and the family. While the disciplines may share approaches and modalities, each retains its identity and the boundaries among disciplines are clearly defined. For example, psychology has aspects in common with social work, spiritual care, psychiatry, nursing, and creative arts modalities. However, like other disciplines, psychology also retains methodologies and approaches in assessment and interventions that are unique to its domain.

Commonly, palliative care is delivered within a consultation model, with palliative care clinicians working in collaboration with the primary medical team to provide the patient and the family with additional levels of *specialized support*.

Palliative care can be provided as the main modality of care, or it can be provided together with disease-modifying treatments. While initially it was mostly made available for patients with cancer, palliative care is now commonly addressing the needs of patients with chronic obstructive lung disease (COPD), congestive heart failure (CHF), HIV-AIDS, renal disease, dementia, neurological disorders and others (Vermylen et al., 2015; Fendler et al., 2015; Shah et al., 2013; Weingaertner et al., 2014; Burns & McIlfatrick, 2015).

Initially focused on adult patients, palliative care is now increasingly available for children and teenagers diagnosed with serious and chronic illness and their families. Pediatric palliative care is recognized as a special field dedicated to supporting the child and the family from diagnosis, throughout treatment and, in the event of the child's death, in bereavement. The overall goals of addressing physical, psychological, and spiritual needs are similar to palliative care for adults. However, caring for children who are ill and approaching the dying process requires specialized training and skills (Wolfe et al. Hinds, & Sourkes, 2011). Alleviating physical suffering, addressing complications of advanced disease, promoting effective communication, and assisting parents with complex and emotionally difficult decision-making are important tasks of palliative care clinicians working with the pediatric population. These require not only medical knowledge of the disease process, but also an understanding of child psychological development, family functioning, and parenting styles. The physical and psychological needs of teenagers and young adults diagnosed with cancer are similarly complex because their developmental stage is characterized by major transitions, as well as the aggressiveness that frequently characterizes the disease (Kuehn, 2016).

To summarize, palliative care has several core principles that guide care delivery in the different settings irrespective of diagnosis and prognosis:

- It is a patient- and family-centered model of care based on a biopsychosocial spiritual understanding of illness and its impact on the individual and the family system.
- It can be provided to patients concurrent with curative and life-prolonging treatment, or independent of those treatments.
- While it includes care for the patient who is at the end of life, it may begin at the time of diagnosis irrespective of prognosis.
- It focuses on identifying and managing sources of discomfort, distress, and suffering while improving quality of life for patients with serious, chronic, and advanced illness, including end of life.
- It actively addresses psychological and psychiatric needs of patients and families by providing assessment, treatment, and coordination of care. It includes grief and bereavement care during illness, during the dying process, and in bereavement.
- It is provided to the patient and the family, in an effort to improve all aspects of quality of life, including relationships, coping, and communication.
- Palliative care is a life-affirming approach. It recognizes and validates individual and family strengths, and it encourages reconnection with sources of meaning and purpose that can support the family system. Palliative care clinicians support positive experiences, connectedness, and personal transformation acknowledging the depths and the richness of human experience, even in the midst of serious challenges.

Generalist and Specialist Palliative Care

All palliative care can be provided through skills at the generalist level and at the specialist level irrespective of the setting of care. It has been argued *that generalist palliative care*, also called "primary" or "basic" palliative care, represents *best practice* for all clinicians working with seriously ill patients. "Best practices" in health care are described as "activities, disciplines and methods that are available to identify, implement and monitor the available evidence in health care" (Perleth, Jakubowski & Busse, 2001).

Because palliative care was initially conceptualized as a medical specialty, these different skill levels have initially been described for physicians. For example, primary care physicians may play an important role in supporting patients with serious illness and their families by providing basic management of pain and other symptoms, as well as depression and anxiety. In fact, the majority of prescriptions for psychotropic medication to treat depression or anxiety in the United States are currently being written by primary care physicians (Cunningham, 2009). Additionally, a systematic review indicated that when primary care physicians are involved in end-of-life care, patients are more likely to die out of the hospital (Kim & Tarn, 2016). These results point to the valuable role that primary care physicians can play in identifying patients with palliative care needs, assisting with clarifying goals of care, decreasing hospitalizations, and identifying preferences for treatment and for end-of-life care (Thoonsen et al., 2016).

Generalist-level palliative care can then be considered best practice for any clinician of any discipline who is caring for a patient with a serious illness, even though they have not received training in specialist palliative care or do not have a primary identity as palliative care providers. In essence, generalist palliative care involves ability to provide treatments that address some of the goals of palliative care.

When specialist palliative care is not available, individual providers with generalist skills can integrate palliative care principles into the care of the patient and the family. Due to limited resources many health-care facilities such as community hospitals do not have access to an interdisciplinary team that can provide specialist care. To illustrate, at a community hospital palliative care may be provided by a physician and a nurse, or by a nurse and a collaborating mental health professional. In rural settings, there may be only one provider for palliative care as well as the medical care of the patient. In whatever form, adopting a palliative care approach should involve a comprehensive and holistic assessment and treatment of the whole person, including the patient's family.

Specialist palliative care, on the other hand, is provided by clinicians who have acquired advanced and specialized knowledge and training to serve the goals of palliative care. Specialist palliative care is ideally provided by an interdisciplinary team that includes providers from various disciplines, each with unique expertise and the ability to collaborate to develop an individual and interdisciplinary care plan. Specialist palliative care clinicians who are part of an interdisciplinary team have obtained special-level competences within their disciplines.

Developing specialist skills involves specific formal training (Box I.2). Recognizing the importance of palliative care in health care, in 2006 the accreditation council for graduate medical education and the American Board of Medical Specialties recognized hospice and palliative medicine as a medical subspecialty. In the United States

> **Box I.2 Generalist (Primary) and Specialty Palliative Care**
>
> GENERALIST (PRIMARY PALLIATIVE CARE)
>
> This type of care is provided by professionals treating patients with serious and advanced illness whose work does not focus primarily on palliative care. For instance, primary care physicians, nursing staff, oncologists, and geriatric specialists can develop generalist palliative care skills through continuing education programs.
>
> A clinician practicing at the generalist level can provide basic management of pain and other physical symptoms (e.g., dyspnea) and emotional distress (e.g., depression and anxiety).
>
> The clinician can also conduct basic discussions with patients and family caregivers about prognosis, goals of treatment, code status, and emotional distress.
>
> SPECIALIST PALLIATIVE CARE
>
> Specialist palliative care is provided by clinicians whose work focuses on providing palliative care it is generally provided by clinicians who have obtained formal training in palliative care and is delivered in the context of an interdisciplinary palliative care team.
>
> Specialist palliative care includes management of refractory pain and other symptoms, as well as management of more complex depression, anxiety, complex grief reactions including complicated grief, and existential distress.
>
> Coordination of care includes addressing conflict about goals or methods of treatment that may occur between the patient and the family, as well as between the patient/family and the treating team.
>
> Specialist palliative care includes addressing ethical questions and concerns.
>
> ---
> (Sources: Gamondi et al., 2012, Quill and Abernethy, 2013, Portenoy, 2014)

the standard for physicians is the completion of a fellowship in hospice and palliative medicine, a subspecialty of ten participating boards. The sponsoring boards are internal medicine, anesthesiology, family medicine, physical medicine and rehabilitation, psychiatry and neurology, surgery, pediatrics, radiology, emergency medicine, and obstetrics and gynecology (Bradley Ruder, 2015; Schafer et al., 2014). The popularity of palliative medicine is rapidly increasing. In the 2017–2018 academic year there were 141 accredited fellowship hospice and palliative medicine programs for physicians (AAHPM, 2017). These fellowship programs focused on developing competence in all eight domains of palliative care.

The Stresses of Living with Illness

Patients' response and adaptation to illness are influenced by multiple factors, including individual coping style, use of defense mechanisms, past experience with illness and death, and grieving style. Response and adaptation are also greatly influenced by the type of illness, stage, treatment course, and prognosis. For example, the threat level implicit in a diagnosis of cancer that is at an early stage and localized is often different from a diagnosis of pancreatic cancer, which generally carries a poor prognosis at the time of diagnosis. Accordingly, disease-related aspects test the patient and the family's ability to adjust to receiving the "bad news" of the diagnosis and engage in active collaboration with medical providers.

A diagnosis of serious illness requires everyone in the family system to integrate the changes imposed by the disease and to minimize the negative impact of these changes. When physical and emotional challenges are not adequately managed suffering can ensue. There may be suffering related to poorly managed pain and other physical symptoms, and suffering related to caregiver distress in family members who are caring for the patient. There is also suffering related to the challenges of interfacing with a medical system that is often confusing to navigate, resulting in the risk of poor communication with medical providers and in decision-making difficulties.

Ineffective communication raises the potential for misunderstandings and conflict within the family and with medical providers. Thus, the importance of the quality of interaction and communication between the patient and the family, and the medical system, cannot be overestimated. Together, these aspects have profound influence on the opportunity for effective collaboration and empowered decision-making.

To summarize, common challenges and stresses facing the patient and the family living with illness are related to the following areas:

- **Disease management and decision-making**
  - choice of medical treatment
  - evaluation of benefits vs. burden of treatment
  - decisions regarding continuing or suspending treatment when illness worsens in spite of treatment, or when side effects from treatment severely affect the patient's quality of life.
- **Physical concerns**
  - pain and symptoms caused by disease
  - pain and symptoms caused by treatment
  - medical comorbidities
- **Psychological concerns**
  - anxiety disorders
  - fear of suffering
  - fear of dying
  - depression
  - suicidal ideation or suicide attempts
  - prior psychiatric illness
  - past experiences of illness
  - psychological impact of treatment
  - demoralization
  - coping with progressive losses and grief
- **Social and family concerns**
  - loss of social role and status

- loss of job and financial stability
- worries about future of the family
- fear of loss of autonomy
- social concerns related to housing, transportation, and insurance coverage
- disagreement with family members and family conflict

• **Spiritual and existential concerns**
- anger at fate or God
- loss of faith
- struggle to maintain meaning
- fear of unknown

• **End of life concerns**
- fear of dying
- desire for hastened death
  ○ fear of loss of control and dignity during the dying process
  ○ fear of unbearable pain during dying

• **Grief reactions during illness and after the patient's death**
- patient's preparatory grief
- family members' grief in bereavement
- complications of bereavement: complicated grief, bereavement-related depression, anxiety disorders, and exacerbation of prior psychiatric illness.

The potential sources of distress mentioned in the preceding are mediated not only by individual and family history, but also by culture. Therefore, each patient and family needs to receive an individualized, comprehensive, and ongoing assessment to determine the appropriate care plan. The ongoing nature of the assessment allows clinicians of the interdisciplinary palliative care team to constantly adjust and refine the care plan to meet the patient's and the family's needs as they change along with the patient's physical, psychological, social, and spiritual conditions. Palliative care clinicians have developed specialized and focused skills in identifying and addressing sources of suffering through careful assessments and interventions. And palliative care provides comprehensive and integrated care for the patient and the family that evolves along the continuum of illness.

The Case for Palliative Psychology as a Specialty

The focus of palliative care on addressing the complex and unique psychological, psychiatric, and existential needs of the patient and the family underscores the importance of ensuring availability of specialized professionals in these areas. The range of psychological and existential concerns experienced by the patient with advanced illness and his or her family, including diagnosing and managing clinical syndromes such as depression, anxiety, and complicated grief reactions, can be effectively conceptualized within the domain of psychology.

In the United States, becoming a licensed psychologist who can work clinically with patients involves obtaining a doctoral degree, either a PhD or a PsyD in clinical psychology or a PhD in counseling psychology. Psychologists who have obtained non-clinical degrees, such as educational or organizational psychology, can pursue specializations in clinical areas. Clinical psychology is described as "the psychological specialty that provides continuing and comprehensive mental and behavioral health care for individuals and families; consultations to agencies and communities; training, education, and supervision; and research-based practice. It is a specialty in breadth—one that is broadly inclusive of severe psychopathology—and marked by comprehensiveness and integration of knowledge and skills from a broad array of disciplines within and outside of psychology proper. The scope of clinical psychology encompasses all ages, multiple diversities, and varied systems" (APA, 2016).

Psychologists working in clinical settings provide expert and developmentally appropriate mental health assessment and intervention to individuals and families across the lifespan. The problems addressed by psychologists range from minor adjustment issues to severe psychopathology. Populations served by clinical psychologists are from all sociocultural and ethnic backgrounds. In summary "psychologists who provide clinical or counseling services assess and treat mental, emotional, and behavioral disorders. They use the science of psychology to treat complex human problems and promote change. They also promote resilience and help people discover their strengths" (APA, 2016).

Many licensed clinical and counseling psychologists have chosen to pursue specialties focused on the assessment and treatment of patients with physical and chronic illness. Clinical health psychology, geropsychology, and rehabilitation psychology are pursued by selecting elective classes during graduate school, as well as externships, internships, and fellowship opportunities offering formal training in these areas. Thus, either during training or because of their practice focus, many psychologists have already acquired basic knowledge and skill for effectively supporting patients with medical illness and their family caregivers.

Clinical health psychology is a specialty that has grown steadily, involving specialized training on the psychological implications of medical illness, both acute and chronic. Rehabilitation psychology focuses on patients with chronic and serious psychiatric illness, physical disabilities, or chronic illnesses. Geropsychology focuses on the impact of the aging process on physical, psychological, and social aspects and on improving quality of life. Geropsychology already includes several components of palliative care. While its scope is focused around the needs of older patients, it does include training in end-of-life care as an expected consequence of aging.

Psychologists working in cancer centers can further specialize in psycho-oncology. Primary care settings can also offer important opportunities for psychologists with the focus on integrating mental health services in primary care. Because many patients diagnosed with a serious illness will continue to receive some aspects of medical care from their primary care physician, primary care psychologists can provide support to the patient and the family by promoting adaptive coping and adjustment to illness, facilitating effective communication within the family and between the patient and medical providers. And they can continue to support patents who are diagnosed with serious illness during the continuum of care (Linton, 2006; Kasl-Godley et al., 2015).

Considering the established role of psychologists in the care of patients who are medically ill, the development of a specialty (i.e., specialized competency in palliative care) can be viewed as a natural evolution. Because of their specialized training, not only in recognizing and addressing psychopathology, but also in facilitating normal development, promoting resilience, and facilitating well-being from a strength-based approach, psychologists can offer an important contribution to palliative care and can become valuable members of the interdisciplinary palliative care team.

Formal training programs (i.e., fellowships) are available to medical and psychosocial professionals who wish to specialize in palliative care. Palliative social work, palliative nursing, and palliative care chaplaincy represent recognized specialties with developed practice guidelines and related competencies (HPCNA, 2014; Altilio & Otis-Green, 2010). These training and certification options are not yet available to psychologists.

However, the complexities of comprehensive and holistic psychological care for the patient and the family receiving palliative care should be adequately conceptualized as a specialty, *palliative psychology*, that is available to licensed psychologists pursuing a career in palliative care. This book, therefore, advocates for palliative psychology to be recognized as an integral component of palliative care and a core discipline within the interdisciplinary team, just like medicine, social work, nursing, and spiritual care.

Unlike existing psychological specialties that may include some training in areas related to palliative care, but are limited to specific populations, palliative psychology is conceptualized in this book as involving specialist psychology competencies in the eight domains of palliative care. Palliative psychology addresses the needs of different populations and age groups. The common denominator among patient groups and populations is a diagnosis of serious illness and the clinician's commitment to relieving the stresses and potential suffering associated with it. This specialist-level competency will allow the palliative psychologist to function as an effective member of an interdisciplinary palliative care team in inpatient, outpatient, and community settings.

How can palliative psychology be defined? This book offers the following working definition: Palliative psychology is a specialty of psychology aimed at relieving physical, psychological, and existential distress and suffering in patients with serious and advanced illness and their family caregivers. Palliative psychology is patient-centered, and it involves the specialized use of psychological assessment and intervention to improve pain and other physical symptoms, as well as psychological distress. Palliative psychology is grounded in a holistic and strength-based approach that aims at promoting psychological well-being for the patient and family caregivers throughout transitions of care, including the death and dying process and in bereavement.

In the United States, psychologists' roles in palliative care have been historically ancillary and not clearly defined. As a result, a small number of psychologists are employed as members of interdisciplinary palliative care teams or as palliative care consultants. Nakajima et al. (2014) conducted a survey of psychologists involved in palliative care of patients with cancer in Japan, investigating psychologists' perception of competence and understanding of their professional role. A study of clinical psychologists working in palliative care in Taiwan described their clinical contributions and challenges (Sheng-Yu, Wei-Chun, & I-Mei, 2015). Studies of psychologists working in palliative care in the United States are not yet available. These could provide important information about the working reality of psychologists involved in palliative care, as well as their perceived competence, training needs, challenges, and levels of collaboration with other disciplines and medical professionals. Currently, there are few formal and structured roles for psychologists in palliative care and end-of-life care, and there are no guidelines defining best practices.

Formalizing palliative psychology as a specialty can promote the development of standardized curricula and practice guidelines. It can allow to better define research areas, increase the number of formal training programs, and facilitate the integration of psychologists into the palliative care team. Ultimately, the goal is to allow patients and families receiving palliative care to be provided with the highest specialized and sophisticated quality of psychological care. Including the psychologist in this important endeavor is an expression of good care.

Palliative Psychology: Generalist and Specialist Levels

It is important to note, however, that lack of a formal palliative care role has not prevented psychologists with the necessary clinical skills from providing needed psychological support to patients with serious illness. To illustrate, a psychologist in private practice can provide elements of palliative psychology to a psychotherapy client who has received a diagnosis of serious illness. The patient may continue seeing the psychologist during medical treatment, transitions of care, and even worsening of illness. If the patient's medical needs require hospitalization, the psychologist may be able to provide ongoing support by visiting the patient at the hospital. Depending on the setting and unique circumstances, regular therapy sessions may be continued. Because of an existing long-term relationship, the therapist may be in a good position to recognize changes in mood and coping skill. With the patient's consent, the psychologist may provide valuable feedback to the medical team about the unique emotional challenges the patient is facing.

The intimacy and trust that develop in the context of ongoing psychotherapy may allow exploration of concerns about illness and dying. As the patient shares the psychological impact of the illness on self and the family, death and dying may become the focus of the therapy. Issues of transference and countertransference for both patient and the therapist may become more prominent and may need to be addressed.

Even though the psychologist described in this hypothetical scenario would not be technically described as a palliative psychologist, important elements of palliative psychology are being provided to support the patient during the course of illness. This level of intervention can be described as *generalist palliative psychology* (Table I.1).

Generalist-level palliative care skills can be considered best practice for all psychologists working with patients with medical illness, both in outpatient or inpatient settings. Generalist-level skills include a basic understanding of the impact of illness on the psychological functioning of the patient and the family; basic ability to provide psychological interventions to address adjustment disorders with depression and anxiety; and the basic ability to recognize and support uncomplicated grief reactions in the patient and the family.

Generalist-level competence can be critically important also for psychologists whose practice focuses on treating patients who are not medically ill, because some patients

Table I.1 **Generalist Palliative Psychology**

Impact of Illness on patient and family	Ability to recognize the different aspects of the patient's and family's life that have been affected by the illness
Assessment and management of psychological distress	Ability to provide psychological interventions to improve symptoms of depression, anxiety, or exacerbation of preexisting psychiatric illness
Recognition of uncomplicated grief reactions	Understanding of what represents a normal grief reaction and ability to support the patient without pathologizing
Communication with medical providers	If requested by the patient and with patient consent, ability to communicate with treating medical team about worsening of mood symptoms, expressed patient's concerns (e.g., difficulty tolerating treatment, pain, etc.), or family conflict that is affecting the patient's mood and coping skills
Countertransference	Ability to recognize and manage countertransference reactions, especially personal grief reactions triggered by working with the patient. Willingness to seek out consultation or supervision to manage own grief or other emotions that may impact on the work with the patient
Death and dying	Ability to provide emotional support to the patient who is approaching death

may develop illness while they are in psychotherapy. Or, the patient's family member may be diagnosed with a serious illness and the impact of these circumstances on the patient and the entire family system may become the focus of therapy. Furthermore, a psychotherapy patient may be facing serious decisions regarding aging parents with chronic illness or approaching end of life. As the aging population continues to grow, these scenarios will become increasingly common.

Elements of generalist palliative psychology can be obtained during psychology graduate training and by attending continuing education courses focused on different aspects of palliative care. For example, the American Psychological Association annual conference frequently offers special workshops on grief and bereavement or on special patient populations affected by chronic medical illness. The Association for Death Education and Counseling (ADEC) offers numerous trainings and a certification program in Thanatology. The American Society for Clinical Hypnosis (ASCH) offers specialty trainings in the use of hypnosis in palliative care. Additionally, collaboration and consultation with primary care physicians, nurses, or oncologists in a clinic or hospital setting can also assist psychologists who wish to develop generalist skills and integrate them in their practice.

In summary, generalist palliative psychology can meet basic psychological needs of the patient facing serious and advanced illness and it is applicable in most settings with different patient populations. The prevalence of chronic and serious illness in today's modern world has created a new imperative for psychologists who wish to provide comprehensive psychological care. Palliative psychology knowledge and skills will add an important dimension to the work of each psychologist practitioner. The following case vignette highlights how generalist palliative psychology skills would have promoted a more therapeutic outcome for the patient and the therapist.

CASE VIGNETTE I.1

Rea is an experienced licensed clinical psychologist with an outpatient practice in a small town. She has been working with a 55-year-old woman diagnosed with borderline personality disorder for about three years, with slow but consistent improvement. The patient and Rea have developed good therapeutic alliance and trust. In therapy, Rea has been effective balancing validation of the patient's distress with boundary setting. This approach has created a welcoming and structured therapeutic environment where the patient's distress is acknowledged, yet not accepted as an excuse for impulsive or explosive behaviors. The regular therapy has allowed the patient to develop self-soothing skills to manage fear of abandonment, reduce impulsivity, and experience overall improvement in the quality of her relationships. The patient lives with her sister and her nephew, but would like more privacy and has been saving money to find her own apartment. After a routine mammogram the patient receives a diagnosis of breast cancer. Further imaging studies show the cancer is metastatic to lungs. The diagnosis creates distress for the patient, who becomes very emotional during the session. She begins chemotherapy treatment and continues seeing Rea, as regularly as her medical condition allows. However, treatment side effects and related medical complications require frequent hospitalizations. Rea visits the patient during the initial hospitalization, but the demands of private practice prevent her from keeping in close contact with her patient. Rea has limited experience working with patients who have cancer and begins considering referring the patient. However, she is unable to identify a suitable referral in her small town. Additionally, she is concerned about triggering feelings of abandonment in the patient. She considers seeking professional consultation, but her schedule is very full and she keeps postponing. Due to further deterioration and progression of illness, the patient becomes unable to continue living with her sister and is admitted to a nursing home. It is agreed that Rea and the patient will continue therapy twice a month in the patient's room at the nursing facility. During the sessions, the patient appears emotionally distressed and spends most of the time complaining about the nursing home staff. She also asks Rea to set up a meeting with her sister "as soon as possible" because she wants to "get things off my chest." Rea feels overwhelmed by the patient's urgent and distressed affect; but she agrees to arrange a family session. However, she does not follow up and is relieved when the patient does not raise the issue again. During the next two sessions at the nursing home, the patient complains of difficulty breathing, pain, and difficulty sleeping at night. Rea focuses on redirecting the patient and encourages her to practice her self-soothing skills. The patient remains distressed and comments that Rea does not "understand what is going on here." This comment is not explored by Rea during the session. She recognizes that a rupture has occurred in the relationship, but feels uncomfortable addressing it outside the setting of the therapy office. Rea becomes avoidant of the patient, uncertain how to continue therapy in light of her ongoing physical deterioration and emotional distress. She feels she lacks the skills to understand the patient's medical condition and is uncertain how to openly address the patient's fears and anxieties. During a particularly emotional moment in the session, the patient bursts into tears and tells Rea, "I am going to die here." Taken aback, Rea quickly redirects the patient and again encourages her to practice the self-soothing strategies they have developed during their work together. Two weeks after that session, Rea returns to the nursing home, where she is told the patient died two days after the last sessions. Rea is shocked by the news and struggles to find closure. In reflecting on the last two months of therapy, she feels she has somehow failed the patient at a time when she needed her most, but she was completely unprepared to deal competently with the situation. As the patient's condition continued to worsen, Rea felt overwhelmed by her distress and demands and progressively became more emotionally detached. She felt the therapy she provided after the patient's diagnosis was not much more than superficial reassuring and redirecting. Yet she was not sure what she could have done differently and decided to seek personal supervision to debrief the case.

Rea, the psychologist in Case Vignette I.1, was a skilled and experienced clinician. She deeply cared for her patient. However, she felt inadequate to meet her patient's needs. The evolution of the therapeutic relationship after the diagnosis of metastatic cancer was explored during her case consultation with a palliative psychologist, resulting in the following considerations.

Outpatient psychotherapy involves a precise and predictable setting, which allows privacy and a high degree of predictability and control. When the patient became hospitalized and then was transferred to a nursing home, the setting changed significantly, and Rea was unsure how to adjust to the change. As a result, she thought she could just continue the sessions with the same clinical focus, thinking that this would allow the patient to feel more in control. In reflecting back during clinical supervision, she admitted feeling overwhelmed by the challenges, and she symbolically "left" the relationship with the patient. She felt that by not acknowledging the meaning and impact of the diagnosis on the patient and on the therapy relationship, she missed the opportunity to be present for her patient on a deeper level. However, she did not know how she could or should have approached the topic without causing more distress for the patient, especially considering her fragile emotional balance.

Additionally, Rea was not familiar with the implication of being diagnosed with metastatic cancer, versus an earlier stage. She also was not aware of how rapidly the patient could deteriorate and what the impact of treatment would be. In an effort to maintain a sense of predictability in the patient's life, she became more directive and continued focusing on helping her practice skills to control suicidal thoughts and explosive behavior. While these interventions were valuable and supported the patient, Rea avoided the entire dimension related to the illness and prognosis.

When the patient stated that Rea did not understand her situation and was "in denial" Rea felt defensive. The patient's comment was interpreted as a manifestation of distress and was not taken at face value. While normally Rea would have explored any statements being offered by the patient, she avoided exploring any comments suggestive of worsening of the patient's condition, or her death. Rather, Rea's therapeutic stance was focused on improving and "fixing."

Rea's countertransference appears to have been anxious avoidance; she dreaded the sessions with the patient but did not explore the meaning of her reaction. In offering the superficial reassurance to the patient that things would be okay if only she would practice her self-soothing skills and control her behavior, Rea prevented the patient from having the opportunity to openly talk about her illness and her impending death with her therapist, whom she trusted. As a result, and perhaps sensing Rea's discomfort, the patient agreed to keep the tone of the sessions superficial and contrived.

Rea felt a sense of shock when she discovered the patient had died soon after the last session. In retrospect, she admitted not allowing the possibility of the patient's death into full awareness. Rea shared that the last few sessions with the patient felt like "a blur" and did not think she had been as present for the patient as she could have been. In her words, "I worked with her for three years and I completely missed the last part of her life."

Rea's grieving process for the death of this long-term patient was characterized by deep guilt, shame, and sadness. She felt that paradoxically she had somehow "bailed" on the patient at her time of need. Her grief appeared disenfranchised: Rea felt she did not have a forum for expressing her grief. Yet she was not sure she "deserved" to grieve or be supported, as she felt she had provided inadequate support to the patient.

The following generalist palliative psychology skills would have been valuable for Rea and her patient:

- understanding of the implications of delivering therapy in medical settings, including how to create a "safe" therapeutic setting in spite of several unpredictable elements
- basic knowledge of cancer, including treatment options, treatment effects, and disease trajectories
- ability to support preparatory grief in patients with advanced illness and patients approaching death
- ability to recognize her own countertransference and grieving process, as important tools in maintaining emotional connection with the patient, as the patient continues to decline and approaches death
- familiarity with interdisciplinary coordination of care and ability to effectively communicate with medical professionals about psychological implications of illness

The previous section and vignette have described generalist-level palliative psychology skills that can greatly benefit the patient and the family. Clinical and counseling psychologists specializing in health psychology, rehabilitation psychology, or geropsychology may already be applying generalist palliative psychology based on their training and experience. Additional generalist-level skills can be developed by attending continuing education training programs focused on palliative care topics.

However, *specialist-level skills* in palliative psychology are necessary for psychologists who have chosen palliative care as their primary field, either as members of an interdisciplinary palliative care team or as palliative care consultants. These specialist-level skills are necessary to meet the patient's *and* the family's evolving needs along the continuum of illness, including treatment, transitions of care, during the death and dying process, and during bereavement, providing care that is continually integrated into the treatment plan.

Specialist palliative psychology involves developing specific competencies in the eight domains of palliative care identified by the *Clinical Practice Guidelines for Quality Palliative Care*. These competencies involve the development of knowledge, skills, and attitudes necessary for a psychologist specialized in palliative care (Table I.2). This competency will enable psychologists to provide services in all settings where patients are receiving palliative care, including hospital settings, inpatient units and outpatient clinics, nursing homes, hospice programs, and in the community. Therefore, specialist palliative psychology requires a focused, formal, and standardized training curriculum that meets standards and follows practice guidelines.

Training in Palliative Psychology

Because palliative psychology is not yet recognized as a specialty, only a few formal and rigorous training programs exist at the time of writing this book, each offering varying levels of depth. The Veteran Administration (VA) Medical Center Interprofessional Fellowship program in Hospice and Palliative Care offers a one-year fellowship for postdoctoral-level psychologists who have the opportunity to function as members of a palliative care team and develop expertise in palliative care and end-of-life care, including hospice. Postdoctoral trainees join other palliative care fellows, including board-certified physicians, advance practice nurses, licensed social workers, chaplains, and post-residency pharmacists.

Trainees participate in inpatient and outpatient activities related to caring for patients with advanced illness, patients approaching death, and their families. This unique setting allows a psychologist to develop the skills necessary to become an effective member of palliative care and hospice teams. The fellows from the different disciplines of medicine, nursing, psychology, social work, chaplaincy, and pharmacy join the core and stable members of the palliative care team. Part of the learning experience is interdisciplinary, where all the fellows attend lectures addressing various aspects of palliative and end-of-life care. Additionally each fellow receives individualized training and supervision within their own discipline.

The Ohio State University has developed a two-year psycho oncology and palliative medicine fellowship program, with a curriculum that addresses specific palliative care competencies for psychologists. The Cambia Palliative Care Center of Excellence at the University of Washington has developed an interprofessional graduate certificate in palliative care open to several disciplines, including psychology. Unlike fellowship programs, this certificate program is open to clinicians who are already licensed practitioners in their community and wish to develop specialized skills in palliative care. The Institute for Palliative Care at the California State University offers trainings on aspects of palliative care open to all professionals in addition to advanced certificate trainings designed for social work, nursing, and chaplaincy. The Center for Palliative Care at Harvard Medical School offers courses in palliative care, open to psychosocial professionals and allied health professionals.

Table I.2 **Specialist Palliative Psychology**

Generalist-Level Skills	Ability to perform at a Generalist Level
Domains of palliative care	Knowledge of the domains and psychologists' role and contribution in each domain
Medical context of advanced illness throughout the continuum including dying process	Knowledge of disease trajectory of common diseases, treatment options, expected psycho-physical changes in end of life, and possible sources of distress for the patient and family caregivers
Prognostication	Understanding of different disease trajectories and of the psychological impact of prognostication on the patient and the family
Cultural Competence	Ability to recognize the impact of cultural factors and to provide psychological interventions that are culturally relevant to the patient and the family
Psychological implications of disease type, stage, treatment, prognosis	Knowledge of psychological impact of different aspects of disease and ability to target needs effectively
Psychological Distress	Ability to diagnose and provide psychological intervention for major depression, anxiety disorders, complicated grief, suicidal ideation. Support patients with serious mental illness.
Pharmacotherapy for pain and symptoms	Familiarity with main classes of medications used in palliative care, knowledge of psychological implications related to use of opioids in advanced illness
Substance use disorder (SUD) in advanced illness	Ability to diagnose SUD in patients with advanced illness and develop integrated treatment approaches with the team
Palliative sedation	Understanding of clinical applications and ethical implications and ability to support the patient and the family
Psychopharmacology	Understanding of psychotropic medications for the treatment of depression, anxiety, and complicated grief and ability to address patients' concerns in therapy
Interdisciplinary teamwork	Knowledge of different team approaches and ability to function effectively as members of an interdisciplinary palliative care team; ability to participate in daily rounds and discussions about ongoing patient care

(continued)

Table I.2 **Continued**

Health-care system	Knowledge of different systems of care and how they impact delivery of palliative care in institutions and in the community
Ethical issues	Understanding of medical decision-making, including goals of care and advance directives and ability to facilitate these conversations with the patient and the family
Individual and Family Therapy	Knowledge and application of psychological therapies relevant for patients with advanced illness and their families. Ability to develop an integrative approach that incorporates different modalities based on needs and goals
Integrative medicine approaches	Familiarity with music therapy, energy-based therapies, clinical hypnosis, imagery, and mindfulness-based approaches for the relief of symptoms. This Includes the ability to work collaboratively with other practitioners when needed (e.g., providing a psychological session jointly with a music therapist)
Teaching and training	Ability to provide education and training on the different components of palliative psychology
Professional self-care	Knowledge of the professional self-care literature and clinical implications; ability to provide staff support; ability to develop a sustainable personal self-care plan

Research fellowships in psycho-oncology are more widespread. These training programs generally allow access to patients with advanced illness and their family in the context of a clinical trial of psychosocial interventions. Clinical research is a natural setting for many psychologists, and it is a role that can significantly contribute to advancement in palliative care.

The role of a practitioner palliative psychologist, however, requires the specialist-level skills that can be utilized directly with patients and families. This is a clinical role that involves becoming part of a palliative care team or functioning as a consultant when their clinical expertise is needed. Currently, physicians, nurses, and social workers with specialized palliative care training and certification can apply directly for palliative care and hospice positions. A similar opportunity is currently rarely available to psychologists.

As mentioned previously, this book calls for the development of a formal and standardized training curriculum available nationally to all psychologists interested in pursuing this specialty. This specialty certification has been available to social workers since 2009 through the National Association of Social Workers (NASW). Additionally, specialty certifications in palliative care are available for nurses and chaplains. Notably, specialty or board certification can facilitate full recognition and integration of a discipline as members of the palliative care team. To date, there is no board certification available to psychologists associated with postgraduate palliative care training. Thus, the recognition of palliative psychology as a specialty recognized by state licensing boards would allow for a national formal training curriculum to be developed. This would ensure that psychologists graduating from the training program meet the highest standards of competence and professionalism.

The palliative care field continues to grow at an impressive rate. However, the needs continue to increase, and palliative care organizations have been calling for more palliative care clinicians (Bradley Ruder, 2015). Although this call primarily applies to physicians and nurses, it is clear that the increase in palliative care needs refers not only to physical needs but also psychological needs. Accordingly, there is an urgent need to formally incorporate the expertise of psychologists in the palliative care field.

The American Psychological Association has been instrumental in promoting the involvement of psychologists in various settings, including medical. However, several barriers related to lack of funding and lack of knowledge regarding the contribution psychologists can offer in palliative care have been identified (Hartmam-Stein, 2001). A statement from APA commented that more psychologists were needed in end-of-life care (deAngelis, 2002). In light of that statement a task force was formed and important clinical papers were published as a result of that impetus. The work of the task force highlighted that despite clinical psychologists' extensive training in assessing, understanding, and treating emotional distress, they are often underrepresented in end-of-life care. Haley et al. (2003) emphasized that while psychologists can offer important support to patient across the life span, this support can become critical after a diagnosis of life limiting illness, in advanced disease and during the dying process, and in bereavement. Certainly, a psychologist would need to develop the necessary knowledge and skills to provide more than general support to a patient and a family facing these challenging circumstances.

This book advocates for involvement of psychologists in palliative care as a whole. Palliative care includes end-of-life care and hospice, but it is not limited to a specific prognostic timeline and it addresses the needs of the patient and the family from the time of diagnosis onward (see also Chapter 1).

Conceptualizing palliative psychology as a specialty is a fundamental step in this direction, as is increasing the number of formal training opportunities. Generalist skills in palliative psychology should become part of the core curriculum for professional psychology programs. Elective classes should be available for students interested in pursuing a career in palliative psychology. Externships and internship rotations providing direct clinical services to patients receiving palliative care, including end-of-life care, should significantly increase. Defining palliative psychology practice guidelines is another important step in the direction of formalizing palliative psychology as a specialty. Such guidelines have not yet been developed in the United States. The European Association for Palliative Care (EAPC) has mobilized efforts in this regard by developing a task force in 2009 to define guidelines for education of psychologists in palliative care. This effort was motivated by the recognition that psychologists lacked a defined role and expected competencies in palliative care. Surveys were conducted regarding the involvement of psychologists in palliative care, and a curriculum was subsequently proposed to facilitate uniform standards of training (Junger et al., 2010; Garamondi et al., 2013; Junger & Payne, 2011).

The proposed curriculum identifies nine areas, based on a framework including knowledge, skills and attitudes, self-reflection, and self-awareness. These areas are: general background and history of palliative care, professional role and self-image, psychological assessment and documentation, counseling and psychotherapy, consultation, supervision and staff support, research, self-awareness and self-care, ethics, and cultural diversity. This European curriculum includes severals areas also covered in the eight domains of palliative care.

Contributions of Palliative Psychology

A person's life can be conceptualized as a developing personal narrative evolving along a storyline. The diagnosis of a serious and life-limiting illness abruptly forces the individual to deal with the unknown and the unfamiliar. Living with illness is a complex process of ongoing adaptation that is demanding and challenging for the patient and the family. In some cases the storyline can be continued, as the disease may be at an early stage or may respond to treatment in ways that suggest a cure may be achieved. If a serious illness is likely to be cured, patients and families may utilize and mobilize emotional and physical resources to cope with treatment and the anxieties and discomfort associated with it. In this scenario, palliative care interventions can effectively help manage symptoms in the various domains that negatively affect quality of life, while disease-modifying treatment is being pursued, with the goals of curing the illness.

It may be argued any diagnosis of serious illness always creates the need to develop a new life narrative, even when the illness can be cured or controlled by medical management of the disease. The profound feeling of uncertainty and vulnerability that the patient and the family may experience as a result of a serious diagnosis affects them deeply. It creates a "rupture" in the fabric of one's life that needs to be processed and integrated on a cognitive and psychological level. And, if the medical intervention cannot help the patient restore the original storyline, it is important to assist the patient and the family in developing a new storyline and establishing a new sense of what is "normal."

As improvements in medical management have resulted in an increase in life expectancy for individuals living with serious illness, patients and providers are similarly confronted by challenges to discover what represents the best quality of life possible and maintaining it for as long as possible. A new life narrative develops to include treatment, interventions, and therapeutic goals. While a cure is not always possible, a healing personal narrative can be a realistic and achievable goal. And an evolving personal narrative can create continued meaningful engagement in life. From this perspective, palliative psychologists can not only facilitate the patient and family's adjustment to the demands of treatment, but also help identify a meaningful and sustaining life narrative.

The breadth and depth of training allows psychologists to have an important role in recognizing and managing the different elements of psychological and existential distress (Ferris et al., 2002; Golijani-Moghaddam, 2014, Nydegger, 1992, 2008; Hartman-Stein, 2001). It is important to note that doctoral training in clinical and counseling psychology *specifically focuses* on clinical assessment and psychological intervention. This involves developing a therapeutic presence constantly balanced by the ability to quickly recognize a pathological process and quickly develop a case conceptualization and treatment plan. Psychologists develop expertise in communication, managing conflict, mediating, and addressing multiple needs and priorities with the highest level of clinical competence. These skills are essential in the palliative care setting. This setting is often unpredictable, with patients' conditions rapidly changing and raising new issues and concerns.

Psychologists' clinical expertise in assessing and treating psychological and existential distress, as well as psychiatric disorders, is especially valuable in the diagnosis and non-pharmacological management of depression, anxiety, delirium, dementia, insomnia, and agitation. Their ability to provide individual and family interventions allows them not only to work with patients individually, but also to include the family and other caregivers, recognizing and respecting cultural, social, and spiritual differences. Cognitive-behavioral and integrative interventions can improve pain and other physical symptoms, such as nausea or dyspnea. Humanistic and meaning-oriented psychotherapy approaches, appropriately modified for the palliative care setting, can promote personal meaning, peace, and connectedness with family members and other loved ones. System-oriented therapy approaches can help the patient and the family resolve conflicts and promote supportive relationships that are mutually sustaining in the face of challenges. Skillful assessment and support of the grieving process for the patient and the family will increase the likelihood that both individual grieving styles and family style will be validated and supported. Additionally, the ability to recognize the development of complications of bereavement will also ensure that grievers receive adequate intervention (Table I.3).

Training in psychopharmacology has become increasingly available for psychologists. Those who have received formal and structured training—for example, by completing a postdoctoral master's degree in psychopharmacology—can engage in a productive dialogue with medical providers. In some cases, and based on state legislation, they can discuss recommendations for psychotropic medications while always working with patients to address barriers to treatment, improve adherence, and minimize burden (see Chapter 3).

The Eight Domains of Palliative Care as a Framework for Specialist-Level Competency in Palliative Psychology

The eight domains of palliative care identified by the National Consensus Project represent a widely accepted framework for competency and best practices in specialist palliative care in the United States. These domains are generally followed by nursing, social work, medicine, and chaplaincy. Thus, they are used as the general framework for this book. Palliative psycholgists are encouraged to review the domains and the associated clinical practice guidelines. The eight domains offer a "common language" to palliative care clinicians, and this book follows this approach to facilitate the conceptual integration of palliative psychology as an emerging specialty. Using this common language while defining the uniqueness of palliative psychology can promote interdisciplinary discussion, collaboration, and growth. It can also promote professional growth for psychologists who have chosen to pursue this complex, rewarding, and rapidly evolving

Table I.3 **Contributions of Palliative Psychology**

Assessment and evaluation	Assessment, diagnosis, case conceptualization, and treatment planning related to • psychiatric disorders • complicated grief • cognitive impairment and decisional capacity • suicidal ideation and risk • crisis intervention • severe grief reactions in the patient and the family
Psychological interventions	• facilitate family meetings • provide evidence-based nonpharmacological interventions for pain and symptom management • provide culturally relevant individual, couple, family, child therapy • provide grief counseling and support • provide grief psychotherapy • provide therapy for complicated grief • provide therapy to patients with personality disorders • evaluate communication within families • validate and support family strengths and coping skills
Care coordination	• contribute to complex case management by providing information and education to different members of the treating team • identify psychological and psychiatric barriers that negatively affect the patient and the family's ability to participate in care • facilitate goals of care conversations • facilitate referrals to psychological and psychiatric resources in the community
Staff education and support	• demonstrate expertise in understanding and addressing issues of burnout, compassion fatigue and conflict in teams. • provide staff debriefing, education, and support • provide training to other disciplines in communication and psychological care of the patient and the family • provide communication skills training for staff

field of palliative care. Following the eight-domain template as a general framework for training programs in palliative psychology, while still creating a curriculum under each domain that is fully representative of psychology, may be desirable.

While professionals involved in palliative care have unique expertise in their respective disciplines, such as medicine, social work, chaplaincy, or psychology, they also should be familiar with all the domains and be able to provide basic interventions in all domains from the perspective of their own discipline. Thus, while psychologists' unique expertise may be primarily expressed in the psychological and psychiatric aspects of care, they would also need to have basic proficiency in all the other domains. This process of developing multiple competencies is comparable to that of palliative care physicians, nurses, chaplains, and social workers pursuing formal training in palliative care. In essence, each of the eight domains of specialist palliative care identifies a broad and essential area that needs to be addressed when caring for the patient with serious illness and the family.

How This Book Is Organized

The following chapters will review selected aspects of the eight domains of palliative care, specifically from the perspective of palliative psychology. For each domain, core competencies for palliative psychology are proposed and discussed in the context of clinical applications. The competencies are described in terms of knowledge, skills, and attitudes that are relevant to the work of a psychologist in palliative care. The clinical vignettes are based on real case scenarios and serve to illustrate clinical applications of palliative psychology in different palliative care settings.

While an extensive discussion of all the areas of knowledge of palliative care is beyond the scope of this book, the main purpose of each chapter is to highlight clinical perspectives and applications. Although each domain of palliative care delimitates specific areas and aspects of care, there is obviously overlap, and the same issue can have implications in several domains.

Because of these overlaps, which reflect the complexity of clinical practice, the same topic is at times presented in more than one chapter, when it can be approached from a different perspective that adds to the overall understanding. To illustrate, grief reactions are discussed in Chapter 3—concerning psychological, psychiatric, and existential aspects of care. Additionally, they are reviewed in Chapter 4 as an important aspect of social care for family caregivers, during illness and also after the patient's death.

The following sections provide a broad description of each domain of palliative care.

1. STRUCTURE AND PROCESSES OF CARE

This domain addresses the what, how, and where of palliative care. It considers the different settings where palliative care is provided and identifies the essential infrastructure for the provision of care. Interdisciplinary teamwork and interdisciplinary assessment of the patient and the family represent key elements of specialist palliative care. Care is provided through the careful and coordinated interdisciplinary teamwork.

A core interdisciplinary team has historically included a physician, a nurse, a social worker, and a spiritual care provider. Optimally, the team will include other specialists, such as palliative psychologists who can provide specialist psychological assessment and intervention. The team conducts comprehensive and interdisciplinary assessments that are integrated into an evolving plan of care addressing the multiple needs of the patient and the family. Palliative care can be provided in different settings (outpatient, inpatient, patient's home, nursing home), and it is the team's responsibility to ensure that assessment and intervention meets the highest standards. Processes of care include recognition of the ongoing needs of the team especially with regard to education and staff support. Thus, the important topic of professional self-care must be addressed.

2. PHYSICAL ASPECTS OF CARE

This domain emphasizes the importance of managing pain and other physical symptoms effectively with the goal of relieving distress and suffering for the patient. It is well recognized that poorly managed pain and symptoms can create not only physical but also psychological and existential suffering. Assessment of pain and symptoms is ongoing and interdisciplinary. Interventions are evidence based and include pharmacological, behavioral, and complementary medicine approaches. Psychologists with specialized knowledge and skills in nonpharmacological interventions for pain and symptoms including hypnosis, imagery, and cognitive-behavioral approaches can add greatly to the interdisciplinary treatment plan.

3. PSYCHOLOGICAL AND PSYCHIATRIC ASPECTS OF CARE

This domain stresses the importance of accurately assessing the psychological impact of illness on the patient and the family. The presence of psychiatric comorbidities and subclinical syndromes is assessed and treated by members of the interdisciplinary palliative care team with specialized skills in this area. Depression, anxiety, and delirium can occur in the context of advanced illness and need to be promptly identified and actively managed. The presence of suicidal ideation needs to be adequately explored, contextualized, and addressed. Patients with preexisting severe psychiatric illnesses such as bipolar disorder or psychotic disorder may experience complex challenges in the face of advanced illness and require specialized psychological and psychiatric care. Clearly, psychologists specialized in palliative care can offer a tremendous contribution to this domain.

4. SOCIAL ASPECTS OF CARE

This domain complements and broadens the third domain by focusing on the patient-family relationship in the context of the complex communications with the medical team. The interdisciplinary team pays special attention to ensuring that discussions about goals of care reflect the patient and the family's sociocultural background and values. The interdisciplinary team should include clinicians that are experts at assessing and managing social distress and providing support to families and children. Special attention is focused on family caregivers and their adaptation to the caregiving process. The stresses of caregiving for a loved one with serious illness are well documented. Assessment and interventions should effectively address caregiver burden by providing adequate psychological support, but also by helping the family identify practical strategies for addressing existing challenges.

5. SPIRITUAL, RELIGIOUS, AND EXISTENTIAL ASPECTS OF CARE

This domain identifies spiritual, religious, and existential needs as essential components of competent and compassionate care. Palliative care clinicians have a responsibility to explore, assess, and manage spiritual pain or distress. While every team member can explore spiritual needs in the patient and the family, specialized assessment and interventions should be provided by a spiritual care professional. Most importantly, the palliative care team should not assume that every patient and family values spirituality or religion or wishes to engage in such explorations or discussions. Palliative care clinicians do not impose their spiritual or religious beliefs, and they do not recommend a particular belief system or practice to the patient and the family.

6. CULTURAL ASPECTS OF CARE

This domain addresses the importance of understanding, respecting and validating the patient and the family's cultural background, practices, and choices. "Culture" is a broad term that not only determines preferences related to health-care decisions, but also affects how a patient and a family understand the meaning and impact of illness, including death and dying. Additionally, a family culture also determines what are considered appropriate behaviors in communicating with medical providers, including what are appropriate manifestations and expressions of grief. The interdisciplinary palliative care team encourages the development of cultural competence in its members. Clinicians' self-awareness allows them to identify their own cultural beliefs and biases in order to avoid imposing such beliefs on the patient and the family.

7. CARE OF THE PATIENT AT THE END OF LIFE

This domain addresses the essential physical, psychological, and spiritual elements of care for the patient who is at the end of life, including the dying process and care of the patient after the death. It emphasizes the importance of supporting the patient and the family at a most sensitive time with pharmacological and nonpharmacological interventions. Allowing for physical comfort and symptom relief in the patient who is dying is essential, as is ongoing supportive education for the family regarding the dying process. It is critical that any spiritual, religious, or secular practices identified by the patient and the family as important be respected and allowed expression. The interdisciplinary palliative care plan includes care for the family after the patient's death and during the grieving process. Ability to provide supportive psychoeducation about the grieving process and its possible manifestations is an important skill for palliative care clinicians. Individuals at risk for developing complications of bereavement should be identified early by the team and receive ongoing psychological care.

8. ETHICAL AND LEGAL ASPECTS OF CARE

Palliative care clinicians should maintain current knowledge of the bioethical and legal aspects of medical decision making. This includes a correct understanding of advanced directives, Do Not Resuscitate (DNR) orders, and use of palliative sedation. This domain addresses the importance of helping the patient and the family express their preferences, wishes, goals, and expectations about medical care in advanced illness and at end of life. This process also involves supporting identified wishes during all transitions of care.

The chapters that follow in this book discuss central aspects of each palliative care domain, identify within each of them specific competencies for palliative psychologists, and present applications for the clinical setting.

References

Altilio, T. & Otis-Green, S. (2010). (Eds.). *Palliative Social Work*. New York, NY: Oxford.

American Academy of Hospice and Palliative Medicine. Hospice and palliative care fellowship programs. http://aahpm.org/uploads/Program_Data_092117.pdf Retrieved on November 7, 2017.

American Association of Colleges of Nursing. (2012). QSEN Education Consortium. *Graduate level QSEN competencies: Knowledge, skills, and attitudes*. Washington, DC: Author.

American Psychological Association. Briefing series on the role of psychology in health care. www.apa.org/health/briefs. Retrieved on October 20, 2016.

Anderson, B. A., Marasco, L. E., Kasl-Godley, J., & Kennedy, S. (2011). Social work and psychology. In T. Altilio & S. Otis-Green (Eds.), *Palliative social work* (pp. 425–431). New York: Oxford University Press.

Blackhall L. J., Read, P., Stukenborg, G., Dillon, P., Barclay, J., Romano, A., & Harrison, J. (2016). CARE track for advanced cancer: Impact and timing of an outpatient palliative care clinic. *Journal of Palliative Medicine*, 19(1), 57–63.

Bradley Ruder, D. (2015). From Specialty to Shortage. Harvard Magazine. https://harvardmagazine.com/2015/03/from-specialty-to-shortage. Retrieved on October 20, 2017.

Burns, M., & McIlfatrick, S. (2015). Palliative care in dementia: Literature review of nurses' knowledge and attitudes towards pain assessment. *International Journal of Palliative Nursing*, 21(8), 400–407.

Center to Advance Palliative Care (CAPC). Definition of palliative care. http://www.capc.org/about/palliative-care/. Retrieved on November 12, 2016.

Centers for Medicare and Medicaid Services (2008). Medicare and Medicaid Programs: hospice conditions of participation. Federal Register, 73, 32087.

Cunningham, P. J. (2009). Beyond parity: Primary care physicians' perspectives on access to mental health care. *Health Affairs*, 28, 490.

deAngelis, T. (2002). More psychologists needed in end-of-life care. *Monitor on Psychology*, 33(3), 52.

Fairman, N., & Irwin, S. A. (2013). Palliative care psychiatry: Update on an emerging dimension of psychiatric care. *Current Psychiatry Reports*, 15(7), 374.

Federal Register (2016). Definitions. Code of Federal Regulations, 3, 418.3. http://www.federalregister.gov/d/2016-1822. Retrieved on November 12, 2016.

Fendler, T. J., Swetz, K. M., & Allen, L. A. (2015). Team-based palliative and end of life care for heart failure. *Heart Failure Clinics*, 11(3), 479–498.

Ferris, F., Balfour, H. M., Bowen, K., Farley, J., Hardwick, M., Lamontagne, C., ... West, P. J. (2002). A model to guide patient and family care: Based on nationally accepted principles and norms of practice. *Journal of Pain and Symptom Management*, 24(2), 106–123.

Gamondi, C., Larkin, P., & Payne, S. (2013). Core competencies in palliative care: An EAPC White Paper on palliative care education—Part 1. *European Journal of Palliative Care*, 20(2), 86–91.

Haley, W. E., Larson, D., Kasl-Godley, J., Neimeyer, R. A., & Kwilosz, D. (2003). Roles for psychologists in end-of-life care: emerging models of practice. *Professional Psychology: Research and Practice*, 34(6), 626–633.

Hartman-Stein, P. (2001). Psychologists trying to overcome barriers to work with hospice patients. *The National Psychologist*, 10(4), 12–13. http://centerforhealthyaging.com/NatPsychArticles/July_August_2001. Retrieved on November 11, 2016.

Hospice and Palliative Care Nurses Association. (2014). *Competencies for the hospice and palliative advanced practice nurse* (2nd ed.). Pittsburgh, PA: Hospice and Palliative Care Nurses Association.
Institute of Medicine. (2015). *Dying in America: Improving quality and honoring individual preferences near the end of life.* Washington, DC: National Academies Press.
Interprofessional Education Collaborative Expert Panel. (2011). *Core competencies for interprofessional collaborative practice: Report of an expert panel.* Washington, DC: Interprofessional Education Collaborative.
Junger, S., & Payne, S. (2011). Guidance on postgraduate education for psychologists involved in palliative care. *European Journal of Palliative Care, 18*(5), 238–252.
Junger, S., Payne, S. A., Costantini A., Kalus, C., & Werth J. L. Jr., (2010). The EAPC task force on education for psychologists in palliative care. *European Journal of Palliative Care, 17*(2), 84–87.
Kasl-Godley, J. E., King, D. A., & Quill, T. E. (2014). Opportunities for psychologists in palliative care. Working with patients and families across the disease continuum. *American Psychologist, 69*(4), 364–376.
Kim, S. L., & Tarn, D. M. (2016). Effect of primary care involvement on end of life care outcomes. *Journal of the American Geriatric Society, 64*(10), 1968–1974.
Kuehn, B. M. Palliative care is for teens, young adults with cancer too. *Medscape.* http://www.medscape.com/viewarticle/860519. Retrieved on March 20, 2016.
Linton, J. C. (2006, Fall). Hospital practice competencies for psychologists. *National Register of Health Psychologists.* http://www.nationalregister.org/pub/the-national-register-report-pub/the-register-report-fall-2006/hospital-practice-competencies-for-psychologists. Retrieved on November 10, 2016.
Menhert A. (2015). Clinical psychology in palliative care. In N. Cherny, M. Fallon, S. Kaasa, R. K. Portenoy, & D. C. Currow (Eds.), *Oxford textbook of palliative medicine* (5th ed.). New York: Oxford.
Nakajima, K., Iwamitsu, Y., Matsubara, M., & Kizawa, Y. (2014). Psychologists involved in cancer palliative care in Japan: A nationwide survey. *Palliative & Supportive Care, 12*, 1–8.
National Consensus Project for Quality Palliative Care. (2013). *Clinical practice guidelines for quality palliative care.* Pittsburgh, PA: National Consensus Project for Quality Palliative Care.
Nydegger, R. (2008). Psychologists and hospice: Where we are and where we can be. *Professional Psychology: Research and Practice, 39*(4), 459–463.
Patel, S. K., Davidson, S., & Folbrecht, J. Communication in clinical psychology. In E. Wittenberg et al. (Eds.), *Textbook of palliative care communication* (pp. 71–78). New York: Oxford University Press.
Perleth, M., Jakubowski, E., & Busse, R. (2001). What is "best practice" in health care? State of the art and perspectives on improving the effectiveness and efficiency of the European health care system. *Health Policy, 56*(3), 235–250.
Portenoy, R. K. (2014). Palliative care: Changing the health care landscape through emerging models. MJHS Institute for Innovation in Palliative Care. Interprofessional Webinar Series. http://www.mjhspalliativeinstitute.org/about-the-institute/news-highlights/. Retrieved on October 10, 2016.
Quill, T. E., Abernethy, A. P. (2013, March). Generalist plus specialist palliative care: Creating a more sustainable model. *New England Journal of Medicine, 368*(13), 1173–1175.
Ryan, K., Connolly, M., Charnley, K., Ainscough, A., Crinion, J., Hayden, C., . . . Wynne, M. (2014). Palliative care competence framework steering group: *Palliative care competence framework.* Dublin: Health Service Executive.
Schaefer, K. G., Chittenden, E. H., Sullivan, A. M., Periyakoil, V. S., Morrison, L. J., Carey, E. C., . . . Block, S. D. (2014). Raising the bar for the care of seriously ill patients: Results of a national survey to define essential palliative are competencies for medical students and residents. *Academic Medicine, 89*(7), 1024–1031.
Sepulveda C, Marlin A, & Yoshida T. (2002). Palliative care: The World Health Organization's global perspective. *Journal of Pain and Symptom Management, 24*(2), 91–96.

Shadd, J. (2008). Should palliative care be a specialty? *Canadian Family Physician, 54*(6), 840–842.

Shah, A. B., Morissey, R. P., Baraghoush, A., Bharadwaj, P., Phan, A., Hamilton, M., . . . Schwarz, E. R. (2013). Failing the failing heart: A review of palliative care in heart failure. *Review of Cardiovascular Medicine, 14*(1), 41–48.

Sheng-Yu, F., Wei-Chun, L., & I-Mei, L. (2015). Psychosocial care and the role of clinical psychologists in palliative care. *American Journal of Hospice and Palliative Medicine, 32*(8), 861–868.

Strada, E. A., & Breitbart, W. (2015). Training psychologists and psychiatrists in palliative care. In J. C. Holland, W. S. Breitbart, P. N. Butow, P. B. Jacobsen, M. J. Loscalzo, & R. M. McCorkle (Eds.), *Psycho-Oncology* (3rd ed., pp. 259–263). New York: Oxford University Press.

Thoonsen, B., Vissers, K., Verhagen, S., Prins, J., Bor, H., van Weel, C., Groot, M., & Engels, Y. (2015). Training general practitioners in early identification and anticipatory palliative care planning: a randomized controlled trial. *BioMedCentral Family Practice, 16*(126).

Vermylen, J. H., Szmuilowicz, E., & Kalhan, R. (2015). Palliative care in COPD: An unmet area for quality improvement. *International Journal of COPD, 10*, 1543–1551.

Voelker, R. (2011). Hospital palliative care programs raise grade to B in new report card on access. *JAMA, 306*(21), 2313–2314.

Weingaertner, V., Schieve, C., Gerdes, V., Schwartz-Eywill, M., Prenzel, R., Bausewein, C., Higginson, I. J., . . . Simon, S. T. (2014). Breathlessness, functional status, distress, and palliative care needs over time in patients with advanced chronic obstructive lung disease or lung cancer: A cohort study. *Journal of Pain and Symptom Management, 48*(4), 569–581.

Wolfe, J., Hinds, P. S., & Sourkes, B. M. (Eds.). (2011). *Textbook of interdisciplinary pediatric palliative care*. Philadelphia, PA: Elsevier.

Palliative Psychology

1

The First Domain of Palliative Care

Structure and Processes of Care

Focus Points

- Palliative care is a system of care delivery focused on preventing, identifying, and managing physical, psychological, social, and spiritual distress in patients living with serious and chronic illness and their families.
- Palliative care is patient- and family-centered care, and it is appropriate from the moment of diagnosis onward.
- Palliative psychology is an emerging specialty for psychologists focused on providing specialist psychological evaluation and intervention to patients and families.
- The most common palliative care models in the United States are institution-based palliative care, community-based palliative care, and hospice.
- Specialist palliative care is based on an interdisciplinary team approach.
- The interdisciplinary team conducts comprehensive assessments and develops care plans that are patient- and family-centered.
- Professional self-care is an important aspect of professionalism and an essential competency for all palliative care clinicians, including palliative psychologists.

Introduction

The first domain of palliative care, "Structure and Processes of Care," addresses the settings and models of care. Competency in this domain also includes a thorough appreciation and understanding of the delivery of palliative care in different settings and an awareness of emerging clinical and research issues in this field. Interdisciplinary teamwork is the cornerstone of specialist palliative care. It allows the development of an integrated plan of care that is the expression of patient and family centered care.

Each member of the interdisciplinary team has a responsibility for maintaining current knowledge of his or her particular discipline and the palliative care field, and the team as a whole provides support as well as educational opportunities for its members. There is a basic recognition of the emotional intensity of palliative care work and the ways it can affect the team. For this reason, addressing the issue of staff support is an essential function of the team. In essence, the first domain of palliative care addresses the physical, cognitive, and emotional infrastructure that allows for the delivery of specialist care.

Competency is not a static construct, but it should reflect a developmental perspective involving ongoing personal and professional development. In its foundation, competency is the result of knowledge, skills, and attitudes (Rodolfa et al., 2005). While the "knowledge" component can be acquired by self-directed study, developing skills and attitudes requires ongoing practice in the field. The ability to function as part of an interdisciplinary team is especially complex, because it also requires the ability to communicate effectively. Box 1.1 summarizes palliative psychology competencies in this domain.

Box 1.1 **Palliative Psychology Competencies in Structure and Processes of Care**

KNOWLEDGE

- history and development of palliative care
- differences and similarities between palliative care and hospice
- current models of palliative care delivery across settings
- barriers related to access and delivery of palliative care
- function of the interdisciplinary palliative care team and professional roles
- risk factors and protective factors for professional burnout; knowledge of interventions that can improve personal and professional well-being

SKILLS

- clearly describe different models of palliative care in different settings
- describe goals and application of palliative care to different patient populations from diverse cultural, social, and religious backgrounds
- facilitate access to palliative care services, coordinating with health-care professionals, patients, and family caregivers
- assess the patient and the family's needs in all domains, from a psychological perspective
- demonstrate active participation in team meetings and offer input about care plan
- integrate psychological assessment into interdisciplinary care plan
- function as a resource for training, education, and staff support
- articulate risk factors and protective factors specific to palliative psychology and develop a sustainable personal self-care plan

ATTITUDES

- respect and sensitivity for cultural values and beliefs of the patient and the family
- focus on mitigating challenges faced by the patient and family caregivers in the different palliative care settings
- appreciation of the values of interdisciplinary teamwork; willingness to rely on team and serve as a resource for team members

Palliative Care Delivery and Outcome Across Settings and Patient Populations

Palliative care can be provided to patients and families in various settings, concurrently with conventional medical treatment, or as the primary or only modality of care. While delivery of palliative care modalities varies according to the local health-care system and resources available, in the United States palliative care is primarily delivered based on three main models or systems of care: hospice, institution-based palliative care (hospitals, outpatient clinics), and community-based palliative care (the patient's home, nursing homes). Confusion still exists among lay people and even clinicians regarding the relationship between palliative care and hospice and understanding the difference and commonality between these two systems of care can provide important direction for clinicians (Strand et al., 2013).

Hospice is not a physical place. It is a health-care system providing specialist palliative care to patients in a home environment, whether in the patient's actual home or an institutional home. Hospice is also a Medicare benefit and is available to patients with a life expectancy of six months or less if the disease follows its expected course. It is a regulated system that over the years has reached an increasing number of patients in the period of time before death. Hospice "provides support and care for persons in the last phases of an incurable disease so that they may live as fully and as comfortably as possible. Hospice recognizes that the dying process is a part of the normal process of living and focuses on enhancing the quality of remaining life. Hospice affirms life and neither hastens nor postpones death. Hospice exists in the hope and belief that through appropriate care, and the promotion of the caring community sensitive to their needs that individuals and their families may be free to attain a degree of satisfaction in preparation for death." (NHPCO, 2014).

Receiving hospice care can be associated with decreased visits to the emergency department and fewer hospital admissions during the end-of-life period (Obermeyer et al., 2015). As hospice care is part of specialist palliative care, it is provided by a core interdisciplinary team including physicians, nurses, social workers, spiritual care providers, home health aides, and volunteers. Integrative medicine approaches including acupuncture, Reiki, music therapy, and art therapy may also be available. Palliative psychologists can be employed by a hospice program as core team members, work in a leadership position to manage provision of psychosocial services (including bereavement), or they may have the role of consultants. While hospice is now more utilized than in the past, barriers to access remain. Instead of receiving hospice care when their prognosis is around six months or less, in most cases patients access hospice when they are close to death. The median of length of stay has not substantially changed over the years and was 18.5 days in 2013 (NHPCO, 2014).

Much has been written about the barriers to accessing hospice services early in the disease process (Aldridge, Carlson et al., 2012). These are related to a knowledge-deficit about the available services on the part of families and also to barriers related to the culture of medicine. The perception that enrolling in hospice signals that death is imminent often deters health-care providers from exploring this option with patients and family members. This can be a result of physician's reluctance to define likely death from disease, as well as inaccurate knowledge of the breadth of services provided. A prognosis of six months or less should not be regarded as defining the date of death and should not deter health-care providers from exploring available services, under hospice, with patients and families (Torres et al., 2016).

Another barrier is related to enrollment policies. Because hospice is a capitated benefit, it is not easily accessible by many patients who are still receiving disease-modifying treatments. Additionally, some hospice programs will require patients to forgo even treatments with a palliative intent, such as palliative chemotherapy to reduce the size of a tumor or control pain, and blood transfusions. Cultural and ethnic barriers include mistrust of the medical system and translate into a much lower utilization of hospice by certain minority groups, such as African Americans, Latino, and Chinese patients. Thus, while hospice represents a high level of specialist palliative care, it is often focused on the very final period of time before death.

Even though it has often been used interchangeably with hospice care or end-of-life care, *palliative care* has a much broader scope. Palliative care as a broad umbrella term includes hospice care, but it can be available to the patient and the family from the moment of diagnosis, regardless of stage of illness, or prognosis. While hospice is a specific benefit for patients with a limited prognosis of six months or less, palliative care can provide supportive care to the patient and the family for years. Palliative care clinicians can become part of the patient care team at any point along the continuum of illness. Many of the practice principles developed in the context of hospice are applicable virtually to all patients receiving palliative care. One of these principles is Total Pain, developed by Cecily Saunders, the founder of the modern hospice movement (Saunders, 1964; Metha & Chan, 2008). Total Pain refers to all the dimensions of pain and suffering that may occur in the context of serious illness: physical pain, psychological pain, social pain, and spiritual pain. Ultimately, the main goal of palliative care is to identify and mitigate all sources of pain and suffering throughout the illness continuum, while promoting quality of life for the patient and the family. Several barriers to early and systematic integration of palliative care also exist, however, and are related to cultural, professional, and system-related factors. These barriers remain despite growing recognition of the value of palliative care in providing additional layers of specialized and individualized support to the patient and the family (Aldridge et al., 2016; Brown et al., 2016; Gidwani et al., 2016; Perrin & Kazanowski, 2015).

As the field of palliative care continues to evolve and become more integrated into mainstream medical care, it is especially important that patients and families not deprive themselves of its beneficial and expert resources, due to the misconception that accepting palliative care means that death is near and their medical care providers have given up hope (O'Rourke, 2015).

THE PALLIATIVE CARE SETTING IN THE UNITED STATES

Institution-based palliative care has grown significantly in the last decade and currently over two thirds of hospitals in the United States have palliative care consultation programs. Institution-based palliative care can be also provided in outpatient clinics, skilled nursing facilities, and nursing homes within a consultative model. There is great variability among the different programs, primarily based on available resources. For example, in smaller hospitals with limited access to resources and specialists in different disciplines, the focus of palliative care may be essentially on pain and symptom management, with limited ability to attend to the complex psychological and spiritual needs of patients and families. On the other hand, larger hospitals with greater resources may have dedicated inpatient palliative care units or scattered beds, where patients can be transferred from other hospital units, including intensive care units. However, hospital inpatient units are generally focused on addressing acute needs that cannot be managed otherwise. Furthermore, institution-based care is generally short-term with limited capability, transitioning patients to the community that continues to provide care.

Community-based palliative care represents a more recent development of the field, where care is provided to patients in their homes. Through the careful integration of institution-based palliative care and hospice, with care in the community, there is potential for specialist-level care to be provided to patients at each stage of illness beginning at diagnosis. Because the development of community-based palliative care is recent, there is still debate about what represents specialist-based palliative care in the community; and there is, therefore, great variability in the quality and intensity of the care provided. Some community-based programs have been created by hospice agencies as a way of reaching patients with needs earlier in the disease trajectory. Some have been created by hospitals as part of their outreach program. They may involve home visits and may be part of a home-based primary-care program. Some programs involve telephonic outreach and support, and some involve the utilization of telehealth approaches. Community-based programs can be led by either physicians or nurses. Despite the variability, there is a common goal of reaching patients where they live: in the home, or the nursing home.

Home-based palliative care can be provided to patients during the course of disease and also during the end-of-life period. While some patients will elect to receive hospice and enroll in a hospice program, others may choose to receive palliative care without hospice services. Home palliative care can then continue to provide physical and emotional support to these patients while they remain at home. A Cochrane review evaluated 23 studies including a total of 37,561 patients and 4,042 family caregivers. Patients included in the studies had malignant or nonmalignant advanced disease no longer responding to treatment. Of the 23 studies examined in the review, 11 were performed in the United States, while the remaining were from Europe, Canada, and Australia. The review concluded that patients receiving home-based palliative care were more likely to experience less symptom burden and to die in the home environment. Family caregivers of patients receiving community-based palliative care reported more satisfaction than those who received conventional care. And, home-based palliative care did not increase grief intensity for family caregivers assessed before the death or 13 months after the death (Gomes et al., 2013). Furthermore, there was no cost increase associated with the provision of home-based palliative care. The authors concluded that although more studies are needed to evaluate cost effectiveness, home palliative care should be provided to patients wishing to die at home because of the associated improvement in symptom control with no negative impact on caregiver grief.

Certainly, as the population ages, chronic illness will increase, and the prevalence of illness burden will represent an important opportunity to offer specialized care to patients in the comfort of a familiar home environment through community palliative care. This may avoid the physical, psychological, and also financial stresses related to multiple hospitalizations.

Preventing hospitalizations through optimal management of pain and physical symptoms, as well as depression and anxiety often associated with advanced illness, is an important and desirable outcome. However, it is also important to ensure that home palliative care is a reflection of the patient and family caregiver's choices and not an imposition based on the assumption that patients will automatically want to die at home. In fact, there are important cultural differences that need to be considered. In some cultures, for example, dying at home is not considered desirable (see also chapter 6). Additionally, remaining at home is often not an option for those patients without a primary caregiver or who cannot receive, due to insurance issues or financial constraints, a sufficient number of home health aide hours to ensure safety.

GENERAL OUTCOMES OF PALLIATIVE CARE

Several studies have assessed quality outcomes in palliative care to determine its effectiveness. Most show improvement in relief of symptoms, and they indicate that palliative care has the potential for improving quality of life in adult and pediatric patients (Chandrasekar et al., 2016; Friedrichsdorf et al., 2015). The majority of studies targeting institution-based palliative care indicate it is associated with improved patient outcome. In particular, it has been associated with improved symptom control, improved satisfaction with care for both patients and families, and decreased burden for caregivers (Ciemins et al., 2007; El-Jawahri, Greer, & Temel, 2011; Gade et al., 2008).

Teno et al. (2004) explored bereaved caregivers' experiences in caring for a dying family member in institutions versus home. Family caregivers who received hospice care at home reported that the patient's physical and emotional needs were better met and the patient was also more likely to be treated with respect. Additionally, their own emotional needs as family caregivers were better addressed through receiving hospice services, creating overall a more positive experience during the patient's dying process.

Research has also been focusing on identifying the potential positive impact of providing palliative care at the time of diagnosis. Temel et al. (2010) conducted a randomized study exploring the impact of early palliative care for patients with metastatic lung cancer. Patients were randomized to standard care alone and standard care plus palliative care interventions. Results showed that patients who received early palliative care interventions in addition to standard care reported significant improvement in quality of life and a significant reduction in symptoms of depression. Patients receiving early palliative care interventions were also significantly less likely to be exposed to prolonged aggressive care (e.g., chemotherapy in the last week of life). For patients who had contact with the palliative care team, the use of IV chemotherapy declined within 60, 30, and 14 days before death. The use of oral chemotherapy was higher within 60 days of death and then was lower as death approached. This was a result of decisions about goals of care made by patients and families who were involved in conversations about preferences, values, and goals. The palliative care intervention facilitated these conversations and allowed patients and families to make informed decisions about their care. In spite of receiving less aggressive care, patients who received palliative care also lived longer by an average of 2.5 months. Overall, while more quality studies are needed, the available evidence indicates that palliative care results in better care for the patient and for family caregivers than does standard care (Cunningham et al., 2016; Dalgard et al., 2014).

The cost-effectiveness of palliative care also has become a focus of outcome measures, and studies indicate that inpatient palliative care can be associated with decreased costs of care (Hughes & Smith, 2014). The impact of community-based palliative care within the Kaiser Permanente system showed that patients who received palliative care had equal survival rates but received better quality of care and communication. An additional outcome was a cost savings per patient of about $7,000 over a three-month period (Brumley et al., 2007). A study of the Compassionate Care Program sponsored by Aetna also indicated improved patient care as well as cost reduction (Krakauer, Spettell, Reisman, & Wade, 2011). Based on this telephonic program, trained registered nurses reached patients with serious illness in their home. As a result of the program, there was an increase in hospice enrollment, and patients received adequate symptoms control and emotional support. Additionally, the program was associated with fewer ICU days, fewer inpatient days, and overall cost savings. Importantly, the cost savings were the result of patients' ability to express preferences about end-of-life care, which, in many cases, was to forgo aggressive care at the end of life.

While quality and satisfaction will continue to drive the development of palliative care, it is important to recognize that economic drivers may also become increasingly relevant. In systems where the provider of care is also the payer, cost avoidance is likely to become an essential consideration. It is important to note that cost control and cost savings *are not* objectives of palliative care, but it may occur as a result of applying medical best practices that carefully consider patients' goals of care.

How can specialist level palliative care result in cost savings? One important component of palliative care is the engagement of the patient and family in sensitive, collaborative, and gradual discussions about expectations and goals of care based on the patient and the family's values and preferences. As a result of conversations related to goal settings and advanced care planning, some patients with serious and terminal illness may decide not to receive disease-modifying therapies when there is little likelihood of benefit but great likelihood of burden. For example, patients with advanced cancer may decide, after conversations with their treating team, that the symptom burden caused by further chemotherapy treatments will likely not extend their life, but will result in poorer quality of life. Or, they may decide that the benefit of living a few weeks longer is not worth the burden of spending that time suffering with debilitating symptoms from treatment side effects. They may decide that they prefer to spend the final weeks or months of life connecting with loved ones and engaging in activities that are meaningful to them with optimal management of physical and psychological symptoms. Furthermore, some patients with advanced cancer may be convinced that continuing chemotherapy may have a curative potential. Being presented with the medical reality that it is not likely to be the case may prompt a difficult but different decision, to forgo disease-modifying treatment in the last weeks of life and to focus on quality-of-life goals and supportive care.

In essence, while cost of care is *never* part of a conversation about goals of care, the cost-saving potential in palliative care may be a result of accurate information and decision making.

As mentioned previously, there are cultural and social variations in the way individuals and families approach medical decision-making. Due to religious and cultural beliefs, some patients will decide to continue receiving aggressive treatments and life-prolonging treatments (e.g., chemotherapy in the last weeks of life; intubation, etc.), regardless of the symptom burden associated with such treatments or the lack of anticipated benefits. Cultural and religious beliefs and family dynamics may also prevent open conversations about goals of care. To be sure, when there are clear cultural or religious factors affecting patient and family decision-making, these should always be respected. And the palliative care team remains committed to supporting them during all transitions.

Adequate coordination of care is also one of the goals of palliative care. When implemented correctly, it may prevent duplication of services. Additionally, a focus on early symptom intervention may prevent hospitalizations allowing the patient to remain in their home or nursing home. Hospitalizations are typically stressful for patients and family and preventing them is a good outcome for all. The financial impact of preventing hospitalizations by adequately controlling symptoms in the home is ultimately cost saving, because the hospital is not only a more expensive setting but also a source of potential infectious complications.

In summary, controlling cost is neither a goal of palliative care nor a focus of the clinical team. However, in a 21st-century environment, the success of a clinical care program is determined not only by the positive clinical outcome, but also by its ability to be sustainable. As a result, the longevity and growth of a clinical program are directly connected to its cost-effectiveness (Cassel et al., 2015).

Where do palliative psychologists fit into this discussion about financial sustainability? For many clinicians, financial considerations in clinical care are not compatible with the ethical image of a mission-driven clinician. This is true for most helping clinicians and certainly for many psychology practitioners. However, not considering the impact of financial considerations on clinical care is detrimental, because it ignores a basic reality, at least in the United States, that the inclusion of additional professionals specialized in palliative care as part of the interdisciplinary team will continue to be affected by issues of financial sustainability.

It is common for members of a palliative care team to recognize the added value offered by psychologists as core team members or consultants, especially when the complex psychological needs of a patient and family present challenges to the team. While a clinical psychologist may bill for services in outpatient programs, many hospitals with palliative care programs have not yet developed a structure that would allow psychologists to obtain reimbursement for services provided to inpatients. Additionally, if the palliative care psychologist bills as a consultant, the cost of the consultation will likely be passed on to the patient, with possible negative repercussions. For this reason, recognizing the presence of financial barriers and developing creative funding and billing practices may help the inclusion of additional professionals, such as psychologists, as core members of the team. Grants specifically designed to enhance psychological support for patients receiving palliative care could support the inclusion of palliative psychologists. In essence, identifying practical strategies to allow the integration of psychologists on palliative care teams in a manner that is financially feasible and sustainable will need to be systematically included in palliative psychology training programs.

EVOLUTION OF PALLIATIVE CARE MODELS IN THE UNITED STATES

Palliative care can be integrated at different times during the illness trajectory; however, clinicians are increasingly advocating for its inclusion at the time of initial diagnosis, at the same time medical therapies focus on modifying the disease and achieving a cure. When the goal of cure cannot be accomplished, medical therapy predominantly focuses on controlling and managing the disease, relieving symptoms and suffering, improving quality of life, and preserving function. If the disease progresses the patient may move into advanced stages of illness and ultimately into the last stages of life. In advanced illness, care becomes focused on allowing patients to live meaningfully, free from physical and emotional distress. Throughout the disease trajectory and as death approaches, palliative care interventions may focus on facilitating meaningful connections with loved ones, on compassionate and supportive life review, and on providing relief from distressing symptoms in the last days and hours of the dying process. After the patient's death, grief and bereavement care for survivors becomes the goal of treatment.

The interpretation and clinical application of palliative care has evolved significantly over the last two decades. Early models did not clearly differentiate between palliative care and end-of-life care. Thus, the comprehensive care of physical, psychological, and spiritual needs was generally not available or presented as an option for patients until medical treatment was suspended due to not being effective, or causing severe adverse effects that could not be tolerated. In this model, palliative care was not initiated until the patient stopped active treatment. This approach limits the integration of palliative care, but it is still the norm in many settings, where a discussion about palliative care is not initiated until the patient stops disease-modifying treatment. In many instances, and especially in the cancer population, patients receive chemotherapy often until a few weeks or sometimes days before they die. As a result, palliative care is often introduced late in the course of the illness, if ever. Figure 1.1 illustrates this approach to palliative care.

The limitations of this model are the following:

1. It encourages abrupt and compartmentalized transitions of care, which can increase suffering for the patient and the family.
2. Because the transition to palliative care is abrupt, it has difficult psychological implications for the patient and the family; it promotes the idea that the medical team is "giving up," and the patient is dying. This can engender profound feelings of abandonment and grief, with a negative impact on quality of life.

Figure 1.1. Palliative care introduced **only** after cessation of disease-modifying treatments. Adapted and modified from Clinical Practice Guidelines, 2009

3. Depending on the timing of referral, patients may not be able to benefit from all the palliative care services available. If the patient is referred late in the course of the illness, when function is severely compromised and there is rapid decline, addressing psychological and existential needs meaningfully becomes more challenging and may be unrealistic.
4. It may promote avoidance of discussion about goals of care on the part of medical providers who may delay involvement of palliative care because they misconstrue it as "giving up."

CASE VIGNETTE 1.1

Lee presents to her appointment at the ambulatory oncology clinic. She is a 45-year-old woman with a diagnosis of peritoneal cancer metastatic to bone and liver, diagnosed several months ago. She comes to the medical appointment with her husband. A CT of her abdomen and pelvis revealed multiple hepatic lesions with progressive disease manifested by interval appearance of new hepatic masses as well an increase in size of three previously identified masses. The CT of the chest is concerning for malignancy. The patient has undergone four cycles of chemotherapy. Despite these treatments, the cancer has spread. Lee's main complaint is shortness of breath with dysphagia and difficulty swallowing pills. She reports pain at a 7 on a scale from 0 to 10 and difficulty walking. She reports feeling "very afraid and anxious," which also exacerbates her shortness of breath. Her husband notes that she seems depressed and "cries herself to sleep every night." The couple have three children, ages 6, 8, and 10. They moved four years ago to a large city from a rural area where they lived with the extended family. The move was motivated by a good job opportunity for the husband, but they miss the support of their previous community. The medical team feels that further chemotherapy is not likely to benefit Lee and will add to her overall symptom burden. However, there is concern that stopping chemotherapy will feel like abandonment to the couple. The patient and her husband agree to a meeting with the palliative care team, and for the first time the topic of goals of care is discussed. A family meeting is arranged with the patient's oncologist, as well as members of the palliative care team (physician, nurse, psychologist, and social worker). The oncologist admits that she would not recommend resuming chemotherapy due to its limited benefit in prior courses. At that point in the meeting, the patient's husband becomes upset and asks, "What are we supposed to do now, then? Are you shipping us out? Are you no longer our doctor?" The oncologist reassures the couple that she will remain available, but suggests that the palliative care team could be more helpful at this point. The palliative care clinicians explain that the team can work actively to help manage pain and other symptoms, as well as help manage the depression and anxiety. They explain that care can be refocused on using all available tools to allow for the best quality of life possible. Lee comments that since the diagnosis she has had no quality of life because the burden of treatment has been so great. She states that she has tolerated the discomfort from the chemotherapy because she thought it would cure the disease. Both patient and her husband comment that they had no idea the treatment had not worked and do not seem aware that the disease has continued to spread in spite of treatment. They feel the news comes as a surprise. The oncologist reminds them of prior conversations when the poor effectiveness of treatment has been discussed. Lee's husband says, "But you never told us it wasn't working." At that point, the patient becomes agitated. She starts crying and keeps repeating, "I don't want to die!" She begins hyperventilating and cannot catch her breath. She looks at her husband and cries, "Help me!" Her husband looks frightened and tries to calm her but is unsuccessful. The psychologist asks permission to approach the patient and help her feel more comfortable. After receiving a nod from the patient, the psychologist sits close to her and uses a hypnotic induction followed by a breathing technique to decrease the level of arousal. Lee responds well to the intervention and becomes calmer. She is able to express that she feels devastated by the news. She also describes her concerns about pain and anxiety, and she mentions she is worried about her children and what she should tell them. Because the patient appears calm, the palliative care physician examines her to assess her pain. After reviewing the patient's medication, he prescribes a new regimen that includes opioids. An antidepressant with antianxiety properties is also prescribed, as well as a low dose of a short-acting benzodiazepine to be used as needed during anxiety exacerbation. The psychologist and the social worker continue the meeting with the patient and her husband after the other team members have left the room and explore the couple's concerns about the children. A follow-up appointment with the psychologist is scheduled for later in the week to initiate regular psychotherapy. After the couple has left the clinic, a debriefing meeting with the oncologist and the palliative care team takes place. The oncologist shares feeling sad and frustrated by the couple's reaction. She admits that vague attempts had been made to suggest to the couple that treatment was not as helpful as initially hoped for, but she did not want to "take hope away from them." Therefore, ambiguous language was used and it appeared that everyone colluded with the desire to avoid discussing a negative outcome. The oncologist further comments that both the medical team and the couple have tried avoiding the discomfort of a conversation about goals of care. As the patient continues working with the psychologist, anxiety and fear of dying become the main focus of treatment. Individual sessions with the patient are followed by couple sessions and family sessions that include the couple's children and the grandparents. Legacy projects are developed for the children and other family members.

In spite of the distress the patient and her husband felt after facing the reality of ineffective treatment, there were positive outcomes after the involvement of palliative care. Lee's pain became more manageable almost overnight and her anxiety also improved within a few days. They continued regular outpatient couple's therapy with the psychologist, with periodic family sessions where the children and the patient's parents also participated. Unfortunately, this couple was introduced to palliative care at a time of crisis, and their initial concern was that they were being abandoned, which triggered anxiety and disappointment. The initial meeting also evidenced previous inadequate communication with the primary medical team and unmet physical and psychological needs that could have been better addressed during the course of disease-modifying treatment. In summary, in a model where palliative care is offered and initiated only after disease-modifying treatments are stopped, palliative care becomes the "instead of," rather than the "in addition to." In the mind of the patient and the family, it is then conceptualized as *instead* of treatment, *instead* of getting better, *instead* of cure, *instead* of hope, *instead* of life. On the other hand, when palliative care is offered "in addition to," it expresses its full potential as offering additional and critical layers of specialized medical and psychosocial-spiritual care to the patient and the family.

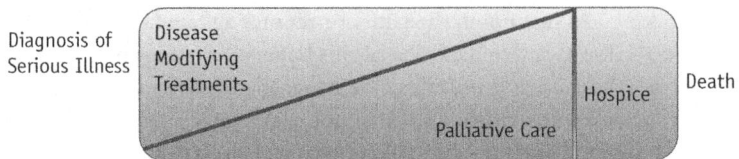

Figure 1.2. Palliative care progressively integrated along the continuum of illness. Adapted and modified from National Consensus Project, 2013

Figure 1.2 shows a model of palliative care delivery presenting several advantages. It includes the progressive involvement of palliative care during disease-modifying or life-prolonging treatments. Therefore, it allows patients and families to benefit from palliative care services along the continuum of care, depending on their needs. It also promotes a more gradual transition of care, where palliative approaches are integrated into the care of the patient as needed, based on their unique circumstances. Furthermore, in this model the patient and the family are introduced to the palliative care team early on, and they can establish relationships and connections.

According to the diagram commonly used to represent the model, the proportion of palliative care services provided to the patient and the family is expected to increase as options for disease-modifying and life-prolonging treatments decrease. Yet it somehow implies that patients and families may have few or no palliative care needs at the time of diagnosis. This is not necessarily accurate, especially when the patient is diagnosed with disease that is already advanced. Additionally, while the patient may not experience distressing pain and physical symptoms, there may be psychological and existential distress; if this sort of distress is not addressed early and adequately managed, it will likely increase and create suffering for the patient and the family.

As research in the last decade has continued to indicate, palliative care interventions can be important at the time of diagnosis to allow for adequate management of physical and psychosocial distress (Bakitas et al., 2009, 2015; Dionne-Odom et al., 2015). Any assumption that patients' palliative care needs steadily and predictably increase as they move along the continuum of illness is generally not reflective of their unique situation and may delay the provision of important support.

According to a more recent model (Figure 1.3), palliative care may be introduced at the time of diagnosis to address any physical, psychological, existential, or spiritual needs the patient and the family may have. It is provided concurrently with all the treatments the patient is receiving, and the transitions are neither predefined nor abrupt. The intensity of palliative care services fluctuate based on the patients' needs, and all

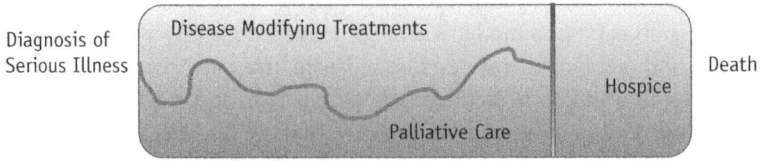

Figure 1.3. Palliative care fully integrated from the time of diagnosis based on patients' evolving needs. Adapted and modified from Amita Health, 2017, https://www.alexianbrothershealth.org/services/palliative-care

needs begin to be assessed at the time of diagnosis. The palliative care team becomes part of the extended care team and the patient and the family can access its resources throughout the continuum of care.

This model presents a model of palliative care delivery that fully reflects the clinical realities of living with serious illness. It emphasizes that patient- and family-centered care requires that all needs be addressed from diagnosis and through the disease continuum. It underscores that ameliorating or palliating any type of distress, be it physical or psychological or spiritual, needs to be a primary goal of care along with the goal of curing or managing the illness. The goal of maintaining or obtaining good quality of life should be prioritized from the time of diagnosis and while the patient receives treatment for a disease. This care must be individualized and the care plan modified to continually adjusts to the patients' evolving needs, including evolving goals of care.

CASE VIGNETTE 1.2

Renee is a 55-year-old woman diagnosed with breast cancer. Imaging studies show that the cancer is localized, and the medical team believes the disease can be cured. Adjuvant chemotherapy is started with the intent to treat for cure. She has successfully tolerated the first chemotherapy treatment and is not complaining of pain or other symptoms other than moderate fatigue for about one week after treatment.

Renee has a preexisting history of panic disorder and major depression, for which she had stopped receiving treatment years ago; however, she is not reporting any symptoms of depression or anxiety. She describes her relationship with her only son, who visits her about once a month, as "complicated." She does not have other immediate family or friends who can provide support. The patient misses her second appointment for chemotherapy treatment; when the nurse calls her at home, she states that she was unable to find transportation to the hospital, but she will try to make the next appointment. The nurse arranges for Access-A-Ride pickup the next day. After the treatment the patient is referred to the outpatient palliative care clinic by her oncologist, who is concerned about her previous history of psychiatric illness, the lack of psychosocial support, and the impact of psycho-social challenges. During an evaluation by the palliative care physician and psychologist, it appears that Renee is experiencing high levels of anxiety about treatment, but she tried to hide it from her oncologist because "everyone is so excited that I can be cured and I don't want to seem ungrateful." The patient also admits that she feels as if she does not really care about being cured and reports feeling "numb" at the idea of living or dying. She also states that she is not sure she wants to start taking medication for depression and anxiety because she heard her son once comment that "only people with a weak mind use antidepressants." She believes the statement was directed at her, even though she never asked him to explain the nature of his comment. After that episode she became more distant with her son and discouraged his attempts to visit more frequently.

Renee agrees to meet regularly with the palliative psychologist for psychotherapy. The sessions take place twice a week and a cognitive-behavioral model is initially followed. During the first session the psychologist illustrates to the patient the relationship between thoughts, emotions, and behaviors, and discusses how this relationship is directly impacting the patient's decision-making process regarding medical treatment. Renee resonates with the model and becomes quite active in therapy. The second therapy session focuses on the patient's relationship with psychotropic medication and presence of cognitive distortions related to her son's comments. Now being familiar with the potential fallacy in making decisions based on assumptions that can prove to be cognitive distortion, the patient admits her depression and anxiety symptoms used to be well managed with medication. She expresses willingness to resume taking an antidepressant with the understanding that her ongoing perception about the medication, as well as any adverse effects, will be addressed in the course of weekly therapy and also discussed with the palliative care physician who is prescribing. Renee is able to continue chemotherapy treatment and her mood improves significantly. Upon the patient's request, her son is invited to join a therapy session. This allows the previous misunderstandings and hurt feelings to be clarified and resolved. As a result, the relationship shifts to being supportive, rather than distant. The patient expresses the desire to continue psychotherapy on a monthly basis to reduce the burden of frequent travel.

Unfortunately, about seven months after the end of treatment, she develops persistent hip pain and a scan indicates the presence of bone metastases. The patient is devastated by the news. The primary medical team recommends a new line of chemotherapy to control spread of disease. Renee is now suffering from moderate to severe pain, nausea, and severe fatigue. She already has a trusting relationship with the palliative care team, and a consultation is arranged. The palliative care physician and the nurse begin actively managing the patient's pain and symptoms, and weekly psychotherapy is resumed. Renee's fear of dying and the difficulty dealing with treatment become the focus of therapy. Additionally, she also questions whether she should continue chemotherapy given the symptom burden, but she decides to "give it a try."

The psychotherapy approach retains some elements of cognitive-behavioral therapy and strategic therapy when dealing with belief system and decision-making. However, a humanistic approach, focused on promoting a sense of connectedness, meaning, and emotional safety, appears to be more appropriate for meeting the patient's needs at this time. A narrative therapy approach is also used to help Renee externalize her anxiety. This approach allows her to develop a more positive attitude toward her life story by recognizing that she is not the problem; rather, "the problem (anxiety) is the problem." Thus, active strategies can be used to solve the different "problems," without undermining her sense of identity. Renee describes herself as "somewhat spiritual" but without any specific beliefs. She shares with the psychologist that at home she has a book of mystical poetry, and she finds it comforting. She asks if she could bring the book to the session. From that day on, the therapy approach once again shifts and becomes focused on nurturing her sense of meaning and spiritual connection. During the therapy session Renee reads a poem slowly, out loud. Subsequently, the patient and the therapist share their thoughts about the impact of the poem. Renee reports that this approach is giving her great comfort and is also calming. Unfortunately, a subsequent scan shows continued spread of disease in spite of treatment. At this point, a meeting is arranged with the patient's oncologist and the palliative care team, and a gentle conversation about goals of care is started. Renee decides to stop chemotherapy treatment, but active symptoms management and psychotherapy continue. With several modifications required by the patient's declining condition, the therapy sessions continue after the patient's admission to an inpatient palliative care unit four months later, where she also died, surrounded by her son and the clinicians who had cared for her.

In this clinical case, the patient had significant psychological/psychiatric needs at the time of diagnosis, which were effectively addressed by a combined approach of medication and intense psychotherapy. Initially, she had few medical needs related to pain and other physical symptoms, as the primary area of distress and suffering was psychological. The early referral to palliative care, even when it was believed that the patient would be cured, was perfectly appropriate. It allowed her to receive the specialized psychological and pharmacological treatment she needed. Additionally, it promoted a trusting relationship with the palliative care team, which became particularly helpful when the patient's condition began to deteriorate. This approach also allowed for continuity of care and prevented a sense of abandonment in a patient who already had limited social support.

CASE VIGNETTE 1.3

Zach is a 58-year-old man who developed persistent back pain, progressive fatigue, and "heaviness" in the substernal region. A CT of the chest ordered by his primary care physician revealed a mass in the right upper lobe with lymphadenopathy in the mediastinum. The primary care physician referred him to an interventional radiologist for a biopsy that confirms a diagnosis of advanced non-small-cell lung cancer. Zach works as an insurance executive, has been married for over 20 years, and has two teenage daughters. He has a history of generalized anxiety disorder for which he takes an SSRI regularly and a low dose of clonazepam as needed for exacerbations of anxiety, prescribed by his primary care physician. The cancer diagnosis comes as a shock to the family.

The oncologist who delivers the diagnosis suggests chemotherapy to control worsening of disease and suggests the patient and the family meet with the palliative care team for additional support during treatment. The physician explains that this is a team of clinicians with specialized skills in managing symptoms of the disease and providing emotional support. The patient and the family are stunned by the diagnosis but agree to meet with the palliative care team. A palliative care consultation is called and a meeting with the family is scheduled for the same day. During the meeting with the palliative care physician, nurse, social worker, psychologists, and chaplain, a thorough assessment reveals that the patient has moderate pain and anxiety. The patient agrees to follow recommendations for pain management, and it is agreed that he will continue seeing his primary care physician for the management of anxiety.

The psychologist and the social worker openly acknowledge that receiving the news of the diagnosis may be overwhelming, but emphasize that they are available for support during the process. The patient and his wife are quiet and say they just want to go home and be with their daughters. At the first treatment appointment four days later, the psychologist and the social worker walk to the infusion suite to greet the patient and his wife. In a kind tone, the wife says, "We appreciate your support, but we are really not interested in talking about this right now. We are very private people and right now we are doing fine." One week later, however, the psychologist receives a phone call from the patient's wife, who is worried about her husband. She explains that since the treatment started he has become increasingly anxious and cannot sleep at night. His primary care physician offered to prescribe hypnotics to help him sleep, but he has refused. The psychologist meets with the couple and normalizes the anxiety the patient is experiencing. She also discusses practical strategies to promote relaxation and decrease rumination.

The psychologist guides the patient in a permissive guided imagery exercise designed to elicit images that can be soothing for him. Zach mentions that he used to love fishing on a lake near his home, and was always calmed by the sense of stillness and quiet. He also remembers that when he went fishing he would listen to a particular piece of piano music by Debussy. With the patient's permission, the psychologist reaches out to a music therapy colleague. With the use of a digital recorder, a guided imagery session is recorded, with the psychologist using the images of fishing and the emotions associated with it by the patient. In the background, the music therapist plays Debussy. The recording is handed to the patient, who starts listening to it several times a day. He also listens to it during chemotherapy sessions and especially when he feels he is becoming anxious and before sleeping. Zach reports feeling more in control and is able to better manage chemotherapy side effects. He continues meeting with the psychologist about once a month, and after each session a new recording is created by the psychologist and the music therapist, with a combination of patient-elicited imagery and music that is meaningful to him.

This case also highlights the benefits of introducing palliative care at the time of diagnosis. The patient and the family may choose not to avail themselves of services, or they may not perceive a need. However, once the connection with the palliative care team is established, they are empowered with the option of reaching out, as in the case described here. It is important to remember that palliative care is not only focused on addressing, but also on preventing suffering. As clinicians are aware, a diagnosis of serious illness does not automatically cause suffering. There is a continuum of distress between the initial perception of psychological discomfort and the development of suffering. Similarly, pain and symptoms, when adequately treated, do not automatically cause suffering. Suffering refers to a kind of mental and spiritual anguish that can make life difficult to bear. By addressing physical symptoms and psychological discomfort early and proactively, palliative care clinicians can effectively prevent the development of suffering in many cases. And when suffering has already developed, they apply the most sophisticated interventions to change the quality of suffering to a manageable experience that can allow room for positive emotions and meaningful connections.

The Palliative Care Assessment: Comprehensive and Interdisciplinary

The domains of palliative care and practice guidelines used as a framework for this book describe the critical role of comprehensive and interdisciplinary palliative care assessment to identify the needs of the patient and family. Assessment in palliative care does not indicate simply an event, but an ongoing process requiring clinicians to continually incorporate new information as the patient's condition evolves with the illness and with medical interventions. Standardized tools can be used, particularly in research settings, to obtain information about certain aspects of the patient's and the family's experience. However, in the psychological assessment, the clinical interview should be considered the gold standard. It allows the clinician to develop quick rapport with the patient and the family. Additionally, the tone of the communication and the direction of the interview can be modified to validate and respect cultural practices and beliefs. This assessment is performed in the context of a relationship, and it offers the opportunity to "join" with the patient and the family, establishing trust and therapeutic alliance.

The psychology clinical interview is a specialized intervention that represents also an opportunity to understand how the patient and the family are interpreting what is happening and what are the values, beliefs, and cultural practices that sustain them or that may be an impediment to their well-being. Palliative psychologists approach the patient from a holistic and strength-based approach. And their assessment skills allow rapid detection of psychological distress that reaches clinical significance. Good clinical interviewing skills are necessary to provide assessments in inpatient and outpatient settings, and in the presence of the team or other family members.

Obviously, the palliative psychology assessment is not provided in a vacuum. Therefore, it should not only address the psychological and psychiatric aspects of care, but also include attention to all basic domains: physical, psychological/psychiatric, social, and spiritual (see Chapter 3). To illustrate, a psychologist should understand the patient's symptom burden created by pain, dyspnea, and others in order to deliver psychological interventions that can effectively target mood. The principles of palliative care reflect collaborative practice and the need for the coordinated work of skilled professionals. No single professional alone can embody expertise in all the domains of palliative care. The importance of this coordination cannot be underestimated; it allows competent management of patients' needs in the different domains, it provides an important forum for case discussion, and it fosters a space where team members can obtain support from each other.

Interdisciplinary communication and collaboration within the team enables clinicians to develop a deep understanding of patients and families' values, beliefs, and needs. It is important to note that at times the patient and the family may disagree on important aspects of care, such as appropriate communication about diagnosis and prognosis, beliefs about life sustaining treatments, and others. Additionally, personal values and beliefs are not immutable and may change, requiring revaluation of care plans and planning. The ability and availability to continually assess the patient's relationship, values, and response to treatment is an essential skill set. The care plan should reflect patient and family values and represent the integration of interdisciplinary input.

Expanding Opportunities for Palliative Psychology

Psychologists interested in expanding their role to include palliative care should first develop a thorough knowledge and understanding of their work setting. The following questions should be considered: What is the general institutional culture that drives the provision of mental health services? For example, is psychology part of a specific service (e.g., psychology or consultation-liaison psychiatry)? Is the psychologist's role understood as a consultant who may be called upon by various staff members in different departments to provide services for patients? How are billing and other financial issues pertinent to the provision of mental health services handled in the institution? For example, can the clinical psychologist bill for inpatient services?

Further, if the hospital/clinic has a designated palliative care team, can the psychologist become involved by offering to assist with patients' and families' psychological needs? Is the psychologist expected to function as part of the team and therefore share information about the patient in the context of regular meetings? If the psychologist functions as an occasional consultant "borrowed" from a different service, (e.g., psychology, psychiatry, consultation liaison psychiatry, or behavioral health), what provisions are made, if any, to support their role in palliative care? What is the level of institutional awareness about the role that psychologists have in the institution and the ways they can contribute to patient care? For example, are various staff members aware of referral criteria that may justify a psychological consult?

Depending on the clinical setting and their assigned roles, palliative psychologists will be required to function within different structures, as well as interface with different professionals, often in the context of an interdisciplinary team of involved clinicians. Institution-based and private or group practice psychologists who wish to provide palliative care need to develop an understanding of the critical aspects of their setting, including challenges and opportunities. Psychologists with inpatient hospital privileges may provide psychological interventions at the bedside; others may, for example, work in a cancer center and develop an outpatient practice. These two modalities allow the involvement of psychologists in palliative care: either as core members of the palliative care team specifically hired for this role, or as consultants, while fulfilling their primary role in a different service or elsewhere.

While specialist palliative care is by definition interdisciplinary, it is important to acknowledge, however, that the presence of an interdisciplinary team is not available in many community settings with limited resources. When this occurs, generally one medical professional, either a physician or a nurse, focuses on addressing the physical domain of care with attention to psychosocial and spiritual needs, including identifying goals of care and communicating with other providers involved in the care of the patient.

This type of scenario may be challenging for a solo psychology practitioner. Thus, it is necessary to collaborate with other providers who have expertise in other disciplines, even if not specifically in palliative care. Collaborative practice and further education in palliative care can help develop skills and implement models of practice even in the absence of a dedicated palliative care team. For example, in a community hospital setting a nurse may have developed expertise in pain and symptom management and may receive consults from the primary team (e.g., oncologists, hospitalists, or internists). A clinical psychologist working in the same setting with a special interest in palliative care may begin collaborating with the nurse on cases requiring pain and symptom control and psychosocial support for both the patient and the family. While the establishment of a dedicated palliative care team may not be a realistic goal in this hypothetical community setting, it is often possible to establish a palliative care focus of practice working with other professionals on individual cases.

Professional Self-Care: An Ethical Imperative for Palliative Psychologists

The importance of staff support and self-care for all palliative care clinicians is also emphasized in the first domain of palliative care. Professional self-care has been increasingly recognized as an essential element for all palliative care clinicians due to the awareness that daily exposure to grief, suffering and death and dying have an impact on clinicians' well-being. Additionally, palliative care involves intense emotional engagement and constant negotiations between patients and family needs with the limitations and demands of the health-care system. Although it is extremely rewarding work, it can also be challenging and stressful.

The ability to develop and maintain professional self-care is a necessary competency for specialist palliative care clinicians, and it is as important as the ability to conduct a thorough psychological assessment to determine patients' and families' needs. Sustaining clinical excellence in palliative and end-of-life care depends on the ability to sustain professional satisfaction and a sense of meaning while providing patient care.

Professional self-care is a complex competence with essential knowledge, skills, and attitudes. It is important to develop knowledge of personal and professional risk factors, and knowledge of appropriate and individualized protective strategies. Self-assessment and intervention skills include the ability to develop a personalized professional self-care plan. The necessary attitudes include viewing self-care as an ongoing practice, rather than an outcome attainable once and for all. Attitudes also include a willingness to engage in a reflective practice of self-awareness and ongoing monitoring of personal motivations, relationship to the work, and responses to stress and grief (Sanso et al., 2015).

In the professional self-care literature, the constructs most commonly utilized to describe the different types of professional stress reactions are burnout, vicarious traumatization, and compassion fatigue. In contrast, personal awareness and mindfulness, exquisite empathy, compassion satisfaction, and resilience have been described among the protective factors that may have a long-lasting positive impact (Kearney, Weininger, Vachon, Harrison, & Mount, 2009; Sanchez-Reilly et al., 2013). Terms indicating professional stress reactions are often used interchangeably, so it may be useful to briefly review them in the context of palliative care. *Burnout* is a stress syndrome manifesting through a combination of emotional exhaustion, depersonalization, and a reduced sense of personal accomplishments (Maslach & Leiter, 1997). Burnout can cause clinicians to feel constantly overworked, unable to meet demands, and therefore discouraged, demoralized, and exhausted. It is specifically related to workplace related stress and is often the result of low job satisfaction, feeling overwhelmed by workload and powerlessness to affect change.

While the provider-patient relationship was initially identified as the source of burnout, current conceptualizations propose that burnout is likely to occur when there is a mismatch between the ethical and professional values held by the individual and those of the organization (Laschinger & Leiter, 2006). The work-related factors that have been shown by research to be primarily associated with burnout are the following: work overload, lack of control, lack of community, lack of fairness, lack of reward, and conflict between the values held by the individual and the values held by the organization. In essence, burnout indicates a condition of physical and emotional exhaustion related to work conditions that are considered challenging and toxic, because of a distressing mismatch between the organization and the individual in several areas. While it can be a significant risk factor for depression and even suicidal ideation, in general the distress lasts for as long as the individual is forced to cope with work conditions that feel unmanageable and unfair. Early studies had described a similar or lower prevalence of burnout in palliative care clinicians compared to other specialties, such as oncology (Peters et al., 2012). However, other studies from the United Kingdom and Canada have begun to indicate a possible increase in level of distress in palliative care clinicians (Berman et al., 2007; Dougherty et al., 2009). A study based on in-depth interviews of 15 palliative care clinicians explored the presence of work stressors to develop a program promoting resilience (Perez et al., 2015). Results from content analysis indicated that the main stressors were related to difficultly managing large caseloads within the time constraints, challenges managing patients' and families' complex and ongoing needs, and challenges managing emotions and professional boundaries.

Palliative care clinicians may be at risk for experiencing post-traumatic stress disorder (PTSD) symptoms (O'Mahoney et al., 2016), especially if they are using avoidant coping as the main strategy. Witnessing refractory suffering in patients also represents a high-risk scenario, which can result in ruptures and conflict within the interdisciplinary team (Swetenham et al., 2011). A study of palliative care clinicians in the United States has indicated a prevalence of burnout of 62% across disciplines (Kamal et al., 2016). Among the predictors of high levels of burnout were being non-physicians (nurses, social workers, and chaplains), working longer hours and weekends, and working for smaller organizations.

In preventing and addressing burnout, it is important to consider not only the factors related to individual clinicians but also organization-related factors. For example, while palliative care focuses on also addressing the needs of family caregivers, current policies do not allow for additional reimbursement to support this complex work with the family system. As a result, while a palliative care or hospice organization may emphasize the importance of providing psychological counseling to the family and may require clinicians to provide these services, the patient caseload may hamper a clinician's ability to provide quality counseling or other services. Providing careful assessment and intervention in the palliative care setting is time consuming, especially when families have complex dynamics or face particular challenges. Balancing efficiency with the desire to provide therapeutic interventions can be challenging, as several individual and family meetings may be needed to truly support the patient and the family. The amount of time needed to satisfactorily address a complex case may affect a clinician's ability to manage an already high caseload. The clinician may begin working longer hours just to meet the daily clinical demands. Alternatively, some begin working on their documentation after they arrive home from work, or just may not complete it.

In the long run, physical and emotional exhaustion can result, as well as cynicism about the mission of the work and the organization. To cope with this challenging situation, clinicians may feel they have no choice but to provide only a superficial level of support in order to meet the demands of the caseload and the required documentation. However, a superficial level of support may not allow clinicians to experience the professional satisfaction they need to continue feeling motivated in their work. In the end, clinicians may feel that even though they want to provide excellent work, they are not being allowed to do so because of the workload demands. In the scenario described here, the clinician has extremely high work demands but little control over how to execute the tasks related to the job. This combination of high demand and low control is a key risk factor.

While organization-related stressors are considered the main contributors to developing burnout, the impact of individual characteristics has also been examined. To illustrate, maladaptive work-related attitudes, such as idealistic expectations on the part of the clinician, can lead to burnout. In the example described above, the clinician's perception about what represents adequate psychological support for a family may become inflexible and based on ideal standards that can only be met in a private practice setting, rather than in a health-care organization. Additionally, if the clinician has the expectation that his or her interventions will always result in positive result for every patient and family, there may be significant disappointment. Interestingly, high levels of idealism and desire to change and improve systems are often typical of less experienced clinicians and have also been described as risk factors for burnout. If the clinician feels that the work demands (clinical, administrative, etc.) outweigh his or her resources, burnout can result. This type of scenario identifies an important area of intervention for professional caregivers who are not merely victims of a toxic system, but may also need to examine whether their perceptions about their professional role should be adjusted to promote adaptation and a sustainable approach to their work.

Compassion fatigue is specifically related to the helping profession. The term was initially used to describe the experience of emergency room nurses in the context of a study of burnout. In response to a highly stressful environment, large workload and ongoing exposure to patients' pain and suffering, distress and traumatic injuries, some nurses appeared to be unable to approach the patients with compassion (Joinson, 1992). They appeared depressed, angry, and detached, and experienced several somatic complaints. Compassion fatigue was subsequently described by Figley (2002) to indicate a clinician's state of physical and emotional exhaustion related to constant exposure to the traumatic circumstances experienced by patients. Compassion fatigue can alter an individual's cognitive schemas and beliefs about the world, causing cognitive shifts and difficulty relating to others. The "relationship" component appears to be the most affected. Compassion fatigue is also known as vicarious traumatization, because the clinician can experience symptoms similar to those of the traumatized patients. Vicarious traumatization describes the emotional distress experienced by clinicians as a result of being continually exposed to images and accounts of traumatic experience of their patients (Pearlman & Saakvitne, 1995). According to the model, this ongoing exposure, coupled with a strong empathic response in the provider, can trigger symptoms similar to PTSD.

Although work and organizational factors at the base of a mismatch between the job and the person are considered at the root of developing burnout, compassion fatigue is considered to be rooted in the patient-provider relationship. In compassion fatigue, the clinician feels depleted, emotionally exhausted, and unable to nurture patients. Unlike burnout, symptoms of compassion fatigue resemble posttraumatic stress disorder (Sabo, 2011).

According to Figley compassion fatigue results from the clinician experiencing both secondary traumatization and burnout. It has also been suggested that high levels of empathy and the provider's empathic response to the trauma and suffering experienced by patients can begin a process that can deplete the emotional resources of the provider (Figley, 2002). This secondary traumatic stress syndrome is similar to PTSD, especially in terms of the somatic experience; in fact, the arousal and avoidance criteria are the same. The key issue is that while in PTDS the individual has experienced trauma personally, in secondary traumatic stress syndrome the clinician is exposed to the patient's trauma through the work. This ongoing and regular indirect exposure to trauma causes sustained arousal and activation of the sympathetic nervous system, resulting in traumatic responses, such as numbing, emotional shutdown, constricted affect, and memory problems. The therapist may experience intrusions of the patient's traumatic narrative during his or her personal life. As a result, the boundaries between work and personal life may become blurred.

A dysregulation of the parasympathetic nervous system has been considered the root cause of compassion fatigue (Baranowsky & Gentry, 2015), with the sympathetic nervous system dominance facilitating the intrusion and codification of the traumatic information in the nervous system. In essence, according to Gentry's conceptualization, the combination of witnessing trauma in patients in conjunction with an overactive sympathetic nervous system and past traumatic experiences can facilitate the traumatization of the clinician. This indirect but chronic exposure to trauma can then create symptoms of compassion fatigue and a situation where the clinician experiences a constant state of arousal and perceives constant threats in the workplace (Box 1.2) Similar to Figley's model, empathy in the clinician is considered the critical element needed to initiate these processes.

The symptoms of compassion fatigue can be described along a continuum of secondary traumatic stress and burnout. Additionally, many of the symptoms are also commonly experienced during grief reactions. In fact, professional caregivers experiencing compassion fatigue may also experience significant grief about the loss of idealism, meaning, and satisfaction in their work.

Box 1.2 **Symptoms of Compassion Fatigue**

- anxiety
- sense of dread
- escape fantasies
- loss of meaning and purpose
- suicidal ideation
- nightmares
- GI distress
- sadness and depression
- difficult relationships with colleagues
- frequent complaining

Interventions

The growing literature on professional self-care indicates that across disciplines, the main challenges are system-related, patient- and family-related, and clinician-related. Addressing only one of the aspects contributing to stress may not result in significant and sustainable improvement. Additionally, clinicians are unique, the same way that patients and families are unique. Circumstances that may represent a risk factor for one clinician may be completely indifferent to another or even promote motivation and determination. To illustrate, while constant exposure to patients' suffering may allow one clinician to experience more compassion and connectedness, it may cause another clinician to feel progressively depleted, and unable to continue engaging in an authentic way. While one clinician may become highly distressed upon hearing he has been criticized by a colleague, another may simply dismiss the event as an expected nuisance in the workplace. Further, while one clinician may feel betrayed and demoralized for not receiving direct acknowledgment from a supervisor for her work, another clinician may interpret this event as an indication of poor leadership skills on the part of the supervisor, rather than a reflection of her worth. Thus, any meaningful professional self-care program for clinicians in an organization requires a careful assessment to identify the specific organizational culture and leadership style, and it should involve a personalized discussion and intervention strategy.

Developing general interventions that can effectively reduce the risk of burnout is challenging and the evidence from available studies is also not compelling. A systematic review examined 58 studies of work-centered or person-centered interventions for healthcare workers (Ruotsalainen et al., 2015). Interventions provided cognitive-behavioral training, combined CBT and relaxation, and organizational interventions, which included changing working conditions, providing organization support, increasing communication skills, and changing work schedule. While each of the interventions provided some decrease in stress levels, the authors concluded that there is low-quality evidence for the benefit of any of the interventions studies, except for relaxation training, for which there was moderate quality evidence. In a small sample of clinicians ($n = 27$), Mindfulness-Based-Stress-Reduction training was associated with a reduction in stress and burnout. Of note, clinicians reported a decrease in judgmental attitudes and an increased ability to understand the patient's experience, which improved the patient-clinician relationship (Dobkin, Bernardi, & Bagnis, 2016).

Similarly, a systematic review examining the impact of psychosocial interventions developed to prevent staff burnout showed lack of improvement of psychological well-being for palliative care staff and highlighted the lack of high-quality research and intervention (Hill et al., 2016). Interventions for decreasing burnout in physicians have been associated with only small effects and have pointed to the need for organization-directed interventions (Panagioti et al., 2017). A systematic review evaluated 20 studies that addressed the impact of strategies designed to promote coping and resilience in oncology and palliative care nurses (Gilman et al., 2015). In this review, promoting connection with the team, providing education focused on developing personal stress management strategies and providing support in processing emotions were helpful interventions.

The Accelerated Recovery Program for Compassion Fatigue (ARP) (Gentry et al., 2002) is based on Figley's model of compassion fatigue attributed to secondary traumatic stress and burnout. It was developed specifically for addressing compassion fatigue in professional caregivers. It consists of five sessions that teach a number of cognitive-behavioral skills to address the different components of secondary traumatic stress and burnout. The practice of relaxation throughout the day and especially while listening to traumatic narratives and witnessing direct effects of trauma and suffering is considered an essential skill to prevent arousal and sympathetic activation. Additionally, the program includes sharing narratives with colleagues in a professional network of support while in a safe and relaxed environment. The goal of the program is not only treating compassion fatigue but also developing compassion fatigue resiliency skills that can protect the professional caregiver during their work. These skills are self-regulation, intentionality, perceptual maturation, connection, and self-care. Studies of ARP have used the three scales of the Professional Quality of Life Test (Pro-QOL) which consists of three subscales: compassion fatigue, secondary traumatic stress, and burnout (Stamm, 2009). Results of using ARP with emergency room nurses has indicated a significant increase in compassion satisfaction scores and decrease in burnout scores (Flarity et al., 2013). Additionally, health-care workers who received facilitator training in the accelerated recovery program reported that applying the resiliency skills learned in the training program helped them manage stress and prevent compassion fatigue (Potter et al., 2013. Others have indicated the potential benefit of interventions aimed at developing resilience in palliative care clinicians (Back et al., 2016; Souba, 2016). Additionally, the use of meaningful ritual on the part of hospice staff was associated with higher levels of compassion satisfaction and lower levels of burnout (Montross-Thomas et al., 2016).

RISK AND PROTECTIVE FACTORS FOR PALLIATIVE PSYCHOLOGISTS

A practicing psychologist in any setting who is unaware of personal risk factors and protective factors will face significant challenges sustaining excellence in clinical work. Thus, as mentioned in the Ethics Code (2002), professional self-care is not conceptualized simply as a desirable option for psychologists but as a professional responsibility and necessary competency.

Palliative care practice is emotionally demanding. It involves constant and attentive engagement with a wide range of emotions experienced by patients and families across the illness experience. Attending to their psychological needs requires clinicians to carefully balance their ability to be emotionally present with the ability to think clinically. Additionally, the complex needs of palliative care patients often involve rapid changes to the psychological treatment plan, as changes in the patient's and family's goals may occur suddenly as a result of changes in the medical condition.

The development of a therapeutic relationship involves creating an emotional human connection, where the necessary engagement reaches different levels of depth, based on patients' and families' needs, preferences, and cultural values. Therapeutic presence involves the therapist's ability to bring the totality of oneself to the clinical encounter with the patient. This includes being present physically, emotionally, cognitively, and also spiritually (Geller, 2013). Different patients will require different levels of emotional engagement and connection, requiring the clinician to be intensely present, yet able to modulate levels of engagement following the patient's lead. This involves constant adjustment of personal energies and ability to hold ambiguity and unpredictability. It is a process that mirrors the constant adjustment required of the patient and the family to cope with the often-unpredictable course of illness and associated unexpected changes.

The length of psychological treatment for the patient receiving palliative care is variable and often unpredictable. It depends not only on the patient's condition and ability to engage in the session, but also on the setting where care is being provided (see also chapter 3). Patients and families often share intimate hopes and fears with the therapist. This intimate sharing can occur during the first psychological session due to a sense of urgency perceived by the patient or imposed by the prognosis. However, the opportunity for a follow-up session may not present itself; the patient may be discharged home or to a different facility. Or, the patient may die suddenly due to a complication of illness. Thus, the clinician needs to hold this ambiguity and combine the ability to be completely present in the moment on multiple levels, with the need to release attachments to plans for future sessions and treatment. Embracing both therapeutic presence and nonattachment at the same time is also an emotionally demanding task from an energy management standpoint.

Palliative psychologists may utilize a variety of approaches and interventions for providing psychological support. However, the clinician "self" is the main vehicle for the delivery of the psychological intervention. The use of the "self" of the therapist involves engaging one's personality, values, sensitivities, empathy, and humanness in the therapeutic encounter through the combination of therapeutic presence and clinical skills. The clinician's therapeutic presence represents the first level of intervention. The ability to establish quick and meaningful rapport with the patient and the family represents the foundation of assessment and treatment planning. Additionally, the effectiveness of psychological interventions is strongly dependent on the therapeutic alliance between the psychologist and the patient more than the actual theoretical framework or specific modality utilized (Benish et al., 2008).

While it is deeply rewarding, the depth of engagement needed requires a significant amount of cognitive and emotional energy and effort. The prominent use of the self is arguably a source of reward for palliative psychologists because it allows for those deep personal connections with patients and family caregivers. However, the complexities of patients' needs and the challenges present can also threaten the clinician's ability to maintain good professional boundaries.

The intensity of the pace and the need to think and act quickly, coupled with complex family dynamics and preexisting conditions such as depression or substance abuse, can become risk factors for work-stress reactions. This may be especially true for psychologists who are new to the field of palliative care and hospice. As other clinical competencies, self-care should be approached in a structured manner, and it will ideally be manifested in an individualized self-care plan. Identifying profession and setting specific risk factors and protective attitudes represent important initial steps in this process (Table 1.1; Box 1.3).

In addition to risk factors common to all palliative care clinicians, psychologists may face risk factors specifically related to their professional role. To illustrate, due to their

Table 1.1 **Risk Factors and Mitigating Strategies for Professional Self-care**

Situation	Possible Negative Outcome	Mitigating Strategies
Perceived pressure to demonstrate added value of psychology	Stress, becoming overly attached to outcome, sense of loneliness and disconnection from team, questioning belonging to team, feelings of inadequacy.	Analyze perception as possible cognitive distortion and "all or nothing" thinking. Focus on collaborative work with other team members.
New to interdisciplinary team dynamics	Becoming overly focused on demonstrating knowledge and experience rather than willingness to learn team culture and become acculturated to IDT work.	Humility and desire to be part of the team. Observing, asking questions, and being willing to tolerate necessary learning curve.
Desire to quickly resolve challenging clinical cases to please team or referring source	Losing focus on the patient and the family. Stress and perception of demands as outweighing resources. Burnout.	Reconnecting with larger and meaning-based personal goals and intentions about working in palliative care.
Stress caused by combination of clinical complexity and system-related limitations	Self-righteousness, entitlement, and frequent complaints about the system, which overshadow clinical focus and achievable goals.	Address cognitive distortions and unsupportive perceptions. Importance of receiving support from colleagues.
Limited access to other palliative psychologists for collaboration and support	Isolation, feeling that one has to do it alone, rationalizing lack of support, trivializing role of support, self-aggrandizing cognitions, and belief that one does not need professional support.	Reality-based approach about palliative psychology being a new specialty. Seek out connections with other psychologists, especially health, clinical, hospital based. Nurture relationship with interdisciplinary team members.
Confusion about role in providing staff support	Taking oneself out of the team and denying one's own need for support. This can generate isolation and burnout.	Recognize difference between role as consultant and team member. Be willing to educate administrators and supervisors about difference.
Difficulty managing demands and expectations from referrals sources	Stress, perception of demands outweighing resources (Gentry, 2002), dissatisfaction, burnout.	Examine perceptions and cognitive distortions; learn boundary setting skills and practice.

Table 1.1 **Continued**

Situation	Possible Negative Outcome	Mitigating Strategies
Unrealistic expectations RE: clinical outcome	Blurring professional boundaries, intrusions into personal life, compassion fatigue.	Frame unrealistic expectations as cognitive distortions and reflect on source of perceived pressure.
Poor boundaries regarding setting limits	Resentment toward the organization and the patient, as well as isolation, burnout.	Reframe boundary setting as necessary skill of mature psychologist. Seek consultation and practice skill through role-playing with other team members.
Making promises to patients and families	Pressure, disappointment, and anger in the patient and the family.	Awareness of countertransference. Reflection on desire to save the patient or becoming the favorite provider; need for validation from patient and the family.
Lack of professional support network	Isolation, inability to detect early manifestations of distress and burnout, as well as compassion fatigue.	Make conscious effort by joining peer supervision groups; join professional list serves.

Box 1.3 **Protective Attitudes**

- avoid becoming overly attached to outcome
- self- versus other validation
- engage in ongoing reflection on the personal motivations for doing the work
- develop a present-focused orientation
- awareness of triggers that can undermine personal and professional well-being
- rely on the team
- nurture collaborative work with team members
- set intentions at the beginning of every day for maintaining a grounded presence
- cultivate the ability to maintain relaxed state in presence of stressors
- establish a routine of self-care practices
- integrate personal check-ins during the workday
- integrate practices and techniques to relieve stress during the workday
- cultivate humility about one's work and recognize personal limitations
- aknowledge mistakes when they occur and determine to learn from them

recent and relatively scant active involvement in palliative care, psychologists may feel or perceive pressure to show the added value of palliative psychology by proving themselves to other members of the palliative care team and other clinicians. They may feel obliged to be available on a moment's notice or to work later than usual to meet the demands. They may also perceive a constant sense of urgency in their work, which can translate into accepting every referral or consult even when their schedule would not allow it. This situation may be particularly difficult for institution-based psychologists who may carry a caseload from another service and function as palliative care consultant when needed.

Psychologists who have not been trained to work as part of the interdisciplinary team will also face a necessary adjustment period. Functioning as a team member is different from acting as an ad-hoc consultant. The team represents an important source of support and professional growth. Interpersonal conflict may develop, but effective communication, professional boundaries, and respect can promote collaboration and facilitate conflict resolution.

Psychologists who are consulted for complex cases may also feel pressured to "fix" or "resolve" a clinically challenging situation. As an illustration, a family may display a high level of dysfunctional communication and conflict, creating distress for the patient and staff. If important medical decisions need to be made that require clarity of communication, the psychologist may be asked to find out "what is going on with this family" and bring some resolution. Or, a family member acting as a health-care proxy agent for a patient who does not have decisional capacity may develop an adversarial position toward the medical team, threatening lawsuits and displaying high levels of distress and anger.

Because of their training connecting with individuals at times of great distress, psychologists can be used a resource for evaluation and for suggestions to develop a plan of care in these challenging scenarios. The focus of the psychologist should, however, remain on evaluating and relieving distress in a holistic manner. If the focus shifts to a desire to "fix" the situation to relieve distress for the team, the psychologist will probably feel burdened with a task that cannot be accomplished by a single individual. This may create unrealistic expectations and disappointment rather than promote a team approach to dealing with the complexity.

Providing staff support can represent an important role for palliative psychologists. They are trained to recognize the impact of intense clinical work on clinician's well-being. Because of their background and training, psychologists may be consulted to provide staff support after the team has faced a difficult case that generated emotional distress. This role can be appropriate for psychologists if they are not core members of the team they are being ask to support. However, if they have also been affected by the distressing situation, they need to recognize their own needs for debriefing and support for their distress. For some, becoming identified as the "go-to person" for staff to debrief a distressing situation may slowly increase stress and possibly even the risk of burnout. It may create a situation where the psychologist becomes unable to express need for support due to being identified as the "expert" in self-care who does not need support because of his or her psychological expertise. A possible negative impact can be disenfranchised grief and isolation.

Although empathy has been identified as the primary vehicle for creating the experience of secondary traumatic stress and compassion fatigue, it clearly remains a fundamental aspect of the quality of the relationship between patient and provider. The key issue may be the ability to modulate empathy and balance it with skills that can be protective for clinicians. "Exquisite empathy" (Harrison & Westwood, 2009) has been described as a protective factor in vicarious traumatization of mental health therapists, allowing clinicians to deeply connect with patients while respecting healthy professional boundaries. It has been defined as "empathic engagement that is discerning, highly present, sensitively attuned, well-boundaried and heartfelt." Thus, the goal is maintaining a deep and intimate connection with the patient and the family, without becoming fused with their pain or the images of their traumatic experiences. Appropriate professional boundaries can allow this kind of empathic attunement without resulting in a counterproductive fusion. Professional boundaries have a behavioral component, a cognitive component, and an affective component, all of which have to be carefully respected for the clinician to maintain well-being as they work with patients who are traumatized.

Self-knowledge is a very important component of a clinician's journey. It refers to a deep knowledge about personal history, unique gifts that are brought to the clinical work, and also unique challenges that one faces. Self-knowledge is a way of reclaiming one's story, acknowledging strengths and vulnerabilities. It allows the clinician to assess his or her personal situation, identifying risk factors and existing stressors. Awareness of stressors, whether related to the work setting or to personal attitudes and behaviors, is an important and necessary first step for the development of a self-care plan.

Self-empathy results from the practice of connecting with oneself and one's vulnerability and practicing self-forgiveness. Clinicians should ask themselves if they are treating themselves with kindness and compassion. Developing a balanced view of skills, abilities, and areas that need improvement will also allow for a development of a balanced view of a work reality. As patients' and families' perception of reality is affected by their thoughts, their emotions, and their worldview, clinicians' perception of reality is also affected by several variables. If a clinician's interpretation of reality is excessively focused on negative elements and negative self-perception, the view and appraisal of the work situation may also be negatively affected. Personal practice, from any contemplative, secular, spiritual, or religious tradition that resonates with the individual clinician and promotes a sense of inner peace, strength, and personal awareness can become a supportive self-care strategy.

The *ability to consciously generate and experience positive mental and emotional states* when needed can prove valuable to help maintain or reestablish a sense of balance in the course of a stressful workday. The use of integrative and contemplative practices based in mindfulness, self-hypnosis, or other forms of imagery can decrease frustration and help change the clinician's internal experience. Strategies focused on reality testing, problem solving and decatastrophizing can help the clinician quickly de-escalate. It is important to be aware of the situations, behaviors, and thought processes that can induce a state of well-being and also change an existing state from distress to harmony.

The clinician can also practice approaching challenges at work with an attitude of curiosity and openness, witnessing a phenomenon without becoming identified with it. Thus, avoiding becoming identified with any negative situation that may arise at work or any negative emotion can be a protective strategy. This approach can be developed by cultivating the stance of an observer and approaching even negative emotions with curiosity and self-compassion. The benefit of avoiding identification with negative emotions, negative situations, or even negative outcomes is a central concept in Eastern approaches to psychological well-being, and also humanistic and transpersonal approaches. The focus on "cultivating" points to a daily practice and a process. For this reason, professional self-care can be described as an ongoing practice.

In addition to a fundamental competence and an ethical responsibility, professional self-care can also be conceptualized as a self-compassion practice. As working in palliative care involves providing compassionate care to patients and families, so is commitment to self-care a way of being truly compassionate to oneself. By committing to self-care, clinicians recognize the importance of maintaining their personal and professional well-being. Pursuing professional self-care is a choice that a clinician can consciously make; it is a manifestation of self-respect, and, ultimately, it can become a way of being.

Because loss is so common to the human experience, palliative psychologists need to recognize their own personal and professional grief and how they are impacted by it. Self-awareness and personal inquiry will allow them to explore their own experience of grief reactions to loss. This personal reflective dialogue also allows exploration and recognition of their own core values and belief system. This is essential for personal development and for developing professional maturity and resilience. Knowledge of one's own relationship with loss and grief and the ability to recognize the impact of personal, social, and cultural variables on how grief is processed is of crucial importance to recognize and manage counter transference reactions. Then it becomes possible to establish a bond with patients and families based upon a compassionate recognition of their grief and ability to honor it, support it, and provide professional guidance and intervention, when necessary. Therefore, exploration of the following areas is particularly beneficial:

- personal loss and grief history
- personal grieving style
- countertransference reactions when witnessing others' grieving process.

Cultivating personal awareness is generally related to understanding of countertransference reactions and represents an important component of psychology training. Clinical supervision during predoctoral and postdoctoral training routinely allows trainees to explore countertransference and personal feelings about patients and their therapeutic work together. The ability to conduct a brief personal mindful inquiry during the workday can become an important aspect of regular self-care. As an example, a psychologist could pause for a few minutes should tension arise during the workday. This moment of personal mindful inquiry may help identify the sources of discomfort. Once identified, the concern can either be addressed, if possible, or symbolically and temporarily placed in a "safe place" by using imagery. This strategy may help clinicians continue functioning during the day, knowing that concerns can be revisited at a later time.

Developing a present-focused orientation can increase the clinician's ability to connect to the present moment, truly existing in the present moment. This strategy will not only benefit clinicians, but also patients and families with anxieties and fear about the future. Being completely involved in an activity in the present moment and giving full attention to the activity of the present moment allows less emotional space for anxiety, depressive thoughts, or worry.

The experience of advanced illness with the associated distress and suffering tests the patient's and family's connection with sources of meaning and purpose. Similarly, ongoing exposure to the pain and suffering in the palliative care setting can test the clinician's sense of meaning. Maintaining an ongoing reflection on what is important, sustaining, and meaningful in the clinician's life can help maintain a sense of balance. In the words of Kubler Ross & Kessler (2000, p. 2), "Consciously or not, we are all on a quest for answers, trying to learn the lessons of life. We grapple with fear and guilt. We search for meaning, love, and power. We try to understand fear, loss, and time. We seek to discover who we are and how we can become truly happy."

The personal relationship with meaning often evolves based on circumstances and emotional states. In the words of Victor Frankl (1959, p. 106), "For the meaning of life differs from man to man, from day to day and from hour to hour. What matters, therefore, is not the meaning of life in general, but rather the specific meaning of a person's life at a given moment." Palliative psychologists recognize the truth of these words because they see it manifested in the clinical setting. Similarly, they recognize that their own personal sense of meaning is closely connected to their personal and professional well-being.

References

Aldridge Carlson, M. D., Barry C. L., Cherlin, E. J., McCorkle, R., & Bradley, E. H. (2012). Hospices' enrollment policies may contribute to underuse of hospice care in the United States. *Health Affairs, 31*(12), 2690–2698.

Aldridge M. D., Hasselar, J., Garralda E., van der Eerden, M., Stevenson, D., McKendrick, K., . . . Meier, D. E. (2016). Education, implementation, and policy barriers to greater integration of palliative care: A literature review. *Palliative Medicine, 30*(3), 224–239.

Back, A. L., Steinhauser, K. E., Kamal, A. H., & Jackson, V. A. (2016). Building resilience for palliative care clinicians: An approach to burnout prevention based on individual skills and workplace factors. *Journal of Pain and Symptom Management, 52*(2), 284–291

Bakitas, M., Doyle Lyons, K., Hegel, M. T., Balan, S., Brokaw, F. C., Seville, J., . . . Ahles, T. A. (2009). Effects of a palliative care intervention on clinical outcomes in patients with advanced cancer: The project ENABLE II randomized controlled trial. *JAMA, 302*(7), 741–749.

Bakitas, M. A., Tosteson, T. D., Lyons, K., D., Hull, J. G., Li, Z., Dionne-Odom, J. N., . . . Ahles, T. A. (2015). Early versus delayed initiation of concurrent palliative oncology care: Patient outcomes in the ENABLE III randomized controlled trial. *Journal of Clinical Oncology, 33*(12), 1438–1445.

Baranowsky, A. B., & Gentry, J. E. (2015). *Trauma practice: tools for stabilization and recovery*. Boston, MA: Hogrefe.

Benish, S. G., Imel, Z., & Wampold, B. (2008). The relative efficacy of bona fide psychotherapies for treating posttraumatic stress disorder: A meta analysis of direct comparisons. *Clinical Psychology Review, 28*, 746–758.

Berman, R., Campbell, M., Makin, W., & Todd, C. (2007). Occupational stress in palliative medicine, medical oncology, and clinical oncology specialist registrars. *Clinical Medicine, 7*(3), 235–242.

Brown, C. E., Jecker, N. S., & Curtis, J. R. (2016). Inadequate palliative care in chronic lung disease: An issue of health care inequality. *Annals of the American Thoracic Society 13*(3), 311–316

Brumley, R., Enguidanos, S., Jamison, P., Seitz, R., Morgenstern, N., Saito, S., . . . Gonzalez, J. (2007). Increased satisfaction with care and lower cost: A result of a randomized trial of in-home palliative care. *Journal of the American Geriatric Society, 55*(7), 993–1000.

Canadian Cancer Society. (2016). Right to care: Palliative care for all Canadians.

Cassel, J. B., Kerr, K. M., Kalman, N. S., & Smith, T. J. (2015). The business case for palliative care: Translating research into program development in the US. *Journal of Pain and Symptom Management, 50*(6), 741–749

Center to Advance Palliative Care. (2014). The case for hospital palliative care. http://www.capc.org/topics/hospital.

Chandrasekar, D., Tribett, E., & Ramchandran, K. (2016). Integrated palliative care and oncology care in non-small cell lung cancer. *Current Treatment Options in Oncology, 17*, 23

Ciemins E. L., Blum, L., Nunley, M., Lasher, A., & Newman, J. M. (2007). The economic and clinical impact of an inpatient palliative care consultation service: A multifaceted approach. *Journal of Palliative Medicine, 10*(6), 1347–1355.

Cunningham, C., Travers, K., Chapman, R., Loos, A., Lawler, E., Liu, S., . . . Ollendorf, D. A. (2016). *Palliative care in the outpatient setting: A comparative effectiveness report.* Institute for Clinical and Economic Review.

Dalgaard, K. M., Bergenholtz, H., Nielsen, M. E., & Timm, H. (2014). Early integration of palliative care in hospitals: A systematic review on methods, barriers, and outcome. *Palliative and Supportive Care, 12*(6), 495–513.

Dionne-Odom, J. N., Azuero, A, Lyons, K. D., Hull, J. G., Tosteson, T., Li, Z., . . . & Bakitas, M. (2015). Benefits of early versus delayed palliative care to informal family caregivers of patients with advanced cancer: Outcomes from the ENABLE III randomized controlled trial. *Journal of Clinical Oncology, 33*(13), 1446–1452.

Dobkin, P. L., Bernardi, N. F., & Bagnis, C. L. (2016). Enhancing clinicians' well being and patient centered care through mindfulness. The *Journal of Continuing Education in the Health Professions, 36*(1), 11–16.

Dougherty, E., Pierce, B., Ma, C., Panzanella, T., Rodin, G., & Zimmerman, C. (2009). Factors associated with work stress and professional satisfaction in oncology staff. *American Journal of Hospice and Palliative Medicine, 26*(2), 105–111.

El-Jawahri, A., Greer, J. A., & Temel, J. S. (2011). Does palliative care improve outcomes for patients with incurable illness? A review of the evidence. *Journal of Supportive Oncology, 9*(3), 87–94.

Figley, C. R. (2002). Compassion fatigue: Psychotherapists' chronic lack of self-care. *Journal of Clinical Psychology, 58*(1), 1433–1441.

Flarity, K., Gentry, J. E., & Mesnikoff, N. (2013). The effectiveness of an educational program on preventing and treating compassion fatigue in emergency nurses. *Advanced Emergency Nursing, 35*(3), 247–258.

Frankl, V. E. (1959). *Man's search for meaning.* Boston: Beacon Press.

Friedrichsdorf, S. J., Postier, A., Dreyfus, J., Osenga K., Sencer, S., & Wolfe, J. (2015). Improved quality of life at the end of life related to home-based palliative care in children with cancer. *Journal of Palliative Medicine, 18*(2), 143–150.

Gade, G., Venohr, I., Conner, D., McGrady, K., Beane, J., Richardson, R. H., . . . Della Penna, R. (2008). Impact of an inpatient palliative care team: a randomized controlled trial. *Journal of Palliative Medicine, 11*(2), 180–190.

Geller, S. M (2013). Therapeutic presence as a foundation for relational depth. In R. Knox, D. Murphy, S. Wiggins, & M. Cooper (Eds.)., *Relational depth: New perspectives and developments* (pp. 175–184). Basingstoke, UK: Palgrave.

Gidwani, R., Joyce, N., Kinosian, B., Faricy-Anderson, K., Levy, C., Miller, S., . . .& Mor, V. (2016). Gap between recommendations and practice of palliative care and hospice in cancer patients. *Journal of Palliative Medicine, 19*(9), 957–963.

Gilman, L., Adams, J., Kovac, R., Kircullen, A., House, A., Doyle, C. (2015). Strategies to promote coping and resilience in oncology and palliative care nurse caring for adult patients with malignancy: A comprehensive systematic review. *JBI Database of Systematic Reviews and Implementation Reports, 13*(5), 131–204.

Gomes, B., Calanzani, N., Curiale, V., McCrone, P., & Higginson, I. J. (2013). Effectiveness and cost-effectiveness of home palliative care services for adults with advanced illness and their caregivers. *Cochrane Database of Systematic Reviews, 6*(6), CD007760.

Harrison, R. L., & Westwood, M. J. (2009). Preventing vicarious traumatization of mental health therapists: Identifying protective practices. *Psychotherapy Theory, Research, Practice, Training*, 46(2), 203–219.

Hill, R. C., Dempster, M., Donnelly M., & McCorry, N. K. (2016). Improving the well-being of staff who work in palliative care settings: A systematic review of psychosocial interventions. *Palliative Medicine*, 30(9), 825–833.

Hughes, M. T., & Smith, T. J. (2014). The growth of palliative care in the United States. *Annual Review of Public Health*, 35, 459–475.

Hui, D., De La Cruz, M., Mori M., & Parsons, H. A., Kwon, J. H., Torres-Vigil, I., . . . Bruera, E. (2013). Concepts and definitions for "supportive care," "best supportive care," "palliative care," and "hospice care" in the published literature, dictionaries, and textbooks. *Supportive Care in Cancer*, 21(3), 659–685.

Joinson, C. Coping with compassion fatigue. *Nursing*, 22(4), 116–120.

Kamal, A. H., Bull, J. H., Wolf, S. P., Swetz, K. M., Shanafelt, T. D., Ast, K., . . . Abernethy, A. P. (2016). Prevalence and predictors of burnout among hospice and palliative care clinicians in the US. *Journal of Pain and Symptom Management*, 51(4), 690–696.

Kearney, M. K., Weininger, R. B., Vachon, M. L., Harrison, R. L., & Mount, B. M. (2009). Self-care of physicians caring for patients at the end of life: "Being connected . . . a key to my survival." *JAMA*, 301(11), 1155–1164.

Krakauer, R., Spettell, C. M., Reisman, L., & Wade, M. J. (2011). Opportunities to improve the quality of care for advanced illness. *Health Affairs*, 28(5), 1357–1359.

Kubler Ross, E., & Kessler, D. (2000). *Life Lessons*.

Laschinger, H. K. S., & Leiter, M. P. (2006). The impact of nursing work environment on patient safety outcomes: The mediating role of burnout/engagement. *Journal of Nursing Administration*, 36, 259–267.

Maslach, C., & Leiter, M. P. (1997). *The truth about burnout*. New York: Josse-Bass.

Metha, A., & Chan, L. S. (2008). Understanding of the concept of "Total Pain": A prerequisite for pain control. *Journal of Hospice and Palliative Nursing*, 10(1), 26–32.

Miller, C. (2016). What is the price of physician stress and burnout? *Medical Economics*. http://medicaleconomics.modernmedicine.com/medical-economics/news/what-price-physician-stress-and-burnout?page=0,2.

Montross-Thomas, L. P., Scheiber, C., Meier, E. A., & Irwin, S. A. (2016). Personally meaningfully rituals: A way to increase compassion and decrease burnout among hospice staff and volunteers. *Journal of Palliative Medicine*, 19(10), 1043–1050.

National Hospice and Palliative Care Organization. (2014). *NHPCO facts and figures hospice care in America*. Alexandria, VA: National Hospice and Palliative Care Organization. Hospice philosophy statement. https://www.nhpco.org/ethical-and-position-statements/preamble-and-philosophy. Retrieved on October 20, 2017.

O'Mahoney, S., Gerhart, J. I., Grosse, J., Abrams, I., Levy, M. M. (2016). Postraumatic stress symptoms in palliative care professionals seeking mindfulness training: Prevalence and vulnerability. *Palliative Medicine*, 30(2):189–192.

O'Rourke, K. M. The evidence for early palliative care in cancer patients. *Medscape* Dec 2, 2015.

Obermeyer, Z., Clarke, A. C., Makar, M., Schuur, J. D., & Cutler, D. M. (2016). Emergency care utilization and the medicare hospice benefit for patients with poor-prognosis cancer. *Journal of the American Geriatric Society*, 64(2), 323–329.

Panagioti, M., Panagopoulou, E., Bower, P., Lewith, G., Kontopantelis, E, Chew-Graham, C., . . . Esmail, A. (2017). Controlled interventions to reduce burnout in physicians. *JAMA Internal Medicine*, 177(2), 195–205.

Paolini, H. O., & Greenwald, M. H. Healers in need of healing cannot heal. http://www.medscape.com/viewarticle/863416_print.

Perlman, L. A., & Saakvitne, K. W. (1995). *Trauma and the therapist: Countertransference and vicarious traumatization in psychotherapy with incest survivors*. New York: Norton.

Perez, G. K., Jaime, V., Jackson, V., Chittenden, E., Metha, D. H., & Park, E. R. (2015). Promoting resilience among palliative care clinicians: Stressors, coping strategies, and training needs. *Journal of Palliative Medicine, 18*(4), 332–337.

Perrin, K., & Kazanowski, M. (2015). Barriers to palliative care consultation. *Critical Care Nurse, 35*, 44–52.

Peters, L., Cant, R., Sellick, K., O'Connor, M., Lee, S., & Burney, S. (2012). Is work stress in palliative care nurses a cause for concern? A literature review. *International Journal of Palliative Nursing, 18*(11), 561–567.

Potter, P., Deshields, T., Berger, J. A., Clarke, M., Olsen, S., & Chen, L. (2013). Evaluation of a compassion fatigue resiliency program for oncology nurses. *Oncology Nursing Forum, 40*(2), 180–187.

Rodolfa, E., Bent, R., Eisman, E., Nelson, P., Rehm, L., & Ritchie, P. (2005). A cube model for competency development: Implications for psychology educators and regulators. *Professional Psychology: Research and Practice, 36*(4), 347–354.

Ruotsalainen, J. H., Verbeek, J. H., Marine, A., & Serra, C. (2015). Preventing occupational stress in healthcare workers. *Cochrane Database of Systematic Reviews, 4*, CD002892.

Sabo, B. (2011). Reflecting on the concept of compassion fatigue. *The Online Journal of Issues in Nursing, 16*(1), 1.

Sanchez-Reilly, S., Morrison, L. J., Carey, E., Bernacki, R., O'Neill, L., Kapo, J., . . . Thomas, J. L. (2013). Caring for oneself to care for others: physicians and their self-care. *Journal of Supportive Oncology, 11*(2), 75–81.

Sanso, N., Galiana, L., Oliver, A., Pascual, A., Sinclair, S., & Benito, E. (2015). Palliative care professionals' inner life: Exploring the relationship among awareness, self care, and compassion satisfaction and fatigue, burnout, and coping with death. *Journal of Pain and Symptom Management, 50*(2), 200–207.

Saunders, C. (1964). The symptomatic treatment of incurable malignant disease. *Prescriber Journal, 4*, 68–73.

Souba, W. W. (2016). Resilience: Back to the future. *JAMA Surgery, 151*(10), 896–897.

Stamm, B. H. (2009). Professional quality of life: Compassion satisfaction and fatigue, version 5 (ProQOL). http://www.isu.edu/~bhstamm. Retrieved on June 18, 2016.

Strand, J. J., Kamdar, M. M., & Carey, E. C. (2013). Top 10 things palliative care clinicians wished everyone knew about palliative care. *Mayo Clinical Procedings, 88*(8), 859–865.

Swetenham, K., Hegarty, M., Breaden, K., & Grbich, C. (2011). Refractory suffering: The impact of team synamics on the interdisciplinary palliative care team. *Palliative and Supportive Care, 9*(1), 55–62.

Temel, J. S., Greer, J. A., Muzikansky, A., Gallagher, E. R., Admane, S., Jackson, V. A., . . . Lynch, T. J. (2010). Early palliative care for patients with metastatic non-small-cell lung cancer. *New England Journal of Medicine, 363*(8), 733–742.

Teno, J. M., Clarridge, B. R., Casey, V., Welch, L. C., Shield, R., & Mor, V. (2004). Family perspectives on end of life care at the last place of care. *JAMA, 291*(1), 88–93.

Teno, J. M., Gozalo, P. L., Bynum, J. P. W., Leland, N. E., & Miller, C. S., Morden, N. E., . . . Mor, V. (2013). Change in end of life care for medical beneficiaries: Site of death, place of care, and health care transitions in 2000, 2005, and 2009. *JAMA, 309*(5), 470–477.

The Irish Hospice Foundation. (2008). Palliative care for all: Integrating palliative care into disease management frameworks. http://www.Hospice-foundation.ie.

Torres, L., Lindstrom, K., Hannah, L., & Webb, F. J. (2016). Exploring barriers among primary care providers in referring patiens to hospice. *Journal of Hospice and Palliative Nursing, 18*(2), 167–172.

2

The Second Domain of Palliative Care

Physical Aspects of Care

Focus Points

- The management of pain and physical symptoms is a major focus of specialist palliative care.
- The psychological pain and symptom assessment identifies psychological factors that modulate the patient's perception of pain and discomfort, affect treatment adherence, and treatment outcome.
- The diagnosis and treatment of comorbid depression and anxiety can improve pain management and overall quality of life.
- Any barriers to the adequate treatment of pain need to be identified and addressed. These can be provider-related, patient-related, and health-care-system related.
- Cognitive-behavioral therapy and integrative medicine modalities, including relaxation, imagery, and clinical hypnosis, can be added to pharmacological management to improve pain and symptoms and to help relieve some distress for the patient and for the family.

Introduction

This second domain of palliative care, the "Physical Aspects of Care," concerns the critically important management of pain and physical symptoms common in serious illness and in end of life. The symptoms experienced may be the result of the specific disease as well as the effects of treatment. Management of these symptoms not only improves physical functioning but also allows disease-modifying treatment to be better tolerated. Additionally, it promotes psychological and spiritual well-being, improving overall quality of life for the patient and family caregivers.

Adequate management of pain and other physical symptoms is essential for preventing the development of suffering. Suffering goes beyond the physical sensation of discomfort by affecting the totality of the patient's sense of meaning and identity. Psychological, social, spiritual, and existential factors are at the interplay of pain and suffering. To illustrate, a patient with advanced cancer who is experiencing poorly managed pain will experience great physical discomfort. Additionally, the patient may begin thinking that the pain will always increase and will become unbearable. This will likely create great anxiety and fear, perhaps creating expectations and images of a horrible and painful death. The combination of unrelieved physical pain and the negative expectations about the future may create a sense of hopelessness and helplessness. This may deeply affect the patient's sources of meaning and purpose, creating suffering.

Addressing psychological and spiritual factors directly can also significantly help manage pain and physical symptoms. For example, the presence of depression and anxiety may continue to create mental and spiritual distress, preventing the patient from experiencing relief even when the physical symptoms are adequately managed.

While the primary management of pain and physical symptoms is pharmacologic, it is often possible to augment the action of medication and reduce the complications of treatment by providing psychological interventions that include integrative medicine modalities. Thus, to maximize the opportunity to reduce physical symptoms and suffering, specialist palliative care integrates pharmacological, psychological, and complementary approaches (Greenlee et al., 2014). This interdisciplinary palliative care plan is the result of a collaborative approach with the patient and the family to provide care that is consistent with the patient's physical and psychological needs, as well as his or her cultural values.

In addition to pain, common physical symptoms in advanced illness and end of life are dyspnea, nausea and vomiting, constipation, fatigue, loss of appetite, delirium, and cognitive dysfunction. Based on the type of illness, a clustering of symptoms is often observed. To illustrate, three symptom clusters have been described in patients with advanced heart failure:

- a distress cluster that includes depression, anxiety, and shortness of breath
- a discomfort cluster that includes pain and a sense of discomfort
- a decondition cluster that includes nausea, fatigue, and drowsiness (Yu et al., 2016).

In patients with advanced cancer, four common clusters have been observed : anxiety-depression, nausea-vomiting, nausea-appetite loss, and fatigue-dyspnea-drowsiness-pain (Dong et al., 2014). In particular, the anxiety-depression cluster has been found to be the strongest predictor of overall quality of life (Dong et al., 2016).

Competencies for Palliative Psychologists

In order to communicate effectively and collaborate with other care providers, palliative psychologists need to develop a good understanding of the physical symptoms most prominent in advanced disease, including the type, frequency, and severity of these physical symptoms, and the medical treatments provided. This information helps guide the psychological assessment of pain and symptoms as it provides the necessary context in which to explore the patients' and families' perceptions and attitudes about the medical treatment. As a result of the comprehensive information obtained during the psychological assessment, a better evaluation of the impact of distress in the physical domain on psychological and spiritual well-being is possible, and specific recommendations can be made for psychological interventions that can be coordinated in an interdisciplinary plan.

As pain is one of the most prominent symptoms encountered, the ability to perform a psychological pain assessment and to use specific interventions for pain are especially important competencies. There is increasing evidence that hypnosis, guided imagery, and relaxation techniques can improve pain and symptoms. Additionally, cognitive behavioral therapy can also help identify and modify or control maladaptive beliefs and thoughts that can interfere with symptom control (Strada & Portenoy, 2015). These noninvasive interventions and strategies are generally welcomed, especially because they are perceived as not adding to the treatment burden. Thus, palliative psychologists with expertise in nonpharmacological symptom relief can significantly contribute to the quality of life for the patient and the family.

A familiarity with basic concepts of pharmacological pain management will allow palliative psychologists to have informed conversations with patients and families, to develop a better understanding of the decision-making processes that occur between them and their medical providers, and to identify beliefs and attitudes about medications that may interfere with adequate management. This aspect is particularly relevant in the context of pain management, as the patient and the family may hold belief and concerns about the use of pain medication that must be addressed as part of the care plan. Furthermore, the presence of psychiatric illness or substance use disorder may complicate management, requiring expert psychological assessment and support. Box 2.1 summarizes competencies for palliative psychologists in the physical domain of care.

Pain and Symptoms in Advanced Disease

As noted previously, serious and advanced illness is characterized by several symptoms that have been reviewed extensively in the palliative care literature (Chai et al., 2014; Goldstein & Morrison, 2013; Matzo & Witt-Sherman, 2015). This section provides clinical considerations about the psychological assessment and management of dyspnea, constipation, and pain.

DYSPNEA

Dyspnea is a common symptom in advanced disease and a particularly distressing symptom for the patient and the family (Kamal et al., 2012).While it has been described as painful breathing, dyspnea is the subjective experience of air hunger, or difficulty moving air in and out of the lungs. It is common in chronic lung diseases, including pulmonary fibrosis, emphysema, chronic airway obstruction, and lung cancer. It is also common in heart failure and neuromuscular disorders that affect breathing muscles. The perception of dyspnea is in part due to activated nerve receptors in the lung and chest that send signals to the brain, resulting in the experience of alarm, arousal, and anxiety. This then causes sympathetic activation, which stimulates the respirator muscles to work harder, often in counterproductive ways.

> ### Box 2.1 Palliative Psychology Competencies in Physical Aspects of Care
>
> #### KNOWLEDGE
>
> - pain and symptoms associated with advanced disease and end of life
> - pain and symptoms associated with treatment
> - basics of pain pathophysiology
> - basics of pharmacological pain management
> - cultural aspects of pain, including barriers
> - knowledge of the role of psychological interventions for pain and symptom management
> - knowledge of evidence about integrative and complementary medicine approaches for pain and physical symptoms
> - pain management and risk assessment in the context of substance use disorder and aberrant drug-taking behaviors.
>
> #### SKILLS
>
> - Conduct a comprehensive psychological pain assessment.
> - Provide non-pharmacological pain and symptom management (e.g., cognitive behavioral therapy, clinical hypnosis, and imagery).
> - Communicate effectively with team about psychological implications of pain and symptoms and possible barriers to treatment.
> - Work with the patient and the family to clarify belief systems and facilitate communication with medical providers.
> - Assess for substance abuse and aberrant drug taking behaviors
> - Develop a psychological care plan for patients with a history of abuse and addiction.
>
> #### ATTITUDES
>
> - cultural sensitivity
> - nonjudgmental approach toward patients' and families' belief systems related to medication use and meaning of pain
> - Integrative mind-set that avoids expressing preferential views toward one particular treatment approach

The end result is often a distressing central nervous system activation, with alarm and anxiety combining to create a self-reinforcing cascade, increasing the distress of dyspnea. Furthermore, in patients with respiratory disorders, depression and anxiety disorders can intensify the distress of dyspnea. They are often comorbid and frequently under-recognized and undertreated (Strang, Ekberg-Jansson & Henoch, 2014).

While sedatives and narcotics have been successfully used to decrease alarm and dyspnea, the use of relaxation techniques and breathing training also can reduce sympathetic activation and can support medication efficacy and enhance a sense of control (Harrison et al., 2016; Mulaski et al., 2009). Additionally, cognitive-behavioral modalities, including thought stopping, cognitive reframing, and addressing cognitive distortions, can be helpful, especially when there are ruminative or catastrophizing negative thoughts. Pulmonary rehabilitation is a comprehensive program involving exercise training, self-management strategies (e.g., breathing techniques), and psychosocial support. While it can be effective in the management of dyspnea, it is a rigorous undertaking and may not be appropriate for patients who have a short life expectancy. Dyspnea in the end-of-life period requires optimal management to avoid distress for the patient during the dying process and for family caregivers.

CONSTIPATION

Constipation is a common symptom in advanced disease and an expected adverse effect resulting from chronic opioid use. It can also occur from disease-related factors (Albert, 2017; Baralatei & Ackerman, 2016). When related to opioid use, constipation is caused by the drug action along the gastrointestinal tract, which causes a decrease in peristalsis and in intestinal secretions. As a result, patients may experience chronic constipation that is difficult to treat, even when stool softeners and laxatives are administered. Constipation is a sensitive issue, and patients may not feel comfortable discussing it with their physicians. Thus they may not volunteer this information unless they are specifically asked. The burden of constipation may be significant, however, ranging from a general sense of malaise, nausea, irritability, and decreased desire to engage in social activities to pain that can become severe and cause the patient to seek emergency care. In attempting to deal with chronic constipation, patients may develop belief systems about what causes constipation, ways to manage the constipation, and the meaning of constipation in relation to the illness. These beliefs are frequently not based on accurate medical information.

A qualitative study that explored symptom burden caused by opioid-related constipation in patients with advanced cancer indicated that constipation negatively affects several areas of quality of life and increases anticipatory anxiety (Dhingra et al., 2013). Palliative psychologists can play an important role by exploring the meaning of this symptom for the patient (e.g., constipation as an indication that the disease is worsening) and understanding how it relates to the patient's suffering. Including family caregivers in these conversations is essential, because they can encourage the patient to report this symptom accurately to the medical team. Medications specifically approved for opioid constipation have been developed.

PAIN

Severe pain is one of the most prevalent and distressing symptoms in patients with advanced disease and in end of life, ranging from 40% to 70% in some diseases (Chang et al., 2007). Adequate management is a fundamental expression of good patient-centered care. Additionally, discussion of pain management has a prominent role in palliative care interdisciplinary team meetings, and it is a fundamental component of discharge planning. The Joint Commission standards recognize the right of all patients to receive pain assessment and management. In palliative care, patients' pain is assessed and reassessed regularly to allow the team to make necessary adjustments to ensure optimal management.

Although pain is common in cancer, it also can be present in other diseases not generally believed to be associated with pain, such as congestive heart failure or chronic obstructive pulmonary disease (COPD). It can also exist independent of the palliative care concerns (van Dam van Isselt, et al., 2014). Poorly controlled pain has several notably negative effects on patients' mood, function, and overall quality of life. Because uncontrolled pain can mimic psychiatric disorders, it is important to clarify the relationship between pain and psychological and psychiatric morbidity for each patient. Common consequences of undertreated pain are anxiety, agitation, depression, and isolation. If not recognized as manifestations of inadequately managed pain, these symptoms can lead to inaccurate diagnoses and unnecessary pharmacotherapy (Box 2.2).

Managing pain in patients with advanced illness can be challenging. It involves a balance between administering sufficient doses of medication to alleviate pain and allowing the patient to maintain the highest level of functioning possible, based on the disease trajectory. While there is general agreement about the importance of managing pain in serious and advanced disease, barriers still exist, and their impact needs to be carefully considered (Table 2.1).

Patient-related barriers. Patients may be reluctant to report pain for fear of the presence of disease, or fear that it means the disease is getting worse. They may be concerned that reporting increased pain will convince physicians to order more tests that may show the progression of disease. Patients may also underreport pain for fear of upsetting their medical providers and being labeled "bad patients" or "drug seeking." They may have a significant fear of addiction and believe they will be labeled addicts by friends, family, or society. Cost of medication may also be a barrier. Because of perceptions and beliefs about pain, patients may hesitate to seek medical attention, they may self-treat with over-the-counter medications, or they may avoid taking prescribed pain medication for fear of side effects.

Health-care-provider-related barriers. These include inadequate training of medical professionals, poor skills in pain assessment, low priority given to pain treatment, lack

---

Box 2.2 **Consequences of Undertreated Pain**

- anxiety
- relationship problems
- agitation
- increased caregiver distress
- depression
- suicidal ideation
- fear
- hopelessness
- isolation
- existential and spiritual suffering
- anorexia
- decreased ability to make decisions

Table 2.1 **Barriers to Adequate Pain Management in Advanced Illness**

Health-care provider	limited training
	fear of adverse effects of opioids
	concerns about promoting addiction
Patient and family caregivers	fear of tests
	fear of medication side effects
	pain as a metaphor for death
	pain as atonement for past actions
	fear of appearing weak if reporting pain
	fear of addiction
	cultural aspects
Health-Care system	cost of medication
	lack of access to adequate care in rural areas

of consistent documentation, concern about controlled substances regulations, fear of toxicity (especially respiratory depression), and fear of patient addiction.

Social and cultural barriers to pain management include lack of access to medical care due to cost concerns. Especially in rural areas, patients may have difficulty with transportation. Some may believe that pain is to be tolerated and should not be "masked" by medication. Inadequate communication by physicians prescribing medication, restrictive regulations of controlled substances, and perceptions about opioid addiction are also significant barriers to adequate pain management. Concerns about opioid misuse and abuse are certainly well founded, but they should not result in undertreatment of pain in patients with advanced or terminal disease. Palliative psychologists can play an important role in identifying cultural and psychological barriers, providing feedback to the team, and developing a collaborative interdisciplinary plan that can effectively address them.

Specialist and interdisciplinary pain management not only benefits the patient, but also improves well-being in family caregivers, who are spared the distress of witnessing a loved one in pain and suffering. Palliative psychologists and other clinicians who also provide bereavement counseling and psychotherapy are well aware of the disruptive impact of witnessing unmanaged pain by surviving family members. The profound feelings of guilt, anger, and helplessness in bereaved family members who believed their loved one suffered with poorly managed pain can prevent them from integrating the loss and engaging in the mourning process. Thus, poorly managed pain is also a risk factor for complicated grief.

Pain management is a common reason for requesting a palliative care consultation. The ultimate goal is to improve the patient's quality of life, maximizing comfort and function and increasing patient satisfaction. Pain assessment in palliative care is an ongoing process and requires constant and careful monitoring of the effect of medication and other treatments so that needed changes to the care plan can be implemented quickly. Palliative psychologists can contribute significantly to the comprehensive and interdisciplinary pain assessment and treatment plan by identifying relevant psychological factors that can create challenging case scenarios (Table 2.2).

Table 2.2 **Pain Management Scenarios Requiring Psychological Assessment and Interventions**

Clinical Scenario	Clinical Implications	Role of the Palliative Psychologist
The patient reports continuous, excruciating pain, despite medication adjustments.	The patient's suffering may be precipitated or worsened by other sources of distress.	Identify sources of psychological, existential, spiritual suffering that are creating mental and psychological anguish for the patient.
Discrepancy between the patient's pain report and that of family caregivers or staff.	The patient's perception of pain may be affected by emotional and social factors occurring *between* pain assessments.	Identify causes of distress but also recognize the presence of any negative beliefs about use of medication by the patient or the family.
The patient holds inflexible beliefs about how medications work alone and in combination with other drugs.	May cause decreased treatment adherence and poor pain management.	Address these beliefs through cognitive restructuring.
The patient is exhibiting aberrant drug-taking behaviors.	This may raise serious concern in the medical team and prevent adequate pain management even if the patient is seriously ill.	Assess risk and develop safety plan, including possible contract; develop comprehensive psychological plan; work with treating team to address risks; recognize concern about pain being undertreated.
The patient expresses psychological distress expressed primarily through physical symptoms (i.e., pain).	Severe pain report continues if the underlying causes of distress are not addressed.	Use nonpharmacological modalities to supplement medication and facilitate emotional expressiveness; recognize cultural factors.

CASE VIGNETTE 2.1

Walter was a 78-year-old man diagnosed with esophageal cancer, status post esophagectomy and gastrectomy, who completed radiation therapy and chemotherapy two years ago. The patient received multiple dilatations of strictures and had a recurrence of the disease three months ago. He refused further treatment and was hospitalized with abdominal pain, nausea, and anxiety. The oncology team requested a palliative care consultation for psychological evaluation of anxiety and distress and discussions of goals of care. The palliative care physician and the chaplain saw the patient initially.

The palliative care evaluation focused on the patient's pain, which was described as severe. He mentioned that he had two siblings, but they were estranged. As he described having some support from a neighbor and his home health aide, he suddenly became anxious and reported difficulty breathing. Initially attributing his anxiety to feelings of loneliness and sadness, the team reassured the patient that support would be provided and that he would not be facing hospitalization alone. Arrangements were made for volunteers to visit the patient. He told the chaplain that he did not need to return because he was not on good terms with God. Over the next couple of days, the palliative care physician increased medication to control pain, but the patient continued to report "11/10" pain. However, nursing staff had reported that he no longer grimaced or complained when they turned him and moved him during the morning hygiene routine. Cleary there was a discrepancy between his pain report and his behavior related to pain. The palliative psychologist was asked to evaluate the patient because he appeared to be anxious and suffering without pain relief. During the psychological evaluation, the patient finally disclosed to the psychologist that he had been carrying a terrible guilt for over 50 years. Driving home when he was 17 after a night out drinking he missed a stop sign and hit a car. The driver was a pregnant woman who died at the scene. Walter was sent to juvenile hall and never drank again; however, he could never process the guilt about causing the accident. He stated that while his memory of the event was blurred because he had been intoxicated, the impact of his actions had affected him deeply and he never felt he deserved a normal life after that. He explained that the guilt "ate" at his body, causing pain that was worse than the cancer. He presented depressed with episodes of anxiety that worsened at night. Further assessment indicated that the patient's guilt had some irrational features, and he described feeling unworthy of any forgiveness and help. Because it was believed his prognosis was in the order of months, a selective serotonin reuptake inhibitor (SSRI) antidepressant was initiated and titrated to effect. The patient also met with the psychologist daily. The psychologist used a cognitive-behavioral approach to process guilt known as "blame pie," which allowed the patient to recognize the presence of several circumstances leading up to the accident. This approach was not meant to minimize Walter's responsibility, but rather to expand his understanding into a more complex story that he could actually learn from. This allowed him to actually listen to his guilt and take action, rather than being simply paralyzed by it. Walter was able to broaden his sense of responsibility and guilt by exploring the circumstances and people who had indirectly contributed to the situation. For example, his father was an alcoholic who encouraged him to drink to show he was an adult. Approaching the event from a broader perspective of a larger narrative allowed him to recognize the larger context for his actions. He decided to document the results of this process in a letter to the editor of a local newspaper, addressing the dangers of teen drinking. His depression improved as a result of medication and psychotherapy, his pain report became more consistent and his pain became better managed.

Psychological Pain Assessment

In approaching pain management in advanced illness, medical professionals will consider several factors related to the patient and the illness to optimize treatment. One important factor is *prognosis*. If this is in the order of months, and the patient wishes to maintain a good level of cognitive function and alertness, it will be critical to promote optimal pain control while minimizing sedation and other adverse effects. While this balance is not easily achieved, it is a major focus of specialist palliative care. The concept of allowing patients to obtain the best quality of life possible for as long as possible truly highlights the fine balance between symptoms control and function. When the prognosis is in the order of months, nonpharmacological pain management strategies can become especially important.

Medical practitioners will also consider the patient's *comorbid medical conditions* affecting the selection of pain medications. Palliative psychologists can help address *comorbid psychiatric conditions*, including depression, anxiety, or severe mental illness, as they will directly impact on pain perception, treatment adherence, side effects, and overall outcome. The psychologist can help explore the patient's and family's *belief system* about the use of medication for pain management. Some express concern early on that using opioid for the treatment of pain will hasten the patient's death. Or they may have heard or read reports about opioid addiction. As a result, patients and family members may associate use of opioid medication, particularly morphine, with death. Palliative psychologists can help assess the *need for information* in this area and provide ongoing supportive education to clarify any confusion about the difference between expert medical use of opioid medication for pain management and symptom control and addiction or hastened death. Training and expertise in recognizing, assessing, and treating addiction and substance use disorder from a psychological and integrative perspective are extremely valuable in the palliative care setting. Additionally, by working closely with the medical providers on the team, psychologists can assess for aberrant drug-taking behaviors and can provide interventions to minimize risk and improve quality of life.

In palliative care, there is often an urgent need to untangle the physical aspects of pain from psychological factors that affect the perception of pain. Therefore, the psychological pain assessment needs to identify not only the physical aspect of the pain experience (e.g., type, duration, location, quality, etc.), but also the relevant psychological, social, and spiritual factors, which can then be incorporated into the interdisciplinary treatment plan. The psychological pain assessment is not only important in identifying different sources of suffering, but also in establishing a trusting and collaborative relationship with the patient and the family (Box 2.3).

Using a self-report measure of pain intensity by asking the patient to rate it ("how bad is the pain?") is a common way of assessing pain. However, because the report of pain intensity does not provide information about all aspects of the pain experience (production, perception, and expression of pain), relying on it alone will prevent the clinician from identifying other factors that may be modulating the perception of pain. Rather, the patient's reported pain intensity may be the result of difficulty expressing emotional distress or suffering in ways other than pain. And it will likely not respond to an increase in pharmacological management. In these circumstances, the patient's report may be inconsistent or variable or may conflict with staff or family, or the patient's behavior may not match the stated difficulty.

The challenge facing the interdisciplinary palliative care team is to translate the meaning of the distress expressed by the patient into clinical targets that can be addressed in the care plan. Especially in complex cases, this requires an ability to reconcile contrasting information and fill in the gaps. Therefore, attention to the psychological impact of

> **Box 2.3 Psychological Pain Assessment**
>
> Pain history
> Onset, past interventions, current pain status
> Characteristics: PQRSTA
>   **P**alliative/Provocative
>   **Q**uality
>   **R**adiation
>   **S**everity
>   **T**emporal
>   **A**ssociative
> Social history
> Psychiatric history
> Substance use
>   ETOH
>   Drugs
>   Smoke
> Current medications
> Pain coping behaviors: active/passive
> Cognitive approaches to pain
>   Meaning of pain (cognitive-emotional)
>   Catastrophizing, overwhelmed, minimizing
> Pharmacological treatment
> Interest in/experience with complementary and integrative approaches
> Mental status
> Strengths
>   Patient
>   Family
>   Spiritual/existential concerns

pain requires more than general and nonspecific psychosocial support. An important role for the palliative psychologist is providing psychotherapy interventions that effectively address the emotional, cognitive, behavioral, and interpersonal aspects of pain. It is important to mention that nonverbal signs of pain can be important when assessing a patient who is no longer verbal. These signs are grimacing, restlessness, tossing in bed, confusion, frowning, agitation, withdrawal, or depressive symptoms.

Focusing attention on psychological factors relevant to the experience of pain in no way minimizes the severity of the patient's distress. In fact, psychological and existential pain can cause excruciating suffering for the patient and should never be underestimated or considered of lesser importance than pain attributed to a physiological cause, such as tumor growth. Rather, uncovering psychological factors and concerns that are impacting the patient's quality of life should prompt active psychological interventions in conjunction with medical management. Several psychological factors are relevant to the pain experience, including beliefs about the meaning of pain, impact of pain on the patient's quality of life, level of adaptation to the illness and its symptoms, presence of mood disorders or other psychiatric disorders, perception of impairment in daily life, sense of self-efficacy, and perceived sense of control. As an example, the meaning and impact of pain are described in the following.

THE MEANING ATTRIBUTED TO PAIN

An exploration of the meaning of pain by the patient can provide important insight into cognitive and emotional processes. The meaning can be concrete when pain is seen as a direct result of the disease or treatment (i.e., pain indicates that the disease is worsening, or that the illness has recurred; treatment is damaging the body; death is closer). The meaning can also be symbolic: that is, the pain can be interpreted as a punishment for past actions, or as an opportunity to learn a psychospiritual lesson, and so on. Beliefs about the meaning of pain that are causing distress to the patient can be reframed in ways that are more supportive or benign. For instance, disease-modifying treatments (e.g., chemotherapy or radiation) can be reframed as powerful allies for the patient against the disease. Physical discomfort can be reframed as an indication of the treatment's aggressiveness and effectiveness. Pharmacological pain management in this context can be seen as necessary to allow treatment to continue to be effective. This kind of reframe in the context of ongoing psychological support can help some patients by removing the element of psychological suffering from the pain experience. As a result, the patient may be willing to interpret treatment and also any necessary pain management in a more positive light.

THE CONSEQUENCES OF PAIN AND THEIR IMPACT

These are unique to each patient and need to be explored. Patients in pain can experience decreased autonomy, decreased enjoinment and quality of life, and challenges to dignity. After obtaining a list of the consequences of pain, it can be useful to ask the patient for a ranking. This can help determine short-term and long-term goals. For example, a patient may report that decreased mobility and impaired physical function are causing distress, but he may also report that the greatest burden is currently caused by opioid-induced constipation. By developing a care plan that is based on the patient's priorities, his or her sense of empowerment and control can be enhanced, promoting hope.

In palliative care, the management of pain is symptomatic. Because pain is the result of the effects of treatment and worsening disease, the underlying causes of pain can be ameliorated but generally cannot be reversed, and thus require ongoing evaluation and management of symptoms for the duration of the patient's life. Although the management of pain in advanced disease is primarily pharmacological, psychological and integrative medicine modalities can have an important supplemental role in providing direct symptom relief and by uncovering and addressing psychological distress that can add to the patient's suffering.

Coexisting with pain and the causes of pain can be challenging, even when pain can be adequately managed. Although the pain can be relieved and managed, the awareness that the underlying pathological process cannot be reversed can be distressing for the patient and the family as constant reminders of the illness. Attention to these thoughts can precipitate or exacerbate fear of the future and fear of dying, and can prevent the patient from experiencing relief—even when he or she does not perceive pain. These are complex situations that may require provision of pain management psychotherapy in addition to pharmacotherapy and broad psychosocial support.

In some situations, the patient may experience exacerbations of pain or pain in new locations that prompt the medical team to order imaging studies to determine the causes of pain. While the patient and family caregivers are waiting for studies to be completed and reviewed, they may be worried by the meaning of pain and experience negative and frightening fantasies. Catastrophizing can occur, compromising coping skills and adaptation. Palliative psychologists can play an important role in containing the patient's and the family's anxiety by helping them redirect their worry in ways that are not disruptive, including identifying strategies for dealing with any negative test results.

In summary, the approach to pain in specialist palliative care is comprehensive, interdisciplinary, and integrative. The goal of relieving pain and preventing or treating suffering involves a complex and ongoing process of assessment, implementation of interventions, evaluation of response, and adjustment of the care plan. The starting point of the care plan for all palliative care team members is the consideration of all available data, including the patient's history, physical examination, and objective studies that can help the medical provider understand the causes of pain. Depending on the patient's disease, level of function, prognosis, and goals, the management of pain includes pharmacological, psychological, and integrative modalities. It should be noted there also exist interventional pain management approaches that can have an important role. These include nerve blocks, neuraxial analgesia, and localized injections of anesthetics. These methodologies have been extensively reviewed elsewhere. The following section briefly reviews basic aspects of pain pathophysiology and pharmacological treatment. Palliative psychologists should aim to continue developing an integrated knowledge of pain assessment and treatment and to maintain an updated knowledge of strategies used in the palliative care setting.

PAIN CLASSIFICATION AND PATHOPHYSIOLOGY

Pain is usually classified based on the following (Bruera & Portenoy, 2010):

- onset and duration (Box 2.3)
- inferred pathophysiology (Box 2.4)
- pattern.

Acute and Chronic

Acute pain has a sudden onset and is of brief duration (Table 2.3). It is usually caused by injury to tissues, including injury from surgery or trauma. Acute pain usually has an identifiable cause, and it is accompanied by signs indicating hyperactivity of the sympathetic nervous system, with increased heart rate and blood pressure and diaphoresis. Pain acuity is not an indication of severity. Acute pain can be the reason a patient without other symptoms seeks medical attention leading to a diagnosis of a serious illness, or it may occur as a result of complications of an ongoing pathological process, such as cancer.

Table 2.3 **Pain Classification Based on Onset and Duration**

	ACUTE	CHRONIC
Onset	Usually sudden	Usually of long duration
Characteristics	Generally sharp and localized but may radiate to other parts of the body	Persistent, may be both nociceptive and neuropathic; qualities and patterns change
Signs and symptoms	Increased blood pressure and heart rate, sweating, facial grimacing and moaning, anxiety, fear	Pain may or may not be acknowledged openly by the patient; overt distress may or not be present; pronounced effect on mood (depressed), and/or presence of anxiety
Goals of treatment	Relief of pain if related to discrete tissue injury or surgery; treatment approach is both pharmacological and nonpharmacological	Relief of pain and ongoing management; treatment approach is both pharmacological and nonpharmacological

Chronic pain does not have a clearly defined onset and is of prolonged duration. The pain can be caused by ongoing inflammation, as in arthritis, or by nerve damage.

Cancer pain is a general category for pain that is usually chronic, caused by disease mass, inflammation, or nerve damage. It can also result from the effects of treatment, such as surgery, radiation, and chemotherapy.

Inferred Pathophysiology

Based on pathophysiology, pain can also be described as nociceptive, neuropathic, or mixed (Table 2.4).

Nociceptive pain is generally well localized. It can be somatic when it affects bones or tissue or visceral when it affects internal organs. *Somatic* pain is often described as aching, throbbing, sharp, pressure-like, or stabbing. *Visceral* pain is frequently described as cramping, squeezing, or gnawing.

Neuropathic pain is a complex process due to multiple mechanisms and it is prevalent in patients with cancer pain. It is defined by the International Association for the Study of Pain as being caused by a lesion or disease in the somatosensory nervous system. Neuropathic pain is not a medical diagnosis but a clinical descriptor. It does not specifically indicate a disease, but it can be present in several medical diagnoses. The key feature is sustained nerve stimulation. This is a result of a reciprocal interaction of pain pathways in the central and peripheral nervous system. Several mechanisms are involved, depending on the type of disease, pathophysiology, or site of the neurological lesion. It is often present as a polyneuropathy caused by chemotherapy agents. It also occurs as a result of radiation therapy, or pressure on nerves or tumor invasion of nerves as in the brachial plexus. Unlike nociceptive pain, neuropathic pain is generally poorly localized and is usually chronic (Cruciani, Strada & Knotkova, 2010; Fallon, 2013).

Table 2.4 **Pain Classification Based on Inferred Pathophysiology**

	Nociceptive **SOMATIC**	*Nociceptive* **VISCERAL**	*Neuropathic*
Pain mechanisms	Tissue injury that stimulates nerve endings	Tissue injury, stretching, or inflammation	Injury or damage to peripheral nerves or central nervous system
Affected areas	Bones, joints, soft tissue	Internal organs	Peripheral nerves, central nervous system
Pain descriptors generally used by patients	Usually well localized and described as sharp, dull, aching, stabbing	Generally poorly localized and described as pressure, aching, stretching, or cramping	Described as tingling, shooting, numbing, electric discharge

Diagnosing neuropathic pain can be challenging, because it is characterized by mixed syndromes and heterogeneous presentations. Assessment of neuropathic pain is also complex because patients describe it differently. It may described as burning, shooting, and numbing, or as lancinating pain. It may even be described atypically as a deep ache. Additionally, the presence of wounds and ulcers and cognitive impairment can also complicate diagnosis.

Mixed pain syndromes are common and are characterized by nociceptive pain related to ongoing tissue damage caused by the disease and neuropathic pain caused by damage to the nervous system.

Pattern

Baseline pain refers to chronic pain that is generally managed by opioid medication provided to patients on a regular schedule or "around the clock" to avoid pain crises. Increasing baseline pain that is caused by the progression of disease needs to be managed proactively to prevent the patient from experiencing disabling pain. When baseline pain management has become inadequate, clinical assessment will allow clinicians to determine whether the baseline pain management regimen has become inadequate and should be adjusted, or if the patient is experiencing breakthrough pain. Any change in pain pattern or lack of response to treatment should prompt consideration of additional psychological re-evaluation to determine whether, in addition to progression of disease, there may be psychological factors that are affecting changes in pain patterns and the patient's response to pain treatment. The presence of depression, anxiety, and existential and spiritual distress can alter the pain threshold and affect the patient's perception of pain (Lahoud et al., 2016).

Breakthrough pain can occur in patients with cancer and non-cancer diagnoses. The initial conceptualization referred to episodes of severe acute pain superimposed on baseline pain. The current understanding considers it an episode of increased pain despite adequate pain control most of the time on a regular opioid regimen (Taylor, 2013). Due to the recognition of breakthrough pain and its potential for creating distress, several drug formulations have been developed over the years to allow for rapid absorption and pain relief. These are used episodically (as needed, or PRN) in addition to the baseline regimen. *Incident pain* is a subtype of breakthrough pain. It is an exacerbation of pain caused by activity or a specific incident, such as a fall.

Pharmacological Pain Management

Published in 1986, the World Health Organization guidelines, known as the WHO Analgesic Ladder, are still considered a valuable approach for the management of pain in patients with cancer (Lahoud et al., 2016; Vargas-Schaffer, 2010). The guidelines are currently also used in non-cancer pain related to advanced illness (Box 2.4). The concept of the analgesic ladder was developed to assist medical providers in the selection and adjustment of pharmacological pain treatments. Based on the WHO ladder, pharmacological management for mild pain (step 1) is generally begun with non-opioids such as acetaminophen, aspirin, and non-steroidal anti-inflammatory drugs (NSAIDS). Non-opioids and weak opioids are recommended for moderate pain (step 2). Strong opioids (e.g., morphine) are used to treat pain that is moderate to severe (step 3). Additionally, based on the guidelines, opioid therapy generally begins with the milder short-acting formulations and progresses, if needed, to the stronger opioids. At any point, based on clinical situations, adjuvant analgesics (e.g., antidepressants, gabapentinoids) may be added to non-opioids or opioids. Adjuvants can be initiated for mild pain and also can be used together with opioids.

Understanding the WHO ladder and its application in practice is valuable for palliative psychologists. They will be able to participate more actively in clinical discussions, not necessarily by discussing medications but by understanding the full range of the patients' experience and their response to medications. Recognizing and evaluating the attitudes that patients develop toward medical treatment (especially pain medication) is particularly important. These can be supportive, or can become dysfunctional and unsupportive of the patient's healing (Matzo & Witt Sherman, 2015). The following content briefly describes the main classes of medication used for pain management in advanced illness, including relevant psychological factors that should be considered by palliative psychologists. (The main sources for this section were Bruera & Portenoy, 2010; Goldstein & Morrison, 2013; Portenoy & Ahmed, 2014; Prommer, 2015; Simmons MacLeod & Laird, 2012.)

Pharmacodynamics is a term used to describe drug actions in the body. Simplified, it refers to *what the drug does to the body*. For example, the pharmacodynamics of opioids on the central nervous system have desirable and undesirable effects. Examples of desirable effects are analgesia and cough suppression. Undesirable effects are euphoria, other mood changes, respiratory depression, and sedation.

Pharmacokinetics can be described as the metabolic processing of the drug. Simplified, it refers to *what the body does to the drug*. This includes the speed of onset and duration of action. The term *half-life* is frequently used to define the time it takes

> ### Box 2.4 **WHO Analgesic Ladder**
>
> #### STEP 1: MILD PAIN
>
> Non-opioids plus or minus adjuvants
>
> - aspirin
> - acetaminophen
> - non-steroidal antiflammatory drugs (NSAIDS)
>
> If pain persists or increases
>
> #### STEP 2: MODERATE PAIN
>
> Weak opioids, plus or minus non-opioids and adjuvants
>
> - codeine
> - hydrocodone
> - oxycodone
> - tramadol
>
> If pain persists or increases
>
> #### STEP 3: MODERATE TO SEVERE PAIN
>
> Strong opioids plus or minus non-opioids and adjuvants
>
> - oxycodone
> - morphine
> - hydromorphone
> - methadone
> - fentanyl

to eliminate (by excretion or metabolic degradation) one-half of a single administered dose. While it is customary to say the drug is elimated in four half-lives, there can be significant variation, as the duration of a single half-life may be altered by many physical circumstances.

OPIOIDS

Opium is the dried powdered mixture of more than 20 chemicals obtained from the unripe seed capsules of the poppy. *Opiate* or *opioid* is a generic term that refers to any agent derived from opium with morphine properties. As a class of medications they attach to multiple natural opiate receptors in the central nervous system, in nerve endings in the periphery, in the gastrointestinal tract, and in the bladder. In addition to analgesia, effects include euphoria, sedation, pupil constriction, respiratory depression, physical dependence, and decreased gastrointestinal motility.

HYDROCODONE AND CODEINE

These are considered the weakest opioid analgesics. Hydrocodone is generally regarded as a more consistent analgesic, but with more sedation. It is available alone or in combination and it is given orally. The onset of analgesic action is 10–30 minutes, with peak analgesic effects 30–60 minutes. The duration of analgesic activity is 4–6 hours and its half-life elimination is 3–4 hours.

OXYCODONE AND OXYMORPHONE

These are more potent opioids generally used as their oral preparations with similar pharmacokinetics. Combination pills are available with acetaminophen and a slow release formulation is available.

MORPHINE

Morphine is a potent analgesic with many formulations that can be given through the oral, parenteral (IV, IM, SC), intrathecal, epidural, and rectal routes with rapid onset of action. Morphine is commonly used in the palliative care and hospice setting because of its versatile delivery, low cost, and accessibility. A time-release oral morphine has a slower onset of action but generally provides pain relief for 8–12 hours. Transition to slow-release morphine is often a first consideration for baseline pain management.

HYDROMORPHONE

Hydromorphone is regarded as 5–10 times more potent than morphine with perhaps better oral absorption. It can be given through the oral, parenteral, and rectal routes. It has similar delivery formulations and kinetics.

FENTANYL

This opioid is 80–100 times more potent than morphine and it is generally not intended for opioid naïve patients (i.e., patients who are new to opioids). It has a more rapid onset of action compared to morphine, causes less hypotensive effects compared to morphine, and it is available in multiple dosage forms. Fentanyl use is mostly by transdermal patch and it can be used in patients with renal failure because it lacks active metabolite. The transdermal patch is gradually absorbed for the first 12–24 hours, followed by constant absorption for 2 days with a dosing interval of 3 days. Accordingly, dosage changes are usually made weekly. Studies have shown that plasma concentration is lower in cancer patients who have cachexia. Heat and elevated body temperature increase the rate of absorption of fentanyl in the patch and decrease the duration of action. Because an increased rate of absorption may result in toxicity, careful monitoring is required. It is important to avoid direct exposure with heating pads, electric blankets, or hot tops. Additionally, it is important to rotate the site with each new patch applied. Family caregivers providing home care to the patient need to receive education about these safety precautions.

METHADONE

Methadone is a potent analgesic that is mainly administered orally. Because of the variable and potentially long half-life (up to two days), it is usually not used for opioid naïve patients, and dosage adjustments must be made with great care. Most patients have heard of methadone in the context of drug addiction and may not be familiar with its use in pain management. Therefore, if the recommendation of switching to methadone is made, some may refuse it because of concerns about the associated stigma. If the medical team feels that methadone would be a good pain management strategy, palliative psychologists may assist the patient by deconstructing their belief and addressing any perceived stigma. It is sometimes useful to remind the patient that not uncommonly medications that have been found effective in one area of medicine are subsequently found useful in additional areas.

ADJUVANTS MEDICATION IN PAIN MANAGEMENT

Adjuvant analgesics are drugs that, as part of the WHO pain ladder, can be added to any step, from non-opioids to weak or strong opoids. The goal is to maintain the step in the pain ladder and avoid the need to progress to stronger analgesics. They can also be used when it is desirable to decrease the amount of opioids because the patient is having significant difficulty managing side effects. They may also be used as primary pain treatment. These drugs were initially approved for use to address conditions other than pain.

Corticosteroids

Corticosteroids have anti-inflammatory qualities and can reduce edema in the areas surrounding tumors. Edema can cause pressure on structures that are sensitive to pain. Corticosteroids can reduce pain from intracranial pressure, and neuropathic pain in spinal cord compression. They are also used to improve nausea, appetite, and the general sense of malaise often described by patients with advanced illness. Among the different corticosteroids, dexamethasone is commonly chosen, because it is less likely to cause fluid retention and has a long duration of action.

Side effects from corticosteroids increase with dose and duration of treatment. They include hypertension, fluid retention, muscle weakness, immunity weakness, and Cushingoid distortions of face and body. Additionally, neuropsychiatric side effects can be significant and range from mild dysphoria to severe depression, anxiety, and even psychosis. Considering corticosteroid-related side effects is important in differential diagnosis when depression and anxiety are considered. Patients who are experiencing anxiety as a result of corticosteroid side effects may describe their symptoms as internal agitation, feeling jittery, or wanting to jump out of their skin. If the onset of symptoms is acute, it is also important to consider superimposed psychosocial causes of distress, especially anxiety (e.g., a family conflict or an upcoming diagnostic procedures that may reveal worsening of illness).

If corticosteroids are considered the cause of the anxiety or the dysphoric affect, the medical providers will evaluate the benefit and burden of continuing to use the drug, determining whether the medication can be stopped, the dose decreased, or an anti-anxiety medication added.

Many patients can benefit from realizing that there is a reason for their symptoms. For most, it is important to recognize that the anxiety they are experiencing is not an indication of poor coping, but rather an expected, though unpleasant, side effect of medication; this can help patients better manage the symptoms. Teaching anxiety-management techniques, including deep breathing and/or progressive muscle relaxation, guided imagery, and self-hypnosis, can be especially useful and can improve their sense of empowerment and control.

Antidepressants

Treatment of pain from advanced illness, especially cancer, generally involves the use of opioids as a first line of treatment for pain that is moderate to severe. Antidepressants can be used to augment pain management, especially when the patient has comorbid depression or anxiety.

TRICYCLIC ANTIDEPRESSANTS

Studies have shown that tricyclic antidepressants have independent analgesic properties. Evidence for the effectiveness of these medications is primarily from studies on chronic, neuropathic pain. Amitriptyline, desipramine, and nortriptyline are commonly used in this setting. As they may also cause sedation, they are generally used at night and may also improve sleep. The anticholinergic side effects from this class of antidepressants may make them difficult to use in older, more frail patients, as well as in patients with urinary retention and glaucoma. Tricyclics are also generally avoided in patients with significant cardiac problems.

SELECTIVE SEROTONION REUPTAKE INHIBITORS (SSRIS) AND SEROTONIN-NOREPINEPHRINE REUPTAKE INHIBITORS (SNRIS)

Because SSRIs have been found to have few independent analgesic properties, they are not generally used to supplement pain management. However, if the existing pain is having a severe impact on the patient's mood, or if the psychological component of suffering is significantly impacting on pain management, there may be a benefit from these antidepressant drugs.

However, SNRIs have been found to have some independent analgesic properties and are used to improve chronic neuropathic pain in patients with advanced illness. Side effects include nausea, increase in blood pressure, insomnia, akathisia, vomiting, and dizziness. Additionally, duloxetine kinetics may affect the kinetics of other drugs, as their metabolism affects the metabolism of other drugs. Venlafaxine appears to be less problematic in this regard, but it is associated with a significant discontinuation syndrome.

Anticonvulsants
This class of medication has been used extensively for the management of neuropathic pain. Gabapentin and pregabalin are generally considered as first-line treatment for neuropathic pain. However, they are generally not utilized in patients who have depression, because they may exacerbate symptoms. Side effects of anticonvulsants include sedation, mental cloudiness, and dizziness.

ADDRESSING OPIOIDS' ADVERSE EFFECTS AND PATIENTS' CONCERNS

Adverse effects often occur during pain management with opioids. These can raise concerns in the patient and the family, or amplify any existing ambivalence about treatment. The management of adverse effects from opioids is primarily pharmacological. The dose can be adjusted, a different agent may be selected, or a specific medication added for the adverse effect. Psychologists should be aware of the medical strategies being used to address adverse effects, as well as the psychological impact of adverse effects on the patient and the family. It is important that patients and families feel that their concerns and questions are adequately addressed by the team. If questions and concerns are quickly dismissed, ambivalence about pain treatment can occur, possibly causing poor treatment adherence and poorly controlled pain. Psychologists can help patients define their concerns and facilitate communications between them and their prescribing physician.

Patients and families often also express concern about fear of developing addiction and especially fear that opioids may hasten the patient's death. Concerns about beginning opioid therapy for pain management should be addressed by providing information in clear and simple language. Misinformation and fear can translate into poor treatment adherence and indirectly contribute to inadequate pain management. It is important that clinicians do not trivialize or quickly minimize these concerns; they should explore the concerns, understand their source, and utilize strategies that will facilitate the development of a collaborative treatment plan that is agreed upon by the patient, the family, and the medical team.

A first level of intervention is providing psychoeducation and clarifying the meaning of concepts such as tolerance, dependence, and addiction. *Tolerance* refers to the need for a dose increase to produce the same analgesic effect. It appears to occur in most patients treated with chronic opioids. In the absence of concerning behaviors on the part of the patient including maladaptive drug-taking behaviors, development of tolerance should not be interpreted as an indication that medication is not being used appropriately. Tolerance is a pharmacological effect of the drug that, in absence of other behaviors, should never be considered addiction.

Physical dependence is also an expected pharmacological effect of the drug. It involves the development of a discontinuation syndrome when the drug is stopped abruptly. Again, in absence of maladaptive behavior, physical dependence is not a sign of abuse or addiction. It is helpful to explain to patients and families that many other drugs carry the potential for physical dependence, such as antidepressants, and certain drugs for hypertension. To use an even simpler and day-to-day example, they could be reminded that even coffee, for many people, causes a discontinuation syndrome, generally in the form of temporary headaches, when stopped abruptly.

Nausea and Vomiting

Nausea caused by opioids is generally addressed by either switching to a different opioid, or by administering antiemetic agents to be used concurrently with the opioid. Patients who are particularly sensitive to the impact of side effects may experience anticipatory nausea even when a different medication is used. Psychological management by teaching patients imagery and self-hypnosis exercises can help manage the anxiety often associated with this symptom.

Respiratory Depression

Decreased respiratory drive is an expected effect of opioids. While it may be desirable in some circumstances, it may become severe and may lead to respiratory failure (elevated levels of blood carbon dioxide). Ultimately, the cessation of breathing (apnea) can result. This can be especially problematic when there is impaired respiratory function and when opioid dosages are increased. Increasing sedation and decreased mental alertness should be considered a potential sign of developing respiratory depression and insufficiency.

Respiratory depression is reversible by administration of naloxone, an opioid antagonist. While patients who have experienced respiratory depression and have been successfully treated may not have a clear recollection of the events, family members may have experienced it as a traumatic and frightening event. In such cases, it is important that medical and psychosocial members of the palliative care team debrief the episode with family members using clear and simple language. Furthermore, it is important to explain what steps have been taken to avoid similar occurrences. Family caregivers who have witnessed management of an episode of respiratory depression or apnea may report intrusive thoughts, nightmares, rumination. Their trust of the medical team may also be affected. Although symptoms of traumatic distress generally resolve, it is important to monitor their duration, severity, and intensity.

Sedation

Patients generally find sedation to be an undesirable adverse effect, especially if they are ambulatory and wish to maintain a high level of function combined with good sense of control. Sedation may affect their ability to drive, to actively engage in daily activities, and it may become a deterrent to medication use. In patients with advanced illness, sedation may interfere with their ability to engage with family members and other loved ones. This can become particularly distressing for family members whose anxiety about the patient's decline is now compounded with the concern about not being able to have quality time due to sedation. Medical professionals generally explain to patients that sedation is in many cases an adverse effect that subsides after several days of continued use. In some cases, the medical team may recommend the use of psychostimulants to counteract sedation and improve overall energy level and mental alertness. Contraindications to psychostimulants need to be carefully considered.

It is important to note that opioid related sedation can be compounded by the use of other medication with sedating effects, such as benzodiazepines prescribed for the treatment of anxiety, or hypnotics prescribed for the treatment of sleep disorders.

Where there is a compounded sedation effect from different medications, introducing the use of nonpharmacological strategies to address anxiety and insomnia may be a valuable addition for improvement of quality of life, and it may at times allow decreasing the amounts of medications. These include clinical hypnosis, imagery, and cognitive behavioral therapy (CBT) techniques (Sage et al., 2008; Marchand, 2014).

As patients approach the end of life, they will generally experience increased somnolence and decreased energy as a result of the illness progression. And, if an increase in pain medication is required, this may also increase sedation, possibly creating confusion and anxiety for family caregivers. Some may fear that medication is preventing the loved one from being alert and that it may hasten death. Conflicts around the use of pain medication may even prompt the need for an ethical consultation. Palliative psychologists can play an important role in preventing these problems by identifying and addressing concerns and distress in family members as early as possible. Also, it needs to be emphasized, having previously established a close working relationship with the family greatly enhances trust and the ability of the palliative psychologist to facilitate the processing of grief and anxiety.

The psychological response to experiencing strong adverse effects is highly individual. While one patient may take the side effect at face value and agree to switch to another class of medication, another patient may attach an especially negative meaning to the experience and develop strong negative attitudes toward medications in general. Some patients may develop and exhibit catastrophizing thinking and develop negative expectations about the effect of a new medication. Palliative psychologists can play an important role in addressing these responses and work effectively with the patient, the family, and the medical team to promote more adaptive coping and facilitate effective pain management. The use of CBT can help identify cognitive distortions related to the action of medication, promote relaxation in the context of a situation that can generate profound anxiety, and generate new ways of thinking about the problem.

CLINICAL HYPNOSIS AS PART OF PSYCHOLOGICAL TREATMENT

An effective approach to pain and symptom management in advanced illness involves the integrated use of pharmacological and psychological strategies, including evidence-based complementary medicine approaches (Cassileth, 2011; Thomas & Weiss, 2000). Among these approaches, clinical hypnosis has received increased attention for its role in supporting improvement of pain and symptoms in patients with cancer (Eimer & Freeman, 1998; Desai, Chaturvedi & Ramachandra, 2001).

While an in-depth discussion is beyond the scope of this book, it is important to mention that clinical applications of hypnosis in palliative care include depression, emotional and existential distress, death anxiety, chemotherapy side effects, fear of medical procedures, hot flashes, and pain (Elkins, 2017; Elkins, Fisher, & Silwinski, 2012; Montgomery, Schnur & Kravits, 2013). If acceptable to the patient and appropriate for the patient, clinical hypnosis can be used in conjunction with pharmacological and procedural treatment in the following ways:

- by making direct suggestions for symptom reduction (e.g., pain, nausea, anxiety)
- as an adjunct to other types of psychotherapy, to deepen insight, or to facilitate relaxation.

Western medicine has long made use of hypnosis. James Esdaile, Jean Charcot, Pierre Janet, Joseph Breuer, and Sigmund Freud all used hypnotic approaches in their practice. In Milton Erikson's words, "Hypnosis is not some mystical procedure, but rather a systematic utilization of experiential leanings—that is, the extensive leanings acquired through the process of living" (Erickson, 1980, p. 224). Hypnosis can be described as a state of attentive, focused concentration with suspension of some peripheral awareness; a state of parallel awareness, with the ability to process information effortlessly on a number of levels simultaneously and as a state of controlled dissociation (Spiegel & Spiegel, 1978). It has also been described as "an animated, altered, integrated state of focused consciousness, that is, controlled imagination. It is an attentive, receptive state of concentration that can be activated readily and measured. It requires some degree of dissociation to enter and become involved in imagined activity, enough concentration for an individual to maintain a certain level of absorption, and some degree of suggestibility to take in new premises" (Spiegel & Greenleaf, 2005, p. 113).

Hypnotic phenomena or trancelike states occur constantly, where the individual is in a state of focused attention directed inwardly. Examples of naturally occurring self-hypnosis are prayer, being completely absorbed in reading a book, watching a movie, road hypnosis, or witnessing something awe inspiring, such as wonders of nature. In all these examples, the individual is focused inward and "forgets" about the current reality but becomes fully immersed in a different reality. In essence, the trance is a state of narrowed or limited external awareness and an expanded or enhanced internal direction and attention. Many practitioners and researchers of hypnosis believe that all hypnosis is self-hypnosis, meaning that it implies active and willing participation of the patients. Patients utilize their own imagination, and they are receptive to suggestions that are acceptable and meaningful to them.

Clinical hypnosis may be particularly suitable for addressing the need of patients in the palliative care setting. Not uncommonly, patients with serious illness describe feeling a sense of alienation as they navigate the medical system and especially after receiving distressing news. They may become completely absorbed in an internal state characterized by negative emotions, and thus are unable to take in or process information from medical providers. They may also become completely focused on the discomfort caused by physical symptoms, which can promote depressed mood and hopelessness. Clinical hypnosis can be used to induce positive and desirable changes in the patients' experience, by shifting attention and using imagination to modify the quality of their physical and emotional experience.

The essential components of a hypnotic procedure are hypnotic induction and hypnotic suggestion. During the induction, the patient is guided to relax, concentrate, and focus attention. Inductions are most effective when they match the patient's style and evoke images or sensations that have a positive meaning for the patients. When the patient has little experience with hypnosis, or there is significant anxiety and difficulty relaxing, inductions can be longer procedures and may include a modified form of progressive muscle relaxation. The hypnotic suggestion involves the verbalization of statements designed to evoke relief from symptoms or experiences that are causing discomfort to the patient.

Hypnosis uses all the sensory modalities: visual, auditory, kinesthetic, and olfactory. The patient is invited to explore his or her experience through all the senses and to become completely part of the experience. During the hypnotic suggestion, the patient is guided to undergo changes in experience, or is directed to focus on certain aspects of his or her experience and ignore others. To this aim, the therapist can use several types of suggestions.

Hypnotic susceptibility has been described as the degree to which an individual responds to hypnotic suggestions. It appears to be a trait-like characteristic that reflects individual differences (Piccione, Hilgard, & Zimbardo, 1989). While high susceptibility to hypnosis has been associated with greater response to pain interventions (Milling, 2008), facilitating a state of focused relaxation with hypnotic elements can benefit most patients and improve quality of life. Palliative psychologists trained in clinical hypnosis can use the session not only to improve symptoms, but also as an opportunity to teach the patient self-hypnosis skills that he or she can continue practicing outside the session. This is especially important in the in-patient setting, where it may be possible to provide only one session to the patient before discharge.

It is important to note that the practice of clinical hypnosis by health professionals and mental health professionals requires a process of structured learning and supervision to ensure competency. This will allow a palliative psychologist to assess whether a patient is appropriate for hypnotic intervention.

CASE VIGNETTE 2.2

Patricia is a 47-year-old Latina who visited her primary care physician after experiencing progressive fatigue, cough, and a sense of heaviness in her chest for about four months. Her symptoms became more prominent after she had the flu and she did not visit the doctor sooner, thinking she was still recovering. Her primary care physician referred her for a CT scan of the chest, which showed two masses in the upper lobe of the right lung and lymphadenopathy. A subsequent lung biopsy confirmed a diagnosis of non-small-cell lung cancer, stage IIIB. The oncologist met with the patient and the husband and told them that surgery was not an option, but he recommended starting chemotherapy, followed by radiation therapy. Prognosis was not discussed. Symptoms of fatigue worsened after the first chemotherapy treatment and she developed neuropathic pain in the upper and lower extremities shortly after the infusion. During the second chemotherapy treatment she suddenly felt her heart rate increase and began sweating profusely. She felt that the hospital room was becoming increasingly smaller and there would not be sufficient air to breathe. She became agitated and stated that the chemotherapy was "killing" her. After a medical evaluation ruled out treatment complications, she was administered an anxiolytic medication and a psychology consultation was requested.

Course of Psychological Treatment for Patricia

Patricia has been married for 20 years and has two teenage daughters. She had been working full-time as a cashier in a supermarket for 15 years, but could no longer work full-time due to the neuropathy, which prevented her from being able to stand and handle grocery items. She described her husband as a good provider but "not very good with emotions." She had a good support network and had been part of a women's group for several years. She went to church regularly with her family. She did not smoke and did not drink alcohol. She denied any use of drugs.

Patricia had difficulty sleeping and anxiety after her mother's death from end-stage congestive heart failure three years prior and was given Alprazolam 0.5 by her primary care physician to be taken two times a day as needed. She had been taking the medication but was not sure it was controlling her anxiety, which had increased significantly after the cancer diagnosis. At the initial session with the palliative psychologist, her husband and daughters commented that Patricia worries "all the time, about everything and anything" and that the situation has worsened after the diagnosis. She became particularly distressed before any follow-up tests.

The psychological evaluation indicates that Patricia is suffering from generalized anxiety disorder, with constant and uncontrollable worry and catastrophizing. She admitted since the diagnosis she had been thinking about the worst-case scenarios. She described her mind as a "tangled web"; even when she was successful in calming a particular worry, another one immediately emerged and she was not allowed any relief. Patricia also suffered from panic disorder. She experienced a panic attack during the second chemotherapy session and was now living in fearful anticipation of another attack. She stated that she wanted to continue chemotherapy but was afraid she would become agitated again.

Patricia was also having difficulty coping with low back pain and neuropathy. The meaning Patricia attributed to the pain was that the cancer was getting worse, and she would die soon. Though the oncologist had explained that neuropathy was a result of treatment and that the low back pain was not related to the cancer, Patricia felt helpless. As a result, she did not take pain medication as prescribed, as she was convinced that it would not help. Her main cognitions about the pain were: "I am overwhelmed by the pain and cannot cope"; "I am in pain because this cancer is very aggressive and there is nothing I can do about it"; and "this is the beginning of the end and it is only going to get worse for me." As a result, Patricia's mood fluctuated between anxious rumination and hopelessness.

When the psychologist explored Patricia's approach toward pharmacological treatment for anxiety, she admitted that alprazolam was only giving temporary relief and she felt tempted to take it more often, which made her feel more anxious about becoming addicted to the medication. The psychologist presented the possibility of considering a medication that would allow ongoing management of her anxiety during the day and offered to discuss this issue with Patricia's oncologist. Patricia felt encouraged and agreed. After a team discussion, the oncologist prescribed escitalopram, 5 mg daily, titrated to 10 mg daily after two weeks. Alprazolam was discontinued after a thorough discussion with the patient.

Patricia's cognitions about pain and her relationship toward pain medication were also addressed in therapy, following a cognitive-behavioral model:

Psychoeducation *about pain and cognitive restructuring*. The psychologist provided a simple description of neuropathy and normalized it as an unfortunate, but common adverse effect of the chemotherapy agents used in Patricia's treatment (Oxaliplatin and Taxotere) and *not* as an indication that the cancer was getting worse. Patricia learned to recognize inaccurate beliefs, cognitive distortions, and maladaptive thoughts about pain and cancer treatment and replace them with more positive and adaptive ones. For example, the cognition that chemotherapy was killing her was explored. Patricia stated that she needed help to continue tolerating treatment and she reframed chemotherapy as a powerful ally that was, however, not always very good at controlling its power. She reframed neuropathy as a consequence that could be managed. Patricia also became progressively aware of how negative thoughts and emotions contributed to her experience of pain.

Patricia's approach toward pharmacological treatment. Therapy uncovered her lack of treatment adherence as a result of feeling overwhelmed and hopeless. The psychologist also discussed with Patricia that gabapentin, the medication she was prescribed for neuropathy, could also help the management of anxiety. Therefore, by taking it as prescribed, she may experience an overall improvement in symptoms and well-being.

Coping skills. Patricia learned self-hypnosis skills to improve relaxation, distraction, and management of anxiety and pain. She developed an imagery exercise where her nervous system was visualized as a factory with hectic energy where everyone worked overtime. She then visualized the Pope visiting the factory and asking everyone to relax, sit down, and listen to his speech. She used this image to become relaxed when she was beginning to feel anxious and upset. She also learned to modify the quality and the location of pain to make it more bearable. For example, she imagined that the sensation of electric shooting was transformed into a deep tissue massage, which made it easier to tolerate. Also, she imagined that all the pain in her body could become concentrated into a small ball of pain that could move downward and stop in her heel, where she did not feel she had much sensation. This also helped her shift her attention and contributed to her sense of control.

Patricia's pain and mood improved as a result of the combined pharmacological and psychological treatment. After her symptoms became better controlled, she raised her deeper concern, which was her unclear prognosis and fear of dying soon. Because she felt more in control physically and emotionally, she was now able to express her sadness and grief. A family meeting with the oncologist was set up with the goal of discussing prognosis. Patricia and her husband were told that her probability of surviving five years was very low, but no one could predict exactly what would happen. While this was difficult news, Patricia felt now empowered to use her physical and emotional energy to spend time creating positive memories with her family. She continued to approach pain and other physical symptoms with a combination of pharmacological and psychological approaches. Her hope for cure shifted to hope for increased physical and emotional well-being and good days with her family. This allowed her to maintain a sense of connection with many sources of meaning and comfort, even as the disease worsened.

CASE VIGNETTE 2.3

Kate was a 50-year-old woman diagnosed two months prior with ovarian cancer metastatic to the bones and was undergoing chemotherapy treatment. She had been unable to work due to back pain and difficulty concentrating, and she was anxious about finances. She was divorced and lived with her 15-year-old son, who had become increasingly withdrawn since her diagnosis. She had been trying to speak with him about her illness, but he had refused to engage and spent most of his time in his room with his door locked. During an argument, he told her that her illness was ruining his life and it would be easier for him if she was dead. Kate felt devastated. She had difficulty reading, which she used to enjoy. Usually optimistic and outgoing, she had been avoiding connecting with friends. For the past month, she had been tearful and anxious. She recognized her illness was serious, and she worried about her future and her son's. Lately, she had been feeling a lack of control over her body and mind. Her thinking process was ruminative, and she admitted feeling hopeless. She admitted to the oncology nurse that she had been fantasizing about dying and wishing she could just not wake up. She denied she would kill herself, not to cause more distress to her son, but she was beginning to think that perhaps he may have been better off without her. She also had been thinking about stopping chemotherapy and letting the disease "run its course." However, her oncologist believed her disease could be managed with treatment. When asked about her rationale for stopping treatment, Kate explained that the disease was taking a bigger toll than she imagined and she was tired of fighting. Kate asked her oncologists if she would meet the criteria for physician-assisted dying, and was disappointed when his answer was negative. At that point the oncologist made a referral to the palliative psychologist, concerned about Kate's distress and suicidal ideation.

Course of Psychological Treatment for Kate
The psychological assessment focused on identifying Kate's sources of suffering in different domains. In the physical domain, she reported back pain that was moderate to severe most days. Her oncologist had prescribed opioids, which had improved her pain; however, she developed persistent constipation. Feeling uncomfortable about discussing this issue with her medical providers, Kate found information online explaining constipation was an adverse effect of opioids. She stopped taking her medication regularly, waiting until the pain was severe to take medication. This approach meant she was in pain most of the time, which negatively affected her mood, creating feelings of hopelessness.

A thorough suicidal ideation revealed that Kate felt helpless about being able to take control of her life and her relationship with her son. When her initial attempts to communicate with him did not succeed, she started feeling like an unwanted burden and began fantasizing about dying so her son could "move on." Kate's depression prevented her from recognizing her son's angry and insensitive remarks as manifestations of his grieving process. Therefore, she became increasingly withdrawn, feeling inadequate and ineffective as a parent.

The psychologist adopted a solution-focused approach in therapy aimed at engaging Kate by identifying strategies that could bring positive change in a very short period of time. Her cognitions about pain medication and the management of constipation were addressed in a comprehensive manner during a meeting with the oncologist and the palliative care nurse. The psychologist's role was to ensure that all of Kate's concerns would be expressed and addressed. On a bowel regimen and an opioid schedule, Kate's constipation improved, as well as her pain level. These improvement had an immediate positive impact on her mood. Kate felt encouraged and accepted an antidepressant to address the feelings of depression and the passive suicidal thoughts. Her son attended several therapy session where the psychologist used an emotion-focused approach to promote communication. He expressed significant anxiety about his mother's illness and fear that she may die. He also felt uncomfortable expressing these emotions to her and had decided to become more distant as a coping mechanism. The psychologist recommended a support group for teenagers coping with a parent with serious illness.

Kate's son found the group supportive and began attending regularly. Kate's mood and level of function improved overall. She experienced periodic exacerbations of anxiety with fear of dying. Learning self-hypnosis and attending restorative yoga classes helped her manage distress. Depression symtpoms became well controlled with psychotherapy and medication. Mostly, the improvement of her relationship with her son and a new sense of closeness greatly enhanced her sense of meaning and hope despite her advanced disease.

References

Albert, R. H. (2017). End of life: managing common symptoms. *American Family Physician, 95*(6), 356–361.
Alexander, J. K., DeVries, A. C., Kigerl, K. A., Dahlman, J. M., & Popovich, P. J. (2009). Stress exacerbates neuropathic pain via glucocorticoid and NMDA receptor activation. *Brain, Behavior and Immunity, 23*(6), 851–860.
Baralatei, F. T., & Ackerman, R. J. (2016). Care of patients at the end of life: management of nonpain symptoms. *FP Essentials, 447*, 18–24.
Bruera, E. D., & Portenoy, R. K. (Eds.) (2010). *Cancer pain.* New York: Cambridge University Press.
Cassileth, B. R. (2011). *The complete guide to complementary therapies in cancer care.* Hackensack, NJ: World Scientific Publishing.
Chai, E., Meier, D., Morris, J., & Bioy, A., & Wood, C. (2006). Hypnosis: Principles of use and benefits in palliative care. *European Journal of Palliative Care, 13*(3), 117–120.
Chai, E., Meier, D., Morris, J., & Goldhirsch, S. (Eds.) (2014). *Geriatric palliative care: A practical guide for clincians.* New York: Oxford.
Chang, V. T., Sorger, B., Rosenfeld, K. E., Lorenz, K. A., Bailey, A. F., Bui, T., . . . Montagnini, M. (2007). Pain and palliative medicine. *Journal of Rehabilitation Research and Development, 44*(2), 279–294.
Cruciani, R. A., Strada, E. A., & Knotkova, H. (2010). Neuropathic pain. In E. D. Bruera & R. K. Portenoy (Eds.). *Cancer Pain.* p. 478–405. New York, NY: Cambridge University Press.
Desai, G., Chaturvedi, S. K., & Ramachandra, S. (2011). Hypnotherapy, Fact or fiction: A review in palliative care and opinions of health professionals. *Indian Journal of Pallliative Care,17*(2),146–149.
Dhingra, L., Shuk, E., Grossman, B., Strada, A., Wald, E., Portenoy, A., . . . Portenoy, R. (2013). A qualitative study to explore psychological distress and illness burden associated with opioid-indiced constipation in cancer pain with advanced disease. *Palliative Medicine, 27*(5), 447–456.
Dong, S. T., Butow, P. N., Costa, D. S. J., Lovell, M. R., & Agar, M. (2014). Symptom clusters in patients with advanced cancer: A systematic review of observational studies. *Journal of Pain and Symptom Management, 48*(3), 411–450.
Dong, S. T., Costa, D. S. J., Butow, P. N., Lovell, M. R., & Agar, M. (2016). Symptom clusters in advanced cancer patients: An empirical comparison of statistical methods on the impact of quality of life. *Journal of Pain and Symptom Management, 51*(1), 88–98.
Eimer, B. N., & Freeman, A. (1998). *Pain management psychotherapy, a practical guide.* New York: Wiley.
Elkins, G. (Ed.). (2017). *Handbook of medical and psychological hypnosis.* New York: Springer.
Elkins, G., Fisher, W., & Silwinski, J. (2012). Clinical hypnosis for the palliative care of cancer patients. *Oncology Nursing,* Cancer Network. http://www.cancernetwork.com/oncology-nursing/clinical-hypnosis-palliative-care-cancer-patients. Retrieved on January 3, 2017
Erickson, M. (1980). *The collected papers of Milton Erickson* (E. Rossi, Ed) Vol IV, Chapter 21. Somerset, NJ: John Wiley & Sons.
Esdaile, J. *Hypnosis in medicine and surgery.* New York: Julian Press, 1846.
Fallon, M. T. (2013). Neuropathic pain in cancer. *British Journal of Anaesthesia 111*(1), 105–111.

Goldstein, N. E., & Morrison, R. S. (Eds.). (2013). *Evidence-based practice of palliative medicine.* Philadelphia, PA: Elsevier.

Greenlee, H., Balneaves, L. G., Carlson, L. E., Cohen, M., Deng, G., Hershman, D., . . . Tripathy, D. (2014). Clinical practice guidelines on the use of integrative therapies as supportive care in patients treated for breast cancer. *Journal of the National Cancer Institute Monographs, 50,* 346–358.

Harrison, S. L., Lee, A., Goldstein, R. S., & Brooks, D. (2016). Perspectives of healthcare professionals and patients on the application of mindfulness in individuals with chronic obstructive pulmonary disease. *Patient Education and Counseling,* doi:10.1016/j.pec.2016.08.018

Kamal, A. H, Maguire, J. M., Wheeler, J. L., Currow, D. C., & Abernethy, A. P. (2012). Dyspea review for the palliative care professional: treatment goals and therapeutic options. *Journal of Palliative Medicine, 15*(1), 106–114.

Lahoud, M. J., Kourie, H. R., Antoun, J., El Osta, L., & Ghosn, M. (2016). Road map for pain management in pancreatic cancer: A review. *World Journal of Gastrointestinal Oncology, 8*(8), 599–606.

Marchand, L. (2014). Integrative and complementary therapies for patients with advanced cancer. *Annals of Palliative Medicine, 3*(3), 160–171.

Matzo, M., & Witt Sherman D. (Eds.). (2015). *Palliative care nursing: Quality care at the end of life.* New York: Springer.

Milling, L. S. (2008). Is high hypnotic suggestibility necessary for successful hypnotic pain intervention? *Current Pain Headache Report, 12*(2), 98–102.

Montgomery, G. H., Schnur, J. B., & Kravits, K. (2013). Hypnosis for cancer care: Over 200 years young. *CA A Cancer Journal for Clinicians, 63*(1), 31–44

Mulaski, R. A., Munjas, B. A., Lorenz, K. A., & Sun, S., (2009). Randomized controlled trial of mindfulness therapy for dyspnea in chronic obstructive lung disease. *Journal of Alternative and Compementary Medicine, 15*(10), 1083–1090.

Piccione, C., Hilgard, E. R., & Zimbardo, P. G. (1989). On the degree of stability of measured hypnotizability over a 25 year period. *Journal of Personality and Social Psychology, 56*(2), 289–295.

Portenoy, R. K., & Ahmed, E. (2014). Principles of opioid use in cancer pain. *Journal of Clinical Oncology, 32*(16), 1662–1670.

Prommer, E. E. (2015). Palliative pharmacotherapy: State of the art management of symptoms in patients with cancer. *Cancer Control, 22*(4), 403–411.

Sage, N., Sowden, M., Chorlton, E., & Edeleanu, A. (2008). *CBT for chronic illness and palliative care.* Chichester, UK: John Wiley.

Simmons, C. P. L., MacLeod, N., & Laird, B. J. A. (2012). Clinical management of pain in advanced lung cancer. *Clinical Medicine and Insights in Oncology, 6,* 331–346.

Spiegel, H., & Greenleaf, M. (2005). Commentary: Defining hypnosis. *American Journal of Clinical Hypnosis, 48*(2-3), 111–116.

Spiegel, H., & Spiegel, D. (1978). *Trance and treatment: Clinical uses of hypnosis.* New York: Basic Books.

Strada, E. A., & Portenoy, R. K. (2015). Psychological, rehabilitative, amd integrative therapies for cancer pain. *UpToDate.* Uptodate.com/contents/psychological-rehabilitative-and-integrative-therapies-for-cancer-pain. Retrieved on February 15, 2017.

Strang, S., Ekberg-Jansson, A., Henoch, I. (2014). Experience of anxiety among patiens with severe COPD: A qualitative, indepth interview study. *Palliative and Supportive Care, 12*(6), 465–472.

Taylor, D. R. (2013). *Managing cancer breakthrough pain.* New York: Springer.

Thomas, E. M., & Weiss, S. M. (2000). Nonpharmacological interventions with chronic cancer pain in adults. *Cancer Control, 7*(2), 157–164.

Van Dam van Isselt, D. F., Groenewegen-Sipkema, K. H., Spruit-van Eijk, M., Chavannes, N. H., da Waal, M. W., Janssen, D. J. A., & Achterberg, W. P. (2014). Pain in patients with COPD: A systematic review and meta-analysis. *BMJ Open, 4*(9), doi: 10.1136/bmjopen-2014-005898.

Vargas-Schaffer, G. (2010). Is the WHO analgesic ladder still valid? *Canadian Family Physician, 56*(6), 514–517.

Yu, D. S. F., Chan, H. Y. L., Leung, D. Y. P., Hui, E., & Sit, J. W. H. (2016). Symptom cluster and quality of life among patients with advanced heart failure. *Journal of Geriatric Cardiology, 13*(5), 408–414.

3

The Third Domain of Palliative Care

Psychological and Psychiatric Aspects of Care

Focus Points

- Assessment and treatment of psychological and psychiatric needs of the patient and the family must be considered an ongoing process throughout the disease trajectory and into bereavement.
- Depression and anxiety are prevalent in advanced illness, increasing the symptom burden for the patient and distress for family caregivers.
- Expression of suicidal ideation should always be followed by a comprehensive suicidal assessment and implementation of a plan for safety and support.
- Grief reactions in the patient and the family should be normalized and supported as well as differentiated from pathological processes such as complicated grief, depression or anxiety disorders.
- Palliative psychologists focus not only on diagnosing the presence of psychopathology but also on facilitating emotional adjustment, connectedness, and healing for the patient and the family.
- Psychological and psychiatric interventions should always take into consideration the patient and family culture and preferences.

Introduction

Specialist palliative care is holistic, expanding beyond the management of pain and physical symptoms, to include careful attention to the psychological and psychiatric aspects of advanced illness. The third domain of palliative care emphasizes it is important to recognize, assess, and treat manifestations of psychological and psychiatric distress in the patient and the family across the illness continuum.

The negative impact of advanced illness on the psychological function of the patient and the family can undermine deeply held values and sources of meaning, family dynamics, an even the integrity of psychological defense mechanisms. Psychiatric disorders can develop or worsen, requiring treatment to reduce morbidity.

The ability to recognize developing distress requires ongoing assessment throughout the experience of illness for the patient and the family. This care needs to continue after the patient's death, during bereavement (see Chapter 4). The provision of nonspecific emotional support can represent an important and valuable expression of empathy and human connection. However, the need to conceptualize a psychological treatment plan based on the type and manifestation of psychological and psychiatric distress requires specialized skills, creating a clear role for palliative psychologists. Depending on the patient's condition, goals, and circumstances, the mode of treatment can be psychological, pharmacological, or both pharmacological and psychological.

Needs in the psychological and psychiatric domain should be conceptualized broadly and holistically. While relieving distress and preventing suffering in the patient is critically important, promoting well-being, connectedness, and a sense of emotional safety in the patient and the family is also an essential component of this domain of care. The complexity of these goals always requires careful balance of the application of advanced clinical skills, with the ability to provide a compassionate and healing presence that honors the patient and the family as the experts in their lives and in determining their goals.

Competencies for Palliative Psychologists

Because of the breadth and depth of their training, palliative psychologists can bring much added and unique value in this domain of palliative care. Competencies include expertise in the assessment, diagnosis, and management of psychological distress and psychiatric syndromes, and an appreciation of how mood disorders such as depression and anxiety manifest in the context of advanced illness. Expertise in differential diagnosis is needed to distinguish between a possible pathological process and normal adjustment to illness that may include profound sadness as part of a grieving process. Additionally, it is important to remember that grief and depression are not mutually exclusive and in some cases they can coexist.

While palliative psychologists always keep their "assessment hat on" to recognize the possible development of a psychological or psychiatric disorder, they relate to patients and families beyond a narrow psychopathology model. This is important, because the complexity of the psychological domain cannot be reduced to diagnoses of anxiety, depression, or cognitive disorders. Palliative psychology is not based on a reductionist approach but rather on an appreciation of the complexity of the human psyche and a willingness to embrace it. The different psychological dimensions should be explored in depth as a unique expression of the humanity of the patient and the family. In essence, palliative psychologists not only focus on identifying distress that can be treated; they actively seek to promote psychospiritual well-being by facilitating a connection with sustaining sources of meaning and purpose. This endeavor requires a comprehensive and holistic understanding of the patient and the family's complex emotional needs, as well as an appreciation for their desire and capacity to engage and experience what is meaningful to them.

Psychological frameworks based on psychospiritual exploration and connectedness, such as positive psychology, transpersonal psychology, and meaning-oriented approaches, can help identify factors that promote a sense of meaning in the midst of suffering. Additionally, integrative and complementary approaches such as clinical hypnosis and creative arts can be valuable in promoting not only well-being for the patient but also allowing for increased connectedness and communication between the patient and the family. Contemplative and mindfulness practices can promote peace and comfort for the patient, family members, and also staff. Applying psychological models that promote positive experience also include use of cognitive-behavioral therapy, interpersonal therapy, narrative therapy, concreteness therapy, and solution-focused approaches and should be part of the repertoire of the palliative psychologist.

There is a great opportunity for positive psychological and spiritual growth for patients with advanced illness and their family caregivers. The overarching goal of psychological care in palliative care is to deeply connect with openness and compassion, as well as clinical expertise. Serious illness can threaten the physical, emotional, social, and spiritual integrity. Specialist psychological support can promote a sense of emotional safety despite advanced disease and even in the context of the dying process. Palliative psychology competencies for this work are summarized in Box 3.1.

Box 3.1 **Competencies for Palliative Psychologists**

KNOWLEDGE

- overall impact of disease type, course, and trajectory on psychological adjustment and family dynamics
- prevalence, manifestations, course, and management of common psychiatric and psychological disorders
- understanding of psychopharmacological treatment
- knowledge of individual and family psychological frameworks and psychotherapy approaches that can address the full range of psychological needs

SKILLS

- provide a safe and therapeutic space for the exploration and expression of cognitive, emotional, social, cultural, and spiritual impact of the illness
- embody therapeutic stance that combines a strength-based approach with diagnostic and treatment expertise
- recognize and diagnose clinical depression, anxiety disorders, delirium, presence of cognitive impairment
- recognize manifestation of existential distress, e.g. demoralization syndrome
- recognize and support grief reactions in the patient and the family
- recognize presence of complicated grief in patients and provide adequate interventions
- promptly identify of risk factors for complications of bereavement in family caregivers
- provide focused supportive interventions, e.g. relaxation and imagery to address procedure-related anxiety
- develop expertise in different psychotherapy frameworks and modalities for individual and family therapy

- develop integrated psychological treatment
- communicate effectively with members of the palliative care team regarding diagnosis and treatment

ATTITUDES

- holistic approach to the patient and the family that considers the needs of the "whole person"
- therapeutic presence supportive of personal growth and healing
- collaborative approach to mental health and well-being that acknowledges unique perspectives and contributions from other team members and disciplines
- unbiased attitude toward use of psychotropic medication in the management of anxiety, depression, and severe grief reactions

The Palliative Psychology Assessment

The palliative psychology assessment represents an important opportunity for exploring the patient and the family from a holistic perspective that focuses on the whole person. According to this approach, while problems must be addressed, a patient does not represent a psychological problem or a medical diagnosis to be solved. Rather, the patient and the family are recognized as unique and irreplaceable. Seeing them in their unique context maintains dignity and promotes healing.

A comprehensive assessment addresses the relevant psychological components of each of the domains of palliative care. The palliative psychologist with knowledge of each of these areas of assessment will explore them based on priorities and goals, without creating unnecessary burden for the patient. While the psychological assessment should be considered as an ongoing process, initial necessary information often must be obtained in a short amount of time by gently guiding the conversation.

Tables 3.1 and 3.2 summarize aspects of the palliative care psychology assessment.

Palliative Psychotherapy

Palliative psychotherapy is specifically used in this book to indicate a general framework for working with patients and family caregivers receiving palliative care. It can be conceptualized as an expression of the biopsychosocialspiritual model of care (Sulmasy, 2002), and it can be described as *holistic* philosophically and *integrative* in methodology, emphasizing the importance of addressing the whole person (Table 3.3).Most psychotherapy theoretical frameworks, including psychodynamic, cognitive-behavioral, humanistic, and existential approaches can be adapted to create a focus for the unique needs of patients with serious illness. An integrative framework allows therapy for each patient to be based on his or her unique needs, medical condition, core cultural values,

Table 3.1 **Characteristics of the Palliative Psychology Assessment**

Characteristic	Clinical Application
It is a flexible framework that can be adapted to different settings and clinical situations.	The assessment can take place in inpatient or outpatient settings, or during a home visit with a hospice patient. Areas of assessment are prioritized based on referral questions and patient's condition.
Assessment is conceptualized as a therapeutic intervention.	The psychologist uses information gathered during the assessment to educate and support the patient at the time of assessment.
There is a collaborative approach to assessment and treatment plan.	Goals and needs identified by the patient and the family are integrated with those identified by the care team and not imposed by the clinician.
Assessment is seemessly incorporated in the clinical interview.	The communication style is conversational and there should not be an abrupt change in affect when the psychologist is assessing mood, etc.
Assessment is equally focused on identifying strengths and sources of distress.	The goal of assessment is not only to recognize sources of suffering, but also and foremost to understand what is important to the patient and the family and what strengths and resources can be validated and mobilized
It includes supportive psychoeducation, cognitive reframes, and description of plan that can encourage the patient and the family and instill hope.	Examples are: normalize grief reactions, reassure family caregivers about their role; acknowledge caregiver distress if present and describe supportive strategies; review impact of depression and anxiety, if present, and describe treatment strategies to improve outcome; summarize results of assessment and briefly describe comprehensive approach.
It emphasizes the role of the team.	The psychologist does not operate in a vacuum but is part of a team, and this is constantly presented to the patient and the family.
Results are documented and shared with the team and other professionals using operational and goal-focused language.	Notes are succinct and operational, clearly delineating problems assessed and psychological plan. Mental status is included.

family structure, and personal preferences. For instance, a psychologist trained in the psychodynamic model may continue to "understand" the patient from that perspective, identifying defense mechanisms and assessing ego-strength. However, the specific psychological modalities and techniques used in each session should be based on the immediate demands of the patient, whether it is the need to manage anxiety, process grief, address difficulty communicating with the medical team, or family conflict. Hence,

Table 3.2 **Areas Covered by the Palliative Psychology Assessment**

Assessment Area	Purpose
Referral question and current concerns	Assess whether the concerns of the referring source (palliative care team or other providers) are shared by the patient and the family and explore their perception of the cause of distress
Medical history and how it has impacted on the patient and the family over time	Gain insight into the context in which the patient and the family have existed and functioned up until this moment
Quality of the relationship with the medical team and presence of challenges or conflict	Critical to assess what aspects of the relationship are supportive or are adding to the stress of the patient and the family. Consider cultural factors.
Family structure, social support, and impact of caregiving	Can help identify the unique strengths of the family system as well as each individual
The patient and the family culture	Assess how it impacts communication, expression of emotions, meaning attributed to illness, understanding of goals of treatment.
Spiritual, existential, religious values	Understand their role in the patient and family life and identify any sources of distress that may warrant a referral to a spiritual care provider for a spiritual assessment
Strengths, coping strategies, and positive emotions that are facilitating the patient and the family adjustment	Understand main psychological defense mechanisms and adaptation style
Psychiatric history and current distress including diagnostic considerations	Past or present history of major depression, anxiety, suicidal ideation, severe mental illness; need for care coordination
Awareness of diagnosis and prognosis	The patient and the family may have a different understanding closely related to cultural aspects of communication
Grieving style in the patient and the family and current grieving process; identification of risk factors	Allows exploration of how grief is understood and expressed; opportunity for psychoeducation
Indication for complementary approaches	Based on institutional availability but also allows facilitation of community resources
Need for community resources	Psychological resources for caregivers and children, religious support, integrative approaches
Psychological plan	Should include immediate goals, short-term goals, and medium-range goals.

Table 3.3 **Principles of Palliative Psychotherapy**

Philosophically holistic	It addresses the needs of the whole person and the family as the unit of care; not focused exclusively on addressing psychopathology
Methodologically integrative	It includes appropriate use of integrative medicine modalities that can provide symptoms relief as well as promote quality of life and well-being; psychotherapy is part of the interdisciplinary care plan; based on clinically sound integration of different frameworks or modalities from different frameworks for the benefit of the patient
Always includes elements of supportive psychoeducation	Patients and families navigating the medical system in the context of advanced illness benefit from receiving information about their emotional reactions, practical ways of improving communication with the treating team, practical ways of controlling the sense of being overwhelmed, and improving communication within the family.
Spirituality is welcomed in the session.	Spirituality and religion can represent important sources of meaning and purpose for patients and can become a focus of therapy. Additional referrals to spiritual care providers can be considered.
Consideration of grief and bereavement	The therapy session can become an opportunity for expressing and processing grief during the illness trajectory.
Focus on emotional safety	A basic goal of psychotherapy in advanced illness is creating a sense of emotional safety for the patient and the family throughout, including the dying process.
Flexible framework	No fixed rules about duration, time of session, and goals
Setting often unpredictable	Requires the therapist to bring a strong therapeutic presence and safety to contain the patient's anxieties
Who is the recipient?	May need to transition to couple or family and even include community members as needed, while preserving the relationship with the patient
Value of single-session approach	Every session should represent a complete gestalt
Rapidly evolving goals of treatment	The medical condition deeply affects goals; sudden changes in prognosis or symptom crises alter psychological treatment
Importance of adjunctive psychological modalities	Integrative medicine approaches

(continued)

Table 3.3 **Continued**

Variable length of session and frequency	From a few minutes, to one hour, or more
End of therapy	Not necessarily acknowledged and often cannot be planned; countertransference work for the therapist
Perception of time	Past, present, and future blend seamlessly
Dual role of the psychologist	Individual therapist and team member; need to provide information about treatment that can help the rest of the team develop and update the care plan

the depth of the therapy session fluctuates, based on the expressed needs. Elements of supportive psychoeducation are generally present in every encounter to address practical questions and concerns about navigating the medical system, as well as to develop optimal ways of communicating with medical providers.

Several resources describing the theory and application of psychological models and psychotherapy are available (Carr & Steel, 2013; Cordella & Poiani, 2014; Watson & Kissane, 2011). Although these have focused on patients with cancer, they can be adapted to patients with other diseases.

A focus on meaning and purpose has always been integral to psychodynamic psychotherapy and humanistic psychotherapy, and especially transpersonal approaches. Thus, for many psychologists, exploring how living with advanced illness has affected the patient's sense of meaning and how their self-esteem and sense of dignity can be preserved or restored already represents a natural extension of their psychotherapy approach. The importance of this focus is also well recognized in supporting loss, grief, and bereavement.

In the last decade dignity and meaning have also emerged in the psycho-oncology and palliative care literature as essential constructs in advanced illness and end of life. This has driven the development of psychosocial interventions supported by outcome studies indicating their potential effectiveness with the palliative care population. As a result, manualized and time-limited interventions such as Dignity Therapy, Meaning Centered Psychotherapy, Meaning-Making Intervention, and Managing Cancer and Living Meaningfully (CALM) Therapy are becoming increasingly available to patients receiving palliative care in various settings. The focus on developing these evidence-based interventions certainly represents an important advancement in improving psychological and spiritual well-being. They can be adapted to diverse patient populations and can be integrated in the broader context of psychological work, including at end of life (Breitbart & Poppito, 2014; Henry et al., 2010; Low et al., 2016; Ramos & Fulton, 2017; Shaw et al., 2017; Sheffold et al., 2015). Ultimately, however, the psychologist's depth of knowledge, clinical skills, and therapeutic presence remain essential in assessing needs and delivering interventions that can address the clinical complexity of the palliative care patient population.

As patients receive palliative care services for variable periods of time, palliative psychotherapy needs to respond to the necessity of caring for the patient and the family in a focused manner, balancing depth and length of treatment with patient-related and system-related factors. These include the patient's pattern of decline, and the settings where the patient is receiving care (i.e., institution vs. home). Thus, palliative psychotherapy is driven by the needs of the patient and the family and is shaped by the often quick evolution of these needs. It is important to remember that as the palliative care setting calls for flexibility, the palliative psychotherapy framework must be flexible as well. The therapist may have the opportunity to work with the patient and the family on a long-term basis, or may only have one focused single therapy session. In the inpatient setting the patient and the therapist may have daily sessions for the duration of the hospitalization or even meet twice a day depending on needs. The frequency can become weekly or monthly after discharge if the patient is followed at home or at a palliative care clinic. Palliative psychologists working as hospice clinicians may also provide psychotherapy in the patient's home during home visits. When feasible and clinically indicated, the clinician can then continue working with family members after the patient's death.

In conventional outpatient psychotherapy, when a family needs both individual and family therapy, it is customary that these services be provided by different therapists. This approach is designed to ensure respect of boundaries and recognizes that different dynamics are at play when working with the entire family versus the individual. The application of this framework to the palliative care setting is generally unrealistic, however. This can be due not only to lack of availability of additional therapists, but also to the need to foster therapeutic results quickly and efficiently. Thus, often the same therapist provides psychotherapy to a patient and the family, jointly or separately. In teams where both a psychologist and a social worker are present, it is possible to provide services separately to the patient and the family, with joint sessions based on need. The psychologist and the social worker can also coordinate care with music therapists and creative arts therapists, if available. This can be extremely beneficial when children need psychological support, whether as patients or as family members.

While any clinical encounter should be focused on the needs expressed by the patient and the family, the role of a palliative psychologist on an interdisciplinary team may be different from that of a practitioner in private practice. The patient's right to lead the session needs to be balanced with what may emerge as urgent clinical needs of interdisciplinary team work. For example, the psychologist may begin providing psychotherapy to family caregivers who are grieving the progressive decline of their loved one. A sudden change in the patient's condition may also suddenly change the prognosis, and the family may resist fully integrating this information because of the emotional distress associated with it. The treating team may express concerns that this disconnect will create further distress for the family, as the death may be perceived as sudden. Or important medical decisions need to be made, and if the family is unwilling to consider them because of distress, ethical dilemmas may arise.

The psychologist in this case needs to carefully consider how to factor the team's concerns and the family's preference about communication and the topics they want to discuss in therapy. Attempting to gently introduce uncomfortable discussions in the therapy session may be a reasonable approach in an effort to support the family. This would not mean that the psychotherapy agenda is determined by the team; rather, it would indicate the psychologist's willingness and ability to embrace and navigate the complexities of the palliative care setting.

The Process and Content of Palliative Psychotherapy

The *therapeutic setting* refers to the space, physical and symbolic, where the therapy takes place. In the palliative care setting the physical space is often unpredictable and may change based on the patient's medical and psychosocial needs. For example, the session can take place in the hospital room, in a clinic exam room, in a space of the emergency department, or in the infusion suite. Sessions can also take place over the phone or, depending on the psychologist's role, in the patient's home. The length can vary depending on the patient's medical condition and needs. For instance, a 15-minute encounter with a hospitalized patient with severe anxiety to help her decrease arousal by using hypnosis can be extremely meaningful and supportive. Most important, it addresses specific needs of the patient "in the moment," and it allows for a deepening of the therapeutic alliance. The patient and the family will feel that the therapist is attuned to real needs and able to provide effective and rapid relief when symptoms occur.

While some patients do not seem particularly affected by the changes in the physical space where therapy is provided, others may become anxious or frustrated, voicing a general sense of lack of control over events in their life. For some patients, whose medical prognosis is unclear, the unpredictability of the setting represents another reminder of the unpredictability in their life. Processing these emotions without attempting to dismiss their disappointment can help patients tolerate increasing levels of ambiguity. Some patients may benefit from reframing the setting as "predictably unpredictable," yet emphasizing the more predictable quality of the symbolic space and the therapeutic relationship.

The predictable component in the palliative care therapy situation is represented by the therapist's therapeutic presence and ability to receive and contain the patients' fears, hopes, emotions—what is on their mind and what is unbearable. While the physical space may change, the symbolic space does not, and this can communicate safety to the patient and have a soothing effect. The therapist's compassionate, nonjudgmental, and welcoming presence is grounded in knowledge, skills, and professional boundaries.

A strong *therapeutic alliance* is essential for good outcomes in psychotherapy, and it may in fact be more important that any specific technique used by the therapist. The ability to "read" the emotional tone of the patient and the family and "tune in" can help establish trust and therapeutic alliance relatively quickly. This can be threatened, however, if there is confusion about the psychologist's role. The patient or the family may incorrectly assume the psychologist has the "power" to affect or change system-related issues, or delay discharge. For example, if the patient has been discharged home with hospice and medical equipment is not delivered as planned, there can be great distress for the patient and the family. Delays in home delivery of medication for hospice patients can also cause great anxiety and alarm. If the psychologist was an integral part of the conversation that led to the decision to enroll in hospice, the family may become angry at him or her for any failures to deliver services as expected.

Palliative psychotherapy involves holding a *multicultural focus*. Every encounter with a patient and family should be conceptualized as a cross-cultural encounter (see also chapter 6) and the particular modalities and interventions used during the session should be chosen on the basis of their cultural relevancy.

Countertransference should be identified and managed. Unrecognized and unmanaged countertransference can threaten the therapeutic relationship. Situations where the patient and the family appear upset or in distress may elicit strong responses in the psychologist. These may include feelings of being overwhelmed, or the desire to avoid contact with the patient and the family, or the desire to "save" them from the distress and suffering. Clinicians with unprocessed grief may become invested in protecting the patient and may be tempted to make "promises" about specific desired outcomes. Even vague but enthusiastic promises to help may be interpreted by a distressed family member as an assurance that the circumstance will evolve as they wish. This can be a set up for disappointment and negatively impact the therapeutic alliance.

Ruptures may occur when working with patients with advanced illness as in any therapy situation. They can occur when there is deterioration in the quality of the communication and the relationship between the therapist and the patient that damages the alliance (Safran, Muran, & Eubanks-Carter, 2011). In dynamic therapy, once a strong therapeutic alliance has been established, there is much emphasis on recognizing ruptures and exploring them with the patient so that damage can be repaired. The same opportunity may not be available in the palliative care setting due to unexpected or sudden events (death, early discharge, or sudden change in the patient's performance status that prevent further engagement in therapy).

If conflict arises between families and the medical team, psychologists must carefully navigate their role on the team and their support for the family. This can become clinically challenging and emotionally trying. The team may expect the psychologist to "fix" the problem and somehow "convince" the patient and the family to cooperate. The family, on the other hand, may expect the psychologist to advocate for them against the team.

Negotiating goals of treatment in palliative psychotherapy involves recognizing the existence of different sets of goals and priorities. Patients are often referred to the palliative psychologist by medical and psychosocial providers with a specific referral question (e.g., evaluate for depression and anxiety; evaluate for suicidal ideation; address high level of family conflict; evaluate a family in distress that is asking the medical team for inappropriate medical interventions). Addressing the referral question is the primary focus initially. Other goals and needs important to the patient and the family may be identified and addressed during the initial consultation, thus determining the focus of any ongoing therapy. It is important to provide feedback to the referral source as soon as possible about the concerns that generated the referral. However, ongoing goals of therapy should be negotiated with the patient and the family based on their perception of need.

Boundaries are an essential component of medical and psychological care with all patients, including patients with advanced illness. These are not expressed by artificial and neurotic distancing, or by a contrived use of a professional persona. Boundaries always represent an expression of high regard. In this setting they represent respect for the patient and the family and preserve their emotional safety. Psychologists are trained to appreciate and respect the importance of boundaries for therapeutic efficacy, rather than self-protection or insulation. In this regard, the issue of touch in therapy has unique characteristics in the palliative and end-of-life care setting. It is common for physicians, nurses, physical therapists and others to touch patients during physical exams. Additionally, holding a patient's hand, gently touching a shoulder, and even occasionally hugging a distressed patient or family member is generally understood as a non-sexual and non-exploitative way of conveying empathy, support, and reassurance. Psychologists' approach to touch in therapy is based on ethical standards, theoretical orientation, and personal style. While the psychodynamic and psychoanalytic approach generally discourages touch that goes beyond a handshake, a humanistic and integrative framework may conceptualize nonsexual touch (e.g., hugging the patient after the death of a family member) as an intervention to promote healing.

Patients with advanced illness are physically and emotionally vulnerable, as are their family members, so every action needs to be based on a rationale that meets the needs of the patient, not those of the clinician. It can be useful to remember the differentiation between boundary crossing and boundary violations (Gabbard & Lester, 2003; Gabbard, 2005). Boundary violations can be sexual or nonsexual, can be harmful to the patient, and are generally repeated patterns. Boundary crossings are generally benign and can be helpful. To illustrate, holding the hand of a bedbound patient expressing grief and fear about approaching death or regrets may represent a boundary crossing for a psychologist, but it can be an important intervention to convey support and understanding. The same could be said for gently touching a patient's shoulder or arm. However, it should not be assumed that touch is expected, or welcome, or interpreted as benign. Most important, the patient should always be asked for permission. Similarly, hugging a family member after the death of the patient can represent a boundary crossing, yet it conveys empathy and support in the moment. However, initiating touch and hugging to convey compassion and human connection without considering the clinical implications can be exploitative and damaging.

The *end of therapy* is commonly referred to as termination. However, this expression has a particularly evocative power when working with a patient with advanced illness, seeming too cold or too close to the anticipated death. In outpatient psychotherapy, the end of treatment is often carefully planned, sometimes idealized, and while its emotional impact on both the patient and the therapist varies, it can be emotionally difficult and require processing. The end of treatment can also be determined by factors that are unrelated to the therapist and the patient and outside of their control, thus it can become a unilateral decision outside of the therapeutic relationship (Gabbard, 2004). For instance, trainees complete their practicum, internship, or postdoctoral training; patients may relocate or change their insurance carrier.

In palliative psychotherapy, beginnings and endings are intertwined, whether explicitly or implicitly, and are contained within the same temporal dimension and sometimes within the same session. Patients' discharge to a different facility or home may occur after only one session with the psychologists. Or, they may die suddenly as a result of a complication of the disease. Awareness of the possibility that every encounter, every session, may be the last should create profound appreciation for the preciousness and uniqueness of every moment of connection with the patient and the family. The goal of every encounter is to provide as much support as possible, identify issues that need addressing, and developing a treatment plan, if possible. A compassionate and attuned therapeutic presence and regard for the patient and the family should be present at every encounter. The psychologist should do what is possible to ensure that every session feels complete, even if others will follow.

Reflecting on the principles of short-term therapy and especially single session psychotherapy may help create the necessary focus in the session with the patient or the family. Many patients can receive effective help from the initial psychotherapy session and experience improvement regardless of diagnosis. Single session psychotherapy can be effective within different theoretical models, including psychodynamic therapy, rational-emotive therapy, Adlerian therapy, strategic hypnotherapy, and Gestalt. Additionally, applying the principles of single session psychotherapy has shown to be particularly helpful in medical contexts, especially when used to guide family meetings where families must make difficult medical decisions (see Bloom, 2001, for a review).

As in most psychotherapy approaches, the therapist's empathy is an important factor in determining the patient's perception that they have been helped. Even a single focused session can help define the situation the patient and the family are facing, explore what solutions have been already attempted, define short-term but specific attainable goals, and delineate a clear plan that can provide emotional safety and hope. This process can be extremely impactful and gratifying even if the circumstances do not allow for another therapy session. Yet this awareness can also engender anxiety in the psychologist who is attempting to reconcile a mindful presence in the "here and now" of the session with a natural hardwired desire to promote healing by planning future sessions and interventions. Thus, the therapist's ability to create a treatment focus during the session needs to be carefully balanced by the ability to suspend an active treatment mode when the patient needs the therapist to bear witness to their suffering or their personal evolution, without problem solving or strategizing.

An ability to internalize and process the unpredictable aspects of psychological treatment and the associated anxieties or feelings of frustration or helplessness is essential. It is part of the personal work of the therapist, and it will allow the psychologist to be fully present for the patient. In essence, an appreciation for impermanence may bring even more depth to the relationship.

Understanding the Role of Psychopharmacology in Palliative Care

Patients with advanced illness are often on complex medication regimens for the management of pain and other physical symptoms. Frequently, these regimens include psychotropic medications (i.e., antidepressants, neuroleptics, sedatives, and hypnotics) for the management of depression, anxiety, cognitive, or sleep disorders. As evidence is increasing for the value of combined medication and psychotherapy treatments in depression and anxiety, psychologists increasingly value the ability to work within an integrative model.

An understanding of the pharmacological management of psychiatric disorders common in palliative care is valuable for palliative psychologists for several reasons. It promotes effective communication and collaboration with medical providers. It enables psychologists to participate more actively in interdisciplinary care that includes medication planning. It also allows for more accurate diagnosis and treatment planning. Perhaps most important, knowledge of psychopharmacology can allow psychologists to improve patient care by helping to identify and address barriers to treatment adherence. These include the following:

- ambivalence about medications
- distressing side effects
- perceived stigma about use of psychotropic medication
- patients' concerns about how the medication will affect them
- confusion about timing of onset of action

In recent years, a growing number of psychologists have pursued informal and formal training opportunities in psychopharmacology. Recognizing the direct or indirect involvement of psychologists in addressing issues related to psychopharmacology, the American Psychological Association (2011) developed practice guidelines to help develop and maintain professional and ethical behavior in this area. According to the guidelines, psychologists' involvement in psychopharmacology can be described along a continuum, ranging from a Level 1–basic to a Level 3. Level 3 applies specifically to licensed psychologists with prescribing privileges, currently available for psychologists practicing in New Mexico, Louisiana, Illinois, Iowa, Idaho, the US Military Health Service, Indian Health Service, and Guam.

Levels 1 and 2 can be especially relevant to palliative psychologists. These levels of involvement and their application to the palliative care setting are conceptualized here as part of generalist and specialist palliative care psychology respectively, and are summarized in Table 3.4.

Level 1 involves a basic knowledge of psychopharmacology similar to what can be developed during a psychology graduate program. This is valuable for all psychologists providing direct clinical services. Psychologists with this knowledge level are generally involved in providing information and psychoeducation. They are aware of general side effects and are able to explore patient's beliefs about medication use. In this capacity, they identify barriers to treatment adherence and can encourage the patient to discuss these issues with the prescribing provider. This basic knowledge and understanding of psychotropic medications can be described as a competency in generalist palliative psychology, and it can be kept current by attending continuing education programs developed specifically for psychologists. Another option is presented by attending psychopharmacology programs developed for different health-care providers, such as primary care physicians and nurses.

Level 2 involves developing not only a broader knowledge base but also a specific focus and understanding of psychopharmacological treatment for a specific patient population. This level of knowledge can be acquired by attending postgraduate trainings in psychopharmacology (e.g., APA-approved postdoctoral master in psychopharmacology) and by attending continuing education programs developed for medical professionals. Specialist-level palliative psychology includes in-depth knowledge of use of psychopharmacology for patients with advanced illness and understanding of the multiple issues that guide physicians' decision to use medication, including prognostic issues, disease-related contraindications, drug-to-drug interactions, and consideration of side effects that could add to the patient's symptom burden. Some prescribing practices are unique to the palliative care setting. For example, the use of psychostimulants

Table 3.4 **Generalist and Specialist-level Involvement in Psychopharmacology for Palliative Psychologists**

Generalist Level	Specialist Level
Knowledge of different classes of antidepressants and basic indications in mood and anxiety disorders in the medically ill; knowledge of main contraindications and side effects	Understanding of pharmacokinetics and pharmacodynamics of antidepressants, benzodiazepines, neuroleptics, and hypnotics
Basic knowledge of benzodiazepines and hypnotics indications; knowledge of main side effects and risk factors	Knowledge of pharmacological treatment of depression, anxiety, and delirium in advanced illness; use of antidepressants and adjuvants in pain management; contraindications for treatment; principles of titration and taper
Ability to recognize the need for a medication evaluation for psychopharmacological treatment	Ability to monitor patients' response to medication and side effects in the context of psychological treatment and actively collaborate with medical providers
Ability to convey basic information to medical providers about patient's relationship with medications, including side effects and other barriers to treatment adherence	Ability to work therapeutically with patients to address concerns about medication use in collaboration with prescriber

for the management of fatigue and depression in patients with advanced cancer especially when the prognosis is less than six months is an accepted practice supported by evidence (Marks & Heinrich, 2013).

Depending on the regulations of the state where they practice, psychologists with adequate psychopharmacology training may develop more collaborative relationship with medical providers and be allowed by law to discuss medication recommendations based on their clinical assessment of the patient (McGrath, 2011). As an example, according to the California Board of Psychology, psychologists with extensive training and experience in psychotropic medications (e.g., a postdoctoral master's in psychopharmacology approved by the American Psychological Association) may discuss medication with a patient and they may suggest a medication to a physician. However, the decision and the responsibility to prescribe is the physician's.

A psychologist's appropriate involvement in psychopharmacology can facilitate the development of an integrative care plan in accordance with the patient's preferences and values regarding medication. Because of their traditional role as non-prescribers, psychologists trained in psychopharmacology may be less likely to generate concerns in the patient and the family about wanting to "fix the problem with a pill." When the use of pharmacological approaches is discussed by psychologists, it can be in the context of a careful clinical assessment, therapeutic alliance, and trust. Additionally, any medication discussion will represent only one component of an integrative and comprehensive care plan focused primarily on the use of appropriate psychological modalities.

To illustrate, if the psychologist's clinical assessment results in a diagnosis of major depression, their assessment will also provide valuable information about the main characteristics of the patient's experience of depression, thus allowing for more targeted treatment. For example, a patient with more endogenous manifestations of depression may benefit more from antidepressant medication with activating qualities. Similarly, a patient who is depressed but also intermittently anxious will benefit from a medication with more anxiolytic characteristics. The patient's level of function, prior experience and response to psychotropics, comorbid medical conditions and current medication regimen of course will always be an important part of these considerations.

CASE VIGNETTE 3.1

Robert is a 73-year-old man diagnosed with advanced COPD, hospitalized for severe dyspnea. He lives alone and has a home health aid four hours a day. He has been divorced for almost 10 years and has two adult children who live in a different state and rarely visit. The medical team requests a palliative care consultation primarily to help clarify the patient's goals of care. The patient does not have advance directives (see Chapter 8), and the medical team feels he is declining rapidly. The team describes Robert as a "difficult patient," "maybe borderline," whose behavior is highly anxious, uncooperative, and irritable. He is also described as highly critical of the medical team's efforts and dismissive of the nurses. The palliative psychologist meets with Robert. He denies any feelings of sadness or depression; however, he is experiencing hopelessness and a sense of helplessness. He also reports vague memory complaints, but he performs within normal limits on a cognitive screen. He is alert and oriented during the interview, his thought process appears linear and he denies perceptual disturbances. Mostly he feels consumed by anxiety and worries, and he admits he feels constantly irritated by the presence of the doctors and nurses because they are a reminder of his physical decline. He is convinced his wife divorced him because of his illness, and he is angry at her for abandoning him. He believes his children could afford to visit him more often but do not care enough. After describing his family situation, he expresses anger and hopelessness. He expresses passive suicidal thoughts. The suicide assessment indicates he does not have clear ideation, intent, means, or a plan, and he does not appear to be at high or imminent risk. The psychologist reports back to the team that the patient is suffering from depression and is also still grieving the end of his marriage. Some clinicians are surprised by the diagnosis because the patient did not appear sad or depressed. When asked previously if he felt depressed, he denied. The psychologist discusses the results of the evaluation and the alternative presentation of depression in older patients. He also comments that he believes the patient would benefit from medication in addition to psychotherapy. He discusses options with the team in the context of the patient's prognosis, which is in the order of months. The palliative care physician prescribes an SSRI, sertraline 25 mg, and the psychologist has six more sessions with the patient before his discharge two weeks later. Because the patient tolerates the antidepressant without significant adverse effects, the dose is titrated to 100 mg daily over the following two-week period. The psychologist uses a combination of interpersonal therapy and a cognitive-behavioral approach to begin addressing the patient's hopelessness, guilt and grief about the divorce, his anxiety about the decline of his health and fear he will not be able to continue living alone. Robert realizes that his resentment has prevented him from reaching out to his children asking them to visit, which has created a sense of abandonment. During the hospital stay, he makes contact with his children and reports they were afraid to visit because he always appeared upset. The combination of frequent psychotherapy and medication allowed the patient to develop a better sense of control and to take actions consistent with the goals he envisioned. His mood improved and one month after discharge, while at home with hospice care, he called the hospital to inform the psychologist and the team he was not longer consumed by anxiety and anger and felt much more comfortable emotionally.

CASE VIGNETTE 3.2

Greg is a 48-year-old patient with colon cancer; his status is post surgery and he is followed by the oncology clinic as an outpatient. He has negative attitudes toward medications of all kinds, especially opioids, which have become necessary to control pain right after surgery. His oncologist has explained to Greg that the cancer had not spread to other organs and that the pain is primarily related to the surgery, but this has not reassured him. Instead, he has become convinced that the need to control pain through medication is an indication of the severity of the illness and that death is near. Greg has a history of generalized anxiety disorder (GAD) and panic disorder, for which he has received pharmacological treatment in the past, but none currently. It appears the anxiety is interfering with his ability to fully process and integrate the information provided by his medical team. He experiences a constant state of worry, alarm, and fear. As a result, he has been feeling out of control and hopeless. He also reports feelings of sadness, which are negatively affecting his motivation to continue treatment. When his oncologist recommends a trial of antidepressants to address anxiety and depression, Greg refuses and becomes increasingly withdrawn. The oncologist requests a palliative care consultation to address pain and anxiety. The patient and the palliative psychologist begin psychotherapy treatment. Greg is able to identify anxiety as the source of much of his distress, but he has developed the belief that it is caused by a personal flaw in his character. Cognitive-behavioral therapy addresses cognitive distortions and deeply rooted beliefs. Imagery and mindfulness techniques are used to promote self-soothing and relaxation and to maintain control during anxiety exacerbations. While respecting the patient's autonomy and preferences regarding psychotropic medication, it becomes clear during the sessions that his refusal is based on fears and misconceptions. Because of his unwillingness to recognize anxiety as a chronic problem requiring management, he is reluctant to take medication for it, even though it has been helpful in the past. Over the course of therapy, he becomes aware that his firm yet untested beliefs about his psychological difficulties are preventing him from making an informed choice and improving his quality of life. Therapy includes several elements of supportive psychoeducation where the mechanism of action of antidepressants is demystified and explained in simple terms. Greg agrees to resume taking medication in conjunction with the breathing and imagery techniques, but remains concerned about side effects. These concerns are regularly addressed in therapy while keeping the oncologist informed. The patient begins to develop a sense that this care coordination is providing a calming effect. And his improved ability to control anxiety and make informed decisions about his care allows him to mobilize the energy necessary for coping with the next phases of treatment.

To summarize, psychologists with training in psychopharmacology can address barriers and resistances in therapy to support the patient during treatment to improve treatment adherence. They are also well suited to discuss and help manage adverse effects that may create difficulty and negatively impact treatment adherence. It can be determined if the side effects are seriously undermining the patient's quality of life, or if more support is needed to allow for stabilization. Helping the patient develop a positive relationship with psychotropic medication, when indicated, can also become an important component of therapy.

Grief Reactions in Patients and Family Caregivers

This section discusses the grieving process for patients and family caregivers *prior* to the patient's death. Chapter 4, social aspects of care, will discuss family caregivers' grieving process *after* the patient's death during bereavement. The decision to divide the discussion about grief into two parts is not intended to create an artificial separation within the grieving process. However, it is important that clinicians recognize the unique aspects of the grieving process in the patient and family caregivers during illness, while recognizing that bereavement can be characterized by additional and new challenges for surviving family caregivers. Furthermore, the structure and availability of bereavement support for family caregivers is also affected by the patient's end-of-life care (e.g., hospice). Palliative psychologists need to be aware of these clinical and system-related factors to guide and support patients and family caregivers appropriately.

At the basis of a patient and a family's encounter with a palliative care team, there is a loss: the loss of health and often the loss of hope for cure or prolongation of life. Therefore grief, whether overtly expressed or quietly experienced, is a constant presence in the lives of patients and families receiving palliative care services. Living with serious and advanced illness brings an ongoing series of physical and emotional losses of different magnitude. These ongoing and often progressive losses may begin at the time of diagnosis and continue with different manifestations and intensity levels throughout the disease trajectory.

A diagnosis of serious illness, even at an early stage, can suddenly change the narrative of the individual and the family life. For some patients, while energies are mobilized to pursue available treatment, there can be a profound sense of loss of continuity and a sense of threat. Furthermore, receiving a diagnosis of illness that is already advanced with limited treatment options can leave the patient and the family feeling stunned by the news and hopeless. Similarly, receiving the news that the disease has worsened or recurred despite treatment can also engender sadness and emptiness, feelings of depression, severe anxiety and fear of abandonment, loss of hope, and even moments of despair.

Grieving in serious illness is a normal response, and it does not represent pathology. Yet, it can cause a wide range of physical, psychological, and spiritual reactions in the patient and family caregivers. Depressed mood, feelings of anxiety, and even intermittent feelings of hopelessness and despair can be part of a grief reaction. An intense grief reaction may also trigger a depressive episode, especially when there is a prior history of depression.

The patient or the family caregiver who is grieving can experience depressive symptoms that generally fluctuate, and they do not eliminate the ability to enjoy the company of loved ones or to look forward to special occasions. In essence, while grief generates mood states that are intensely painful, the patient and the family retain the capacity to experience moments of pleasure, joy, hope, and connectedness. Self-esteem remains generally intact and, while patients and family caregivers may feel a sense of responsibility and even guilt for past behaviors (e.g., a patient may feel guilt about not stopping smoking; a caregiver spouse may feel guilt about not trying harder to convince the patient to seek medical care for concerning symptoms), they generally do not describe irrational guilt. Generally, symptoms of acute grief that are in reaction to bad news (e.g., news that the illness is incurable; news that the patient's life expectancy is short) may improve as a psychological and spiritual support plan is undertaken and the patient and the family gradually adapt emotionally to their situation.

Supporting the patient's and the family's grief reactions is a mandate for all palliative care clinicians. The intensity and structure of psychological support for grief reactions depend on the patient's and the family's needs and preferences. While grief can be intensely painful, it represents a normal process of adaptation. For some, channeling the emotions of grief into creative expressions such as music, poetry, or legacy projects can be part of a psychotherapy session and also the result of interdisciplinary work with music therapists and art therapists. Psychological interventions range from support, to supportive counseling, to psychotherapy. The palliative psychologist can accompany and gently guide and inform, but cannot decrease the amount of sadness the patient and the family are experiencing. Therefore, it must be emphasized that grief during illness and end of life is not a pathological process that needs to be resolved. Rather, it is a normal manifestation of human experience that needs to be supported. The provision of psychological intervention during the grieving process will not eliminate the sadness of grief and the pain of imminent loss for the patient and family caregivers, but it can make it bearable. Therefore, it is important to provide a reassuring and compassionate therapeutic presence, where the therapist is comfortable being in the presence of grief, resisting any temptation to fix, change, or negate the experience. However, assessment of grief reactions should be ongoing for recognizing whether the patient's or family caregivers' grief is becoming disabling and unmanageable and whether a pathological process (e.g., depression) has developed.

Grief-related terminology is described in Table 3.5 based on current conceptualizations. While technical terms are generally not used with patients and families, it is important that palliative care clinicians use a common language that also reflects the current literature and research.

Table 3.5 **Grief-Related Terminology**

Grief	Normal reaction to any significant loss; physical, cognitive, psychological, and spiritual manifestations experienced as a reaction to loss.
Bereavement	The state of having experienced the death of someone close and the grieving process associated with it
Mourning	The psychological process of integrating the pain and implications of the loss that allows gradual adaptations to the death; also refers to the outward manifestation of grief through culture-based practices
Family caregivers' anticipatory grief	The grief experienced by family members who have a loved one with advanced illness before the death; usefulness of this conceptualization has been recently questioned in the grief literature
Patients' preparatory grief	The grieving process experienced by patients with advanced illness before they die. Despite the term, the grieving process does not necessarily allow patients to prepare for death.
Complicated Grief (see chapter 4) a.k.a. Prolonged Grief Disorder a.k.a. Persistent Complex Bereavement Disorder (proposed by DSM-5 as diagnostic entity for further study; criteria not to be used clinically)	A multitude of severely distressing symptoms, including psychiatric presentations indicating that the griever is symbolically "stuck" and the integration of the loss is not occurring; complicated grief requires professional interventions

Anticipatory grief and preparatory grief both have been used in the literature to describe the grieving process occurring prior to the patient's death. The patient and the family grieve, together or separately, overtly or silently, for the shared losses of their family life and experience. Yet, each also grieves personal losses.

The grieving process experienced by patients with advanced illness approaching death was initially named *preparatory grief* by Kübler-Ross (1997) who described it as a process allowing patients who are terminally ill to prepare themselves for the impending death. Grief reactions in family members have been historically named *anticipatory grief*.

While these constructs—anticipatory grief and preparatory grief—are still used in the literature and by most palliative care and hospice clinicians, the validity of their assumptions has been questioned. Family caregivers with high levels of anticipatory grief (grief prior to the death of the loved one) were believed to somehow face a less problematic bereavement process. Instead, studies have indicated that high levels of anticipatory grief are not protective factors in bereavement, but may actually represent a risk factor for complicated grief, especially for caregivers who felt poorly prepared during caregiving (Nielsen et al., 2016). Deconstructing the function of anticipatory grief makes sense clinically. Family caregivers do not have a set "amount" or intensity of grief they need to process. Grieving more intensely before the death of their loved one does not mean they will experience less intense grief afterward. Rather, grief reactions can become unmanageable at any time, and it is critical that family caregivers be supported in a manner that is consistent with their needs, which are always evolving (Moon, 2015).

A similar discussion applies to the richness and complexity of the terminally patient's grief (aka *preparatory*). Grief in advanced illness is part of the complex set of a patient's psychological and spiritual responses; while it may serve a preparatory function for some, this does not apply to everyone. A patient's grief can unfold opportunities for personal exploration and growth, and it may allow for the development of a sense of peace about dying. But it also presents several challenges, which may prevent adaptation or preparation for death. Describing all patients' grief as preparatory reveals an inherent assumption about the function of the grieving process for each patient. Yet, such an assumption appears to be limited, preventing the clinician from developing a full appreciation of the patient's experience. And it does not reflect the complexity of the clinical and sociocultural reality of different patient populations.

A patient's grieving process is in fact the result of many factors related to the disease, awareness of prognosis, psychological makeup, and availability of support (see Strada, 2013a, for a review). For instance, a patient who is diagnosed with illness that is advanced and receives a prognosis of months may nonetheless be unwilling to entertain the possibility of death. Rather, he may mobilize energies to pursue treatment that is offered to him, even when the likelihood of benefit is small. Other patients may face several psychosocial challenges in addition to those brought by the illness and may remain in crisis mode until near death. Other patients may not openly grieve, or even allow themselves to feel sadness for their circumstances. It would also be incorrect to assume that the patient who is not openly grieving with her family (or is not acknowledging death) will automatically experience emotional alienation or worse quality of end-of-life care. The key point is, every patient and family story is unique and nuanced. A palliative psychologist should embrace the complexity of the clinical work, avoiding assumptions about the function or progression of a grieving process.

Supporting the grieving process in a patient with advanced illness consists in recognizing and validating the values, beliefs, and personal stories that are sustaining and can create a sense of emotional safety. For some patients, becoming involved with their family caregivers in legacy projects based on life review can involve meaningful and positive reflection and can promote a sense of peace and completion (Allen et al., 2008). However, the grieving process can be particularly difficult for patients who have little or no family or social support system. In this case, the clinicians of the palliative care and hospice team may represent an important, if not the only, source of emotional support. Using art therapy modalities as additional tools or as the main approach can facilitate expression and understanding that bypass words and conceptualizations, and thus can be particularly healing (Hartley, 2013). Many palliative care and hospice clinicians are also aware of the value of music therapy for many patients in promoting connectedness between the patient and the family caregivers and also in facilitating processing of difficult emotions, including grief.

In essence, supporting the grieving process in patients who are seriously ill requires presence, sensitivity, and creativity on the part of the clinician. It also requires an appreciation of the need to release preconceived notions and formulations in order to be truly able to bear witness to the patient's story.

Adopting a nonpathological approach to normal grief or sadness does not mean that the support provided can then be sporadic, casual, and superficial. When psychological intervention is part of the treatment approach, it should be delivered in a planned, focused, and consistent manner, and the session frequency should be based on the patient's needs.

CASE VIGNETTE 3.3

Randy was a 56-year-old woman admitted to the hospital with severe pain and distress. Eight months prior, she was diagnosed with stage IV colorectal cancer that had metastasized to the liver and the lungs. Chemotherapy was initiated at the time of diagnosis but stopped due to the patient's declining health. Randy lived with her partner of three years. About three weeks prior to the hospitalization, she had enrolled in hospice. Two weeks later she became dissatisfied with the care and disenrolled from hospice. At the hospital, both she and her partner appeared distressed, and a palliative care consultation was requested for pain and emotional distress.

During the meeting with the palliative care nurse and psychologist, the patient shared she was very anxious and felt her partner was not supportive enough at home. Randy was diagnosed with bipolar disorder, and her symptoms had been controlled with a commination of medication (olanzapine) and weekly therapy. According to her partner, Randy stopped treatment when she was diagnosed with cancer, and he described her behavior as "out of control." The patient admitted feeling sad and angry about the cancer diagnosis and the limited treatment options. She explained that her mood was volatile and she often lashed out at her sister and her partner. After every argument, she would become deeply depressed, fearing her partner was going to leave her. These thoughts triggered suicidal ideation, leading to alternating crying spells and anger. While she had never attempted suicide, she admitted threatening to kill herself in order to obtain more attention from her partner, who had become progressively distant. Her physical function had decreased significantly over the past two weeks and she had become bedbound. The psychologist and the nurse discussed that resuming medication and regular psychotherapy could help manage symptoms and relieve distress. The patient agreed and commented that she expected to be discharged home and planned to re-enroll in hospice. The partner was quiet and after the meeting he asked to speak with the clinicians privately. He described feeling overwhelmed, exhausted, and angry with the patient for the emotional outbursts. He stated that he had no intention of caring for her until her death. He also stated that he had no intention of taking her home and that the apartment was his property and he had paid for all expenses. He planned to tell the patient that his work schedule no longer allowed him to care for her at home and that she would be safer in a facility. He asked the palliative care clinicians to help him deliver the news to the patient to support her. This unfortunate development was discussed at a palliative team meeting. It was discussed that attempting to convince the distressed and resentful partner to care for the patient at home may be not only damaging to the patient emotionally, but potentially also unsafe. Considering the patient's limited life expectancy, lack of social support, and fragile emotional state, it seemed that caring for her at the hospital was indicated. The palliative care clinicians and the patient's partner gathered in the patient's room, and he explained his intentions not to take her home. As anticipated, she became distressed and asked her partner to pay for a nurse to provide her with 24-hour care, but he refused, saying he could not afford it. The patient became agitated and started complaining of severe pain. It was decided it would be best to end the meeting. The nurse and the psychologist remained in the room with the patient. Medication was administered to the patient to reduce agitation, but she remained upset. The patient remained hospitalized on the oncology floor, and was followed daily by the palliative care team. Her pain became well managed. Olanzepine was resumed to control her anxiety and agitation with good outcome. Randy felt profound grief for the end of her relationship, as her partner never returned to the hospital to visit. Aware that she was dying, she felt her life had unraveled before her eyes and could not understand how her partner could abandon her. The palliative psychologist met with the patient daily to help her process grief and distress. With her psychiatric symptoms controlled, the patient expressed the desire to reconcile with her sister, and the psychologist facilitated a positive meeting between them. The daily psychotherapy sessions focused on practicing self-soothing techniques, releasing anger about the partner's behavior, and developing positive images not only about her life, but also related to her belief in the possibility of life after death. Her grieving process was intense, and several issues remained unresolved and distressing. However, by managing pain and psychiatric symptoms and providing daily psychological support, it was possible to create physical and emotional safety in her dying process.

Clinical Depression in Advanced Illness

Although the presence of depressive symptoms is common in serious illness and at end of life, clinical depression is a pathological process and should not be considered an expected consequence. Clinical depression is associated with increased morbidity, reduced quality of life, and reduced autonomy. Most important, it is also associated with increased risk for suicide and desire for hastened death, attempted suicide, and completed suicide (Fairman, Hirst & Irwin, 2016; Rosenstein, 2011). Conversely, patients with cancer receiving palliative care with lower depression scores and higher levels of hopefulness have been found to be more likely to trust their physicians. This is important, as trust can be considered a critical component of effective communication and care (Tanco et al., 2017).

In most patients, the clinical presentation of depression is not as dramatic as the presentation with a pain crisis or hyperactive delirium. A patient who is depressed may present as withdrawn, uninterested in engaging, lethargic, and may even deny emotional distress. This presentation should not prevent clinicians from appreciating the extent of the patient's suffering. Depression represents a psychosocial and spiritual crisis, and clinicians need to be as proactive in treatment as they are treating pain and other distressing physical symptoms. Depression may not only prevent a patient from receiving important support from sources of meaning and purpose (e.g., spiritual and religious beliefs, family and community), it can also deprive the patient and the family of the opportunity to connect with each other at perhaps the most sensitive time in their lives. Thus, treatment needs to address specific goals and be evidence-based, integrative, and respectful of cultural norms (Ishyama, 2003).

Clinical depression is prevalent in advanced illness. In patients with cancer, there is a higher association of depression for oropharyngeal, pancreatic, breast, and lung cancer. The prevalence in pancreatic cancer has been estimated between 33% and 76%, with a suicide risk that is 11 times higher than in the general population (Turaga et al., 2010).

Depression in also prevalent in patients with non-cancer diseases, including end-stage renal disease, Parkinson's disease, advanced heart failure, and end-stage AIDS. For instance, a prospective study of 662 patients with heart failure diagnosed with major, minor, or no depression during hospitalization and followed for five years indicated that major depression was associated with a higher risk of mortality. In fact, results indicate that major depression is an independent risk factor for all-cause mortality in patients with heart failure (Freedland et al., 2016a). In the same patient cohort, major depression was also an independent risk factor for multiple hospitalizations (Freedland et al., 2016b).

Depression is also prevalent in patients with COPD, affecting around 40% of patients. Here, diagnosis is especially challenging because of significant symptom overlap (Stage et al., 2006). Depression is these patients is associated with higher levels of disability, poorer quality of life, and overall morbidity (Maurer et al., 2008). It has been estimated that less than one-third of patients with COPD experiencing depression or anxiety receive adequate treatment (Yohannes & Alexopoulos, 2014).

There is an association between depression and the type of coping strategies patients employ to adjust to incurable illness. In patients with incurable cancer, coping strategies based on acceptance and emotional support were associated with better mood scores and quality of life. On the other hand, coping strategies based on denial and self-blame were associated with a worse outcome (Nipp et al., 2016a).

Depression in advanced illness affects both the patient and the family and can impact the complex family dynamics that are established in the process of caregiving. A study of family caregivers of patients with incurable cancer showed high levels of depression and anxiety in caregivers (Nipp et al., 2016b). In particular, the study found an association between the caregiver's coping style, the patient's goals for treatment, and depression/anxiety. Acceptance-based coping was associated with less caregiver depression. Caregiver depression was also higher when the patients (with incurable cancer) reported that their goal for treatment was cure. While this discussion is focused on recognizing and managing depression in patients, it is important to recognize risk factors and the presence of depression in family caregivers. Interventions to support caregivers can facilitate their role and prevent the development of complications of bereavement (see Chapter 4). In particular, receiving focused support during the patient's end of life by receiving hospice care has been associated with a reduction in caregivers' depressive symptoms (Ornstein et al., 2015).

Palliative psychologists should be aware of professional and attitudinal barriers to timely diagnosis and treatment:

- belief that depression in advanced illness and end-of-life is an expected, normal development
- diagnostic challenge of differentiating expected emotional distress and grief reactions from major depression (a psychiatric disorder); the focus on differential diagnosis may discount the clinical reality that grief and depression may co-occur and both should be addressed
- overlap of neurovegetative symptoms in depression and advanced illness, which can complicate diagnosis and possibly result in over- or under-diagnosing depression
- fear of medicalizing and over-pathologizing grief in advanced illness and end of life, resulting in attempts to normalize depression rather than treat
- knowledge deficits about the appropriate use of psychotropic medication, including drug-drug interaction, adverse effects, and fear of adding to the patient's burden by adding another medication
- lack of experience providing psychotherapy and integrative medicine interventions.

MEDICAL AND PSYCHOSOCIAL RISK FACTORS

The presence of risk factors can increase the patient's vulnerability to developing depression and should be noted in the treatment plan (Box 3.2). The patient's mood and adaptation to circumstances should be closely monitored for prompt identification of changes. Important risk factors include the following:

A prior history of depression should warrant early psychology evaluation to gather information about past treatment (both pharmacological and psychological) and the patient's response. Past hospitalizations for depression, past suicidal ideation, and past suicide attempts are particularly concerning. Even though the patient may not be currently symptomatic, careful assessment should be ongoing, with particular attention to suicidal ideation.

Poorly controlled pain and other physical symptoms can cause distress, mimicking psychiatric disorders. Uncontrolled pain is a common cause of depressed mood in patients with cancer and other advanced illness. The association between poorly managed pain, anxiety, and depression has been found in different cultures (Li et al., 2017). Therefore, before proceeding with any diagnostic considerations related to depression or anxiety, it is important to ensure that pain and symptoms are optimally managed. Poorly controlled pain is also greatly feared by patients as they approach death, and it is associated with requests for hastened death. Thus, adequate control of pain in advanced disease is a crucial component of treatment and can lead to alleviation of depressive as well as anxiety symptoms.

Box 3.2 **Important Risk Factors for Depression in Advanced Illness**

- prior history of depression
- poorly controlled pain and other physical symptoms
- spiritual and existential suffering with loss of meaning and purpose
- significant family conflict
- history of complicated grief

Psychosocial-spiritual factors, including existential and spiritual suffering, significant family conflict, or a history of complicated grief factors, can trigger a major depressive episode or worsen depression.

Medical conditions that can precipitate or worsen depressive symptoms include the following:

- *Metabolic abnormalities*: hypercalcemia, anemia, decreased vitamin B-12, and electrolyte abnormalities, particularly hyponatremia.
- *Endocrine abnormalities*: hyper- or hypo-thyroidism, hyper-parathyroidism, adrenal insufficiency, Cushing's syndrome
- *Inflammatory cytokines*: studies have shown that inflammatory cytokines such as interleukin 6 and TNF-alpha have been associated with depression in healthy individuals and patients with medical illness, including cancer, advanced chronic kidney disease, and end-stage renal disease (Breitbart et al., 2014; Taraz, Taraz & Dashti-Khavidaki, 2014; Oliveira Miranda et al., 2014).
- *Neurologic abnormalities*: brain tumors and metastases can mimic or cause depressive symptoms. In particular, right-sided and frontal lesions are associated with mood symptoms.

Medications can also mimic or cause depressive symptoms. Steroids, benzodiazepines, beta blockers, some antibiotics, and several chemotherapy agents are particularly noteworthy. In addition, patients may have highly individual reactions based on drug interactions.

DIAGNOSTIC CONSIDERATIONS

In palliative psychology, the clinical interview represents an important tool with a unique role. It offers the opportunity to obtain information about the patient's symptoms and provide supportive psychoeducation and a hopeful reframe during the same meeting. To accomplish these goals, the palliative psychologist needs to develop a quick rapport with the patient and the family, develop a quick working conceptualization of the case, and also provide comfort and hope during all interactions. Accordingly, the clinical interview in the palliative care setting can then be conceptualized as a *therapeutic assessment* (Strada, 2013b), where the psychologist skillfully blends sophisticated assessment with psychotherapeutic presence and interventions.

If validated tools are used in conjunction with the clinical interview, they should be relevant to the palliative care setting and not be burdensome for the patient and the family. The Hospital Anxiety and Depression Scale (HADS) is frequently used in inpatient and outpatient settings, including palliative care (Ziegler et al., 2011). The HSCL-20, MHI-5, and PHQ-9 have been studied in patients with cancer and have shown to have good psychometric properties (Johns et al., 2013; Possel & Knopf, 2013). Other well-known tools, such as the Beck depression inventory, have limited usefulness in the palliative care setting due to the focus on somatic symptoms of depression. Because any one symptom alone does not diagnose a major depressive episode, the palliative psychologist will consider the range of symptoms, severity, and subjective perception of distress experienced by the patient.

The DSM-5 criteria for depression (APA, 2013) include psychological and somatic symptoms (e.g., weight loss is considered a somatic symptom, whereas guilt is a psychological symptom). As a general principle, depression assessment in advanced illness should focus on the psychological symptoms, to avoid overdiagnosing based on common overlap between somatic symptoms of depression and symptoms of advanced disease (Table 3.6). In exploring the presence of symptoms, it is important to carefully consider the unique circumstances of each patient. This can help the clinician contextualize symptoms and understand their meaning for the patient. This is important not only to avoid interpreting symptoms of advanced disease as a sign of depression, but also to avoid automatically and inappropriately excluding somatic symptoms from a depression diagnosis. The experienced clinician will approach assessment and diagnosis through an appreciation of the clinical complexity and will avoid oversimplifications.

This section discusses the symptoms of depression based on the DSM and considers their relevance to patients in the palliative care setting. According to the DSM-5, depression diagnosis can be considered when the patient has experienced *five or more of*

Table 3.6 **Difference Between Grief Reactions and Depression in Patients with Advanced Illness**

Clinical Presentation	Grief	Depression
Predominant affect	Feelings of sadness and loss, focused on pain about leaving loved ones or the opportunity to complete life projects	Persistent depressed mood Inability to anticipate happiness or pleasure
Intensity	Emotions can range from sadness to moments of despair, but may also include positive affect	The patient's affect does not seem to fluctuate or respond to positive stimuli from the environment, e.g., visits from loved ones.
Duration	Fluctuates	Persistent
Presence of positive emotions	Positive emotions and even humor can be present.	The patient appears constantly unhappy and unable to feel different emotions.
Thought content	Can be focused on ensuring that family members are cared for	Negative, with and feelings of hopeless; rumination
Self-esteem	Generally preserved	Feelings of worthlessness and self-deprecation are common.
Thoughts of death and dying	May be caused by physical suffering, or desire to take control of one's life	Death is wished as a result of feeling worthless, undeserving, or unable to cope

the following symptoms for a period of two weeks, and one of the symptoms is either depressed mood or loss of interest:

Depressed mood most of the day, nearly every day, as reported either by the patient or noticed by others. For example, the patient may describe feeling sad, feeling like crying continuously, or feeling empty and unable to care about anything. Children and older patients may instead report feel irritable rather than sad. Their affect and behavior may also present as irritable and with acting out.

Markedly diminished interest or pleasure in activities the patient used to enjoy engaging in. Loss of interest or pleasure should obviously be explored with regard to activities that the patients can still perform, not activities they used to perform, even if in the recent past. Depending on the patient's current performance status, this range of activities can be limited but still meaningful and supportive, such as looking forward to a favorite TV show, a visit from grandchildren, or reading religious scriptures. If the patient loses interest in these activities, though still physically and cognitively able to perform them, depression should be considered a possibility.

Significant weight fluctuations (weight loss when not dieting or weight gain or decrease or increase in appetite nearly every day). Weight loss or gain is considered a somatic symptom of depression. Significant weight loss is a common symptom of advanced disease and may not be relevant to a depression diagnosis. However, it is important when evaluating a patient at earlier stages of disease who has lost a significant amount of weight as a result of chemotherapy and radiation, and is now continuing to lose weight, in the absence of obvious medical reasons.

Insomnia or hypersonmnia nearly every day. Hypersomnia is frequently associated with worsening disease and approaching end of life. Therefore, per se it would not be a relevant symptom. However, the experienced clinician will be able to determine whether the patient's hypersomnia is a result of progression of illness, or if the patient is sleeping or keeping her eyes closed most of the time as a way of disconnecting from the environment.

Psychomotor agitation or retardation nearly every day. Psychomotor agitation can be present in delirium or as a medication side effect. The patient can present restless, unable to sit or lie in bed, pulling at clothes, or moving his or her hands continuously. However, if the patient is not delirious and is not taking medication that can cause agitation (e.g., corticosteroids), it may be the result of worries, anxieties, and ruminations caused by depression or anxiety, or both. Psychomotor retardation may manifest with slowed movement and speech, which can also be a consequence of advanced illness.

Fatigue, tiredness, or loss of energy nearly every day is common in advanced illness. Usually, patients who are not depressed describe fatigue and loss of energy as physical aspects related to medical treatment, or evolution of the disease, but they generally retain the ability to appear engaged in some of the activities that are meaningful to them.

It is also possible that, as a result of approaching death, the patient is experiencing an adaptive progressive emotional withdrawal from meaningful activities and even from loved ones. This may be in conjunction with progressive fatigue and lack of energy. Unlike depression, this process can feel ego-syntonic to the patient and may not cause distress or a desire to modify the situation. The goal of treatment in this case may become focused on helping the patient and the family preserve a supportive relationship, even when it involves allowing the patient the emotional space to be less engaged.

Feelings of worthlessness or excessive or inappropriate guilt nearly every day represent an important psychological symptom of depression. However, it is important to contextualize the cause of guilt. For example, patients who had a role of provider in the family may express guilt for not being able to care for the family. This guilt may be accentuated when caregiver distress or difficult family dynamics cause family caregivers to openly complain about the negative impact of their loved one's illness. A patient who is not depressed is generally receptive to reassurance by family members, and their attention can be redirected toward more positive thoughts. This is generally not the case when a patient is depressed and generally not receptive to interventions aimed at improving his or her mood.

Diminished ability to think or concentrate, or indecisiveness, nearly every day (e.g., the patient appears easily distracted, complains of memory difficulties). A diminished ability to think or concentrate is common in advanced illness and can also be associated with increasing doses of pain medications. However, difficulty concentrating can also be caused by negative thoughts and hopelessness, or triggered by unmanageable grief and fear of dying.

Recurrent thoughts of death that cannot be simply described as fear of dying. A patient with depression may experience passive suicidal ideation (i.e., without a specific plan), or may formulate a specific plan for suicide, or may even attempt suicide. The manifestation and meaning of this symptom, however, need to be expanded when working with a palliative care population. It is important to note that a desire for hastened death in patients who are seriously ill can be present not only as a manifestation of depression, but can be the expression of a terminally ill patient's choice to determine the moment of his or her death. This aspect is further described in the next section.

SUICIDAL IDEATION

The presence of suicidal ideation should always be assessed in patients who are depressed. It is important to differentiate between fleeting and passive wishes for death at times of pronounced distress, especially after receiving difficult news, and active suicidal ideation, which involves formulation of a plan and the presence of means to complete the suicide. Establishing a trusting relationship with the patient and the family is especially important to promote open and effective communication, and a collaborative approach to ensure safety. Risk factors for suicidal ideation and suicide should be carefully explored (Box 3.3). In assessing a patient who admits to occasional thoughts of suicide, it is important to also identify factors that are protective and would deter the patient from attempting suicide.

The most effective assessment strategy involves asking the patient clearly and directly whether she has been thinking about ending her life. Palliative psychologists should be aware of attitudinal barriers assessing suicide in patients who are seriously ill. Some clinicians are concerned that raising the question of suicidal ideation may actually worsen the patient's mood and may even trigger thoughts of suicide. There is, however, no evidence to support this concern. Patients who have thoughts of suicide often feel relieved when offered the opportunity to share their concerns. Any expression of suicidal ideation should be followed by a thorough suicide assessment. The clinician should inquire about ideation, plan, intent, and means. Leading questions (e.g., "you are not thinking

> *Box 3.3* **Risk Factors for Suicide in Patients with Advanced Illness**
> - poorly controlled pain
> - advanced stage of illness
> - mild delirium
> - mental status changes with poor impulse control
> - prior psychiatric history and or prior suicide attempts
> - family history of suicide
> - substance abuse
> - recent bereavement
> - lack of or inadequate social support
> - hopelessness

about suicide, are you?") should be avoided, as they may indirectly communicate that the clinician is not willing to contemplate this possibility. Based on the assessment, the clinician can then determine the risk level and develop an interdisciplinary plan focused on promoting safety, but also on providing the patient with the necessary psychological and pharmacological support. Several validated assessment tools are also available and can be used to supplement the clinical interview. In particular, the Schedule of Attitudes towards Hastened Death is widely used and is considered a valid and reliable tool (Bellido-Perez et al., 2017).

Suicidal ideation that occurs in depression can improve with treatment. For instance, in a large group of patients with advanced AIDS who were also depressed, desire for hastened death was associated with depression, and it decreased dramatically in those patients whose depression responded to antidepressants treatment (Breitbart et al., 2010). It has also been suggested that treatments specifically targeting hopelessness may decrease desire for hastened death (Rosenfeld et al., 2014).

It is important to note that desire for hastened death in patients who are terminally ill is not only associated with depression, anxiety, or other mental disorder (Wilson et al., 2016). At the time of the writing of this book, five US states have legalized physician-assisted dying via legislation, and one state has legalized it via court ruling, whereby terminally ill patients with a prognosis of six months or less can legally receive a prescription for a lethal dose of narcotics to end their lives. A discussion of this topic is beyond the scope of this book. However, palliative psychologists should be aware of the important distinction between physician-assisted dying (which remains illegal in most of the United States) euthanasia (illegal in the United States), and palliative sedation, which is a legal and ethical medical practice for patients with intractable physical suffering (see also Chapter 7).

PHARMACOLOGICAL TREATMENT CONSIDERATIONS

The first step in addressing depression involves managing any uncontrolled symptoms, especially pain, as these can generate severe distress and hopelessness, which can mimic depression. A number of randomized trials and meta-analyses, especially in patients with cancer, have indicated that SSRIs and SNRI antidepressants are relatively safe and moderately effective. The choice of an antidepressant is based on a number of factors, especially the available time frame for treatment based on the patient's prognosis, side-effect profile, target symptoms, patient's past treatment response, and coexisting medical conditions. Additionally, pharmacological properties (e.g., half-life, potential for drug-drug interaction, and availability of liquid formulation when the patient cannot swallow) should also be considered (Marks & Heinrich, 2013).

Because of their delayed onset of action, SSRIs and SNRIs are not indicated for patients with a prognosis of days or weeks, as they may only add to the symptoms burden without an effect on depressive symptoms. Instead, due to their rapid onset of action and favorable side-effect profile, *psychostimulants* are occasionally used in palliative care to improve fatigue and depressive symptoms in patients with a short prognosis. Psychostimulants can improve mood, apathy, fatigue, psychomotor slowing, appetite, and promote a sense of well-being. Attention can improve in patients experiencing cognitive deficits. They are avoided in patients with delirium and are used with caution in patients with heart disease (Kerr et al., 2012).

While positive results have been reported with electroconvulsive therapy (ECT) for the most severe cases of depression (Rasmussen & Richardson, 2011), it is rarely used in the palliative care setting because it is considered an invasive procedure requiring general anesthesia and causing significant side effects.

PSYCHOLOGICAL APPROACHES

Psychological approaches should always be integrated in the management of depression because they can contribute to effective management, are not invasive, and do not add to the patient's symptoms burden (Farah et al., 2016). The framework, type, and frequency of these interventions is determined by patient-related and illness-related factors, including prognosis, personal values and preferences, and clinical setting. Additionally, the quality of the patient's depression should be considered to determine which intervention or combination of interventions is most appropriate. Different psychotherapy approaches, including cognitive-behavioral, interpersonal, and narrative therapy, can be used to improve symptoms of depression when the patient is able to engage in therapy. Similarly, positive life-review approaches (e.g., dignity therapies) and meaning-oriented approaches (e.g., meaning-centered psychotherapy) can promote a sense of purpose and can decrease depressive symptoms.

A palliative psychologist should also be prepared to provide insight-oriented psychotherapy, exploring how the patient's experience, relationships, unconscious conflicts, and even fantasies have contributed to his or her current emotional state. For some patients, there is great value in exploring unconscious conflict and the behaviors they have developed to protect themselves from painful or intolerable emotions, even as they approach end of life. Therefore, the palliative psychologist will be able to choose and provide interventions that match the patient's needs and personal style. All of this does not mean that the palliative psychologist will follow a random approach, providing a meaningless patchwork of interventions. Rather, a practice-based knowledge of different psychotherapy approaches will allow a palliative psychologist to provide truly integrative psychological treatments, based on clinical competence.

The Anxiety Continuum in Advanced Illness

Anxiety can be described as a mood state characterized by apprehensive anticipation of future negative events or danger. While anxiety is closely related to fear, there is an important difference. Fear generally has an identifiable cause (e.g., fear of upcoming surgery, fear of side effects from treatment, fear of dying); anxiety may or may not be related to identifiable causes, and the patient may simply report general worry and mental suffering without a specific trigger. Fear is more frequently associated with surges of arousal, thoughts of imminent danger, and escape behaviors. Anxiety, on the other hand, is associated with avoidance behaviors and muscle tension and hypervigilance in preparation for future danger (American Psychiatric Association, 2013)

While symptoms of anxiety are common and expected in serious and advanced illness, it is important to differentiate between temporary symptoms of anxiety and the development of an anxiety disorder. Transient anxiety can be adaptive and even help the patient and the family mobilize necessary energies while navigating the medical system and pursuing treatment options. When anxiety is not clinically significant, the level of arousal returns to baseline after the perceived threat or danger is controlled or neutralized, and the patient can continue functioning. However, when it becomes persistent and significantly interferes with the patient's psychosocial functioning, the presence of an anxiety disorder should be considered and assessed. Additionally, if a patient experiences anxiety that is nonadaptive and interferes with function, management is necessary even if the clinical presentation does not meet the full criteria for an anxiety disorder.

The burden of untreated anxiety is significant and can cause great suffering for the patient and the family. Untreated anxiety can increase the patient's interest in a hastened death; it can decrease the patient's ability to understand and process clinical information that is relevant to decision-making; it can undermine the relationship with the medical team and decrease trust; it decreases trust in adequate symptom control at the end of life; additionally, it is associated with the belief that they will be offered ineffective therapies (Spencer et al., 2010).

CLINICAL MANIFESTATIONS OF ANXIETY

Anxiety can present with psychological, cognitive, behavioral, and autonomic/physical symptoms (American Psychiatric Association, 2013). Physical symptoms include diaphoresis, diarrhea, nausea, dizziness, tachycardia or tachypnea, palpitations, chest discomfort, and gastrointestinal distress. Psychological symptoms include feeling edgy or irritable. Cognitive symptoms include worrying, hypervigilance, catastrophizing, and rumination (Table 3.7).

In anxiety there is considerable interplay of physical and psychological symptoms. To illustrate, fear of death is a psychological symptom of anxiety, while shortness of breath can be a physical symptom. However, physical symptoms can be linked to

Table 3.7 **Clinical Manifestations of Anxiety**

Emotional	Cognitive	Behavioral	Physical/Autonomic
Feeling edgy	Constant worry	Avoidance	Diaphoresis (profuse sweating)
Sense of impending doom	Obsessions	Compulsions	Dizziness
Terror	Catastrophizing	Suspiciousness	Tachycardia, tachypnea
Agitation-exhaustion cycle	Inability to process information	Psychomotor agitation	Nausea

psychological symptoms. For example, patients with lung cancer or respiratory illnesses can experience shortness of breath as part of the illness. Fear that the illness may be worsening can cause anxiety, which in turn, may increase shortness of breath, thus creating a complex clinical picture with overlap of physical symptoms of illness, physical symptoms of anxiety, and psychological symptoms of anxiety. As a result, the patient may experience increased arousal and distress that can evolve into a sense of lack of control. Understanding the different manifestations of anxiety is therefore important not only for accurate diagnosis, but also for a focused approach that targets symptoms.

MEDICAL CAUSES OF ANXIETY

Medical conditions and medications can mimic, precipitate, or worsen anxiety. Anxiety is associated with specific diseases, such as hyperthyroidism, COPD, or lung cancer. Undertreated pain and poorly controlled dyspnea are well-recognized causes of anxiety. Corticosteroid treatment can cause restlessness, insomnia, agitation, depression, and mania. So can antiemetics and stimulant drug intoxication, including any disorder associated with a confused state (e.g. delirium).

Palliative psychologists should pay special attention to anxiety associated undertreated pain (see also Chapter 2). Patients in pain are often anxious and agitated with high levels of anticipatory anxiety even when pain is relieved. If they have experienced severe pain, or undertreated pain, they may fear that the relief will only be temporary. Some family caregivers may also experience anxiety about the patient taking pain medication regularly to manage their pain, expressing worry they will develop addiction or that the medication will hasten the patient's death.

If it is believed that a medication (e.g., corticosteroids) is contributing to the patient's anxiety, the medical team will evaluate whether the agent can be discontinued and replaced. In general, it is important to educate the patient and the family about the causes of anxiety, especially in sudden onset. Patients may worry that anxiety is the result of a personal failure and may begin to experience helplessness. Awareness of external causes can allow reframing the meaning of anxiety, promoting the ability to detach and objectify the symptom, and improving mastery and management.

PSYCHOSOCIAL AND SPIRITUAL FACTORS ASSOCIATED WITH ANXIETY

Existential distress and uncertainty about the future in the face of advanced illness; spiritual crises, doubt and loss of faith; difficult relationships with the treating team; and practical concerns related to finances or insurance coverage are all factors that can contribute to creating or worsening anxiety for the patient and the family. Additionally, fear of dying and fear of uncontrolled symptoms at the end of life can also increase anxiety and suffering. Anxiety can also develop as a conditioned response to an aversive stimulus. For instance, patients may begin experiencing nausea before the chemotherapy session. The anticipatory anxiety related to having experienced nausea after chemotherapy treatment in the past creates the expectation that nausea will be present and can actually induce nausea even without the stimulus.

DIAGNOSTIC CONSIDERATIONS

As noted previously, when anxiety has become a disorder rather than indicating a temporary reaction to a threatening situation, the patient continues to experience a high level of arousal and threat even when the levels of threat should decrease. For instance, for many patients with cancer, the thought of an upcoming follow-up scan that could possibly show recurrence of disease may understandably generate intense worry and situational anxiety. Cancer survivors may report that the longer they remain disease free or the longer their disease is successfully controlled by the treatment, the more anxious they become about upcoming follow-up tests and waiting for the results. If the scan is negative however, many patients are generally able to experience some degree of relaxation and relief and may not think about the next follow-up. Or, they may occasionally think about it but are able to refocus on enjoying life and connecting with loved ones. Others may use forms of adaptive denial and successfully erase from their awareness the thought of the next scan or the thought of a possible recurrence. On the other hand, patients with an anxiety disorder may not experience any decrease in their arousal level and may focus on worrying about the next procedure, concerned that it may show recurrence of disease.

Anxiety disorders that are most commonly observed in the inpatient and outpatient palliative care setting are: panic disorder, generalized anxiety disorder, and post-traumatic stress disorder (American Psychiatric Association, 2013). *Adjustment disorder* with anxiety is characterized by severe symptoms that develop within three months of an identifiable stressor (e.g., receiving a diagnosis of serious or advanced illness). *Generalized anxiety disorder* is characterized by ongoing, excessive, and uncontrollable anxiety and worry that lasts for at least six months and significantly impacts the patient's psychosocial functioning. *Panic disorder* is characterized by recurrent panic attacks, worry, avoidance behaviors, and apprehension about future attacks that significantly impairs psychosocial functioning. A *panic attack* is a sudden onset of intense anxiety and fear, often accompanied by shortness of breath and palpitations, usually lasting 15 to 20 minutes. *Post-Traumatic Stress Disorder* (PTSD) is characterized by reexperiencing a traumatic event with nightmares, intrusive memories, and hypervigilance. Patients with PTSD also experience avoidance and numbness. As with adjustment disorders, patients may develop PTSD after receiving news of a diagnosis of advanced illness, news of a limited prognosis, or after life-threatening complications of treatment that required aggressive medical management, including admission to ICU.

Patients should be routinely screened for the presence of anxiety symptoms. It is important to note that a patient may not recognize, acknowledge, or verbalize anxiety. The clinician should observe the patient's behavior, affect, or speech that may be indicative of anxiety. The use of brief screening tools, such as the Patient Health Questionnaire for Anxiety and Depression (PHQ), is appropriate, provided it does not increase burden for the patient. Additionally, simple screening questions can be routinely incorporate in the clinical interview:

- Do you feel jittery, nervous?
- Do you ever feel like you cannot stop worrying?
- Do you ever wake up in the middle of the night with negative thoughts that worry you?
- What do you think about most of the time?

The goal of the psychological assessment is to identify the contribution of different manifestations of anxiety (i.e., psychological, physical, autonomic) to the patient's overall experience of distress and suffering. To illustrate, a patient may describe primarily physical symptoms of anxiety that do not appear to be triggered by or linked to any particular thought or situation. Other patients describe that their mind is constantly focused on playing negative narratives, mental scripts, and imagery that fuel and worsen anxiety. Some patients resonate with the idea that anxiety creates a sort of *mental movie* with a negative plot and an even more negative outcome. By paying constant attention to the negative mental movie, they find themselves in a constant state of arousal and negative anticipation.

PHARMACOLOGICAL TREATMENT CONSIDERATIONS

The management of anxiety in patients with serious illness is driven primarily by the patient's prognosis and goals of treatment and it generally focuses on symptom relief. Pharmacological agents are chosen based on goals, life expectancy, and side-effect profile. If the patient's life expectancy is greater than two to three months, treatments may include antidepressants (e.g., SSRIs such as escitalopram, citalopram, and sertraline, or SNRIs such as venlafaxine and duloxetine) or gabapentinoids (e.g., gabapentin). Antidepressants are also used if the patient has comorbid depression. Additionally, when anxiety is severe, the short-term use of benzodiazepines may result in more manageable levels of arousal, allowing nonpharmacological interventions to be introduced effectively. Benzodiazepines (e.g., lorazepam or alprazolam) are usually considered the drugs of choice for the management of acute anxiety and management of anxiety at the end of life (Marks & Heinrich, 2013).

The risks associated with benzodiazepine use (dependence, oversedation, confusion, falls) are well known and are particularly concerning in older and debilitated patients. Benzodiazepines can also cause paradoxical agitation in patients with dementia or brain injury. While it is reasonable to have concerns about dependence, the judicious use of benzodiazepines, combined with adequate psychosocial support and psychological interventions, has an important role in relieving the suffering caused by severe worry or persistent arousal. If anxiety is associated with an emerging confused state (e.g., delirium) a neuroleptic (e.g., haloperidol) is also considered (Caruso et al., 2013). Anxiety associated with terminal delirium is generally managed with a neuroleptic, and a benzodiazepine is added when there is severe agitation (see Chapter 7).

PSYCHOLOGICAL AND INTEGRATIVE MEDICINE APPROACHES

Depending on the patient's life expectancy, psychological and integrative approaches may be effective and should always be considered as a first-line treatment, if possible, or in conjunction with pharmacological treatment. The palliative psychology treatment plan should be comprehensive and yet focused, targeting goals based on the acuity and severity of psychological distress. The palliative psychotherapy framework is integrative, and it allows the palliative psychologist to use different approaches at different times, based on the patient's goals and target symptoms. Cognitive-behavioral therapy can improve the patient's sense of control, self-confidence, and coping by addressing cognitive distortions and automatic negative thoughts that can precipitate and worsen anxiety. Complementary and integrative medicine approaches, such as clinical hypnosis, guided imagery, and music therapy, can similarly increase the patient's empowerment by decreasing arousal and promoting relaxation and positive imagery (Bradt et al., 2011; Brugnoli, 2016; Greer et al., 2010). Research on the use of acupuncture in the palliative care setting is limited, but there is indication that it can be effective in reducing symptoms of anxiety, as well as pain, depression, and nausea in patients receiving hospice care (Romeo et al., 2015). Other mind-body and energy-based approaches, including massage and Reiki, have limited supportive evidence currently, but they are acceptable to some patients to promote comfort and relaxation.

CASE VIGNETTE 3.4

Manuel was a 48-year-old Latino man with end-stage renal disease receiving dialysis four times a week. After presenting to the emergency department with severe abdominal pain and agitation, stating he wanted to stop dialysis treatment so he could die; he was admitted for management of pain and agitation, and a palliative care consultation was requested. Manuel had a history of alcohol and drug use that began in his late twenties, which caused him to be arrested. He completed a drug rehabilitation program and worked at a hardware store for a few years but lost the job when the store went bankrupt. In the following years, he supported himself with occasional jobs, lived with different friends, and resumed his use of alcohol and drugs. Manuel was raised in a lower-middle-class family with both parents working in a local factory. The father had been an alcoholic and physically abusive toward his wife and the children. His older brother Luis had left home when Manuel was 13 and currently worked as a paramedic. The relationship between the patient and his brother was strained, but he had been appointed as the health-care proxy agent. A year prior, Manuel entered rehab and began attending 12-step meetings, and was in sustained recovery afterward. At the hospital, the palliative care team met with Manuel and his brother, and recommendations were offered to improve pain management. The patient complained that his nephrologist was unwilling to take his pain seriously due to his past history of drug use. With everyone's agreement, it was decided that after discharge he would be followed in the outpatient palliative care clinic. During the meeting, he denied being suicidal, but admitted being tired of receiving dialysis and commented that his wish to die had been increased by the severe pain. He agreed to meet with the palliative psychologist to discuss his wishes to stop treatment and die.

Course of Psychological Treatment for Manuel

The initial psychology session focused on continuing to build rapport and assess Manuel's needs and risk level (i.e., assess for suicidal ideation and decisional capacity; assess risk level for drug misuse or abuse in the context of pain management). The patient denied suicidal ideation, did not have a history of suicide attempts, and stated that he never considered taking actions to end his life. However, he complained of depressed mood, fatigue, difficulty concentrating, and overall lack of motivation. He also reported feeling guilty about his past drug use and feeling that he had wasted his life. To maintain his recovery, he continued to attend daily meetings and speak with his sponsor on a daily basis. He explained that guilt and negative self-image were often the main topics of discussion, and that his sponsor had warned him that these negative feelings could trigger a relapse. Manuel did not exhibit aberrant drug-related behaviors and stated that his pain was well managed with his current regimen, which included opioid medications on a regular schedule. He considered the burden of dialysis challenging, both physically and emotionally.

The psychologist framed the psychotherapy sessions as an opportunity for safely exploring options without pressure, so that Manuel would be able to make an informed and empowered decision about medical treatment and his life. The patient particularly resonated with the term "empowered," as he admitted feeling powerless to control his life and addiction. The psychologist also discussed that depression may interfere with Manuel's ability to make a fully informed decision and recommended addressing this in therapy.

The possibility of adding an antidepressant was discussed during the subsequent palliative care team meeting. The lack of data and evidence regarding safety and efficacy of antidepressants in patients with end-stage renal disease was a concern. However, the team thought that because the patient's depression was severe, consideration could be given to a medication trial, if acceptable to the patient, and in the context of constant monitoring for adverse effects. Manuel agreed with the plan and sertraline, 50 mg daily, was initiated. In addition, he attended psychotherapy twice a week.

Pschotherapy was delivered, following primarily a narrative approach, to address Manuel's guilt and sense of being a failure. *Re-Authoring* conversations allowed him to develop and consider alternative narratives about his life. His long-standing struggle with addiction was externalized as the problem that had mostly impacted on Manuel's life. At the same time, he began considering his recovery as evidence of his unwillingness to give up on himself and his ability to use the vision of a better life as a source of motivation. His brother Luis attended several sessions, which allowed the use of the *outsider witness* technique to the therapy conversations. Luis expressed guilt about leaving home when Manuel was young and depriving him of support. To Manuel's surprise, Luis also praised his brother's strength and resilience, further helping develop an alternative narrative for Manuel's life. Witnessing the progressive shift in Manuel's mood, self-perception, and newfound hope over three months of psychotherapy was a powerful and moving process. He stated that he now felt able to make decisions about dialysis not from a place of depression and defeat, but from a place of empowerment and peace. He continued treatment and psychotherapy for the following eight months, and then concluded that dialysis had become too physically burdensome. After reflecting further and discussing with his brother and the palliative care team, he decided to stop treatment and receive hospice care at his brother's house. He asked the palliative psychologist if therapy could be continued at home. Weekly therapy continued at home, where Manuel died three weeks after stopping dialysis.

References

Allen, R. S., Hilgeman, M. M., Ege, M. A., Shuster, J. L., & Burgio, L. D. (2008). Legacy activities as interventions approaching the end of life. *Journal of Palliative Medicine, 11*(7), 1029–1038.
American Psychiatric Association. (2013). Diagnostic and statistical manual of mental disorders (5th ed.). Washington, DC: American Psychiatric Association Press.
American Psychological Association. (2011). Practice guidelines regarding psychologists' involvement in pharmacological issues. *American Psychologist, 66*(9), 835–849.
Bellido-Perez, M., Monforte-Royo, C., Tomas-Sabado, J., Porta-Sales, J., & Balaquer, A. (2017). Assessment of the wish to hasten death in patients with advanced disease: A systematic review of measurement instruments. *Palliative Medicine, 31*(6), 510–525.
Bloom, B. L. (2001). Focused single-session psychotherapy: a review of the clinical and research literature. *Brief Treatment and Crisis Intervention, 1*, 75–86.
Bradt, J., Dileo, C., Magill, L., & Teague, A. (2011). Music intervention for improving psychological and physical outcomes in cancer patiens. *Cochrane Database of Systematic Reviews.* doi: 10.1002/14651858.CD006911.pub3
Breitbart, W. S., & Poppito, S. R. (2014). *Individual meaning centered psychotherapy for patients with advanced cancer: A treatment manual.* New York: Oxford University Press.
Breitbart, W., Rosenfeld, B., Gibson, C., Kramer, M., Yuelin, L., Tomarken, A., . . . Schuster, M. (2010). Impact of treatment for depression on desire for hastened death in patients with advanced AIDS. *Psychosomatics, 51*(2), 98–105.
Breitbart, W., Rosenfeld, B., Tobias, K., Pessin, H., Ku, G. Y., Yuan, J. & Wolchok, J. (2014). Depression, cytokines, and pancreatic cancer. *Psycho-Oncology, 23*, 339–345.
Brugnoli, M. P. (2016). Clinical hypnosis for palliative care in severe chronic diseases; a review and the procedures for relieving physical, psychological, and spiritual symptoms. *Annals of Palliative Medicine, 5*(4), 280–297.
Carr, B. I., & Steel, J. (2013). *Psychological aspects of cancer.* New York: Springer.
Caruso, R., Grassi, L., Nanni, M. G., & Riba, M. (2013). Psychopharmacology in psycho-oncology. *Current Psychiatry Reports, 15*(9), 393.
Cordella, M., & Poiani, A. (2014). *Behavioural oncology.* New York: Springer.
Fairman, N., Hirst, J. M., & Irwin, S. A. (2016). *Clinical manual of palliative care psychiatry.* Arlington, VA: American Psychiatric Association Publishing.
Farah, W. H., Alsawas, M., Mainou, M., Alahdab, F., Farah, M. H., Ahmed, A. T., . . . LoBlanc, A. Non-pharmacolgical treatment of depression: A systematic review and evidence map. *Evidence Based Medicine, 21*(6), 214–221.
Freedland, K. E., Carney, R. M., Rich, M. W., Steinmeyer, B. C., Skala, J. A., & Davila-Roman, V. G. (2016a). Depression and multiple rehospitalization in patients with heart failure. *Clinical Cardiology, 39*(5), 257–262.
Freedland, K. E., Hesseler, M. J., Carney, R. M., Steinmeyer, B. C., Skala, J. A., Davila-Roman, V. G., & Rich, M. W. (2016b). Major depression and long-term survival of patients with heart failure. *Psychosomatic Medicine, 78*(8), 896–903.

Gabbard, G. O. (2004). *Long-term psychodynamic psychotherapy: A basic text*. Washington, DC: American Psychiatric Press.
Gabbard, G. O. (2005). Patient-therapist boundary issues. *Psychiatric Times*, 22(12). http://www.psychiatrictimes.com/articles/patient-therapist-boundary-issues. Retrieved on June 11, 2017.
Gabbard, G. O., & Lester, E. O. (2003). *Boundaries and boundary violations in psychoanalysis*. Washington, DC: American Psychiatric Publishing.
Greer, J. A., Park, E. R., Prigerson, H. G., & Safren, S. A. (2010). Tailoring cognitive-behavioral therapy to treat anxiety comorbid with advanced cancer. *Journal of Cognitive Psychotherapy*, 24, 294–313.
Hartley, N. (2013). *End of life care: A guide for therapists, artists, and art therapists*. London, UK: Jessica Kingsley Publishers.
Henry, M., Cohen, S. R., Lee, V., Sauthier, P., Provencher, D., Drouin, P., . . . Mayo, N. (2010). The Meaning-Making intervention (MMI) appears to increase meaning in life in advanced ovarian cancer: a randomized controlled pilot study. *Psychooncology*, 19(12), 1340–1347.
Ishiyama, F. I. (2003). A bending willow tree: A Japanese (Morita Therapy) model of human nature and client change. *Canadian Journal of Counselling*, 37(3), 216–231.
Johns, S. A., Kroenke, K., Krebs, E. E., Theobald, D. E., Wu, J., & Tu, W. (2013). Longitudinal comparison of three depression measures in adult cancer patients. *Journal of Pain Symptom Management*, 45(1), 71–82.
Kerr, C. W., Drake, J., Milch, R. A., Brazeau, D. A., Skretny, J. A., Brazeau, G. A., & Donnelly, J. P. (2012). Effects of methylphenidate on fatigue and depression: a randomized, double blind, placebo-controlled trial. *Journal of Pain and Symptom Management*, 43(1), 68–77.
Kübler-Ross, E. (1997). *On death and dying: What the dying have to teach doctors, nurses, clergy and their own families*. New York: Scribner Classics.
Li, X. M, Xiao, W. H., Yang, P., & Zhao, H. X. (2017). Psychological distress and cancer pain: results from a controlled cross-sectional survey in China. *Scientific Reports*, 7. doi: 10.1038/srep39397
Low J., Serfaty M., Davis S., Vickerstaff V., Gola, A., Omar, R. Z., . . . Jones, L. (2016). Acceptance and commitment therapy for adults with advanced cancer (CanACT): Study protocol for a feasibility randomized controlled trial. *Trials*, 17, 77.
Marks, S., & Heinrich, T. (2013). Assessing and treating depression in palliative care patients. *Current Psychiatry*, 12(8), 35–40.
Maurer, J., Rebbepragada, V., Borson, S., Goldstein, R., Kunik, M. E., Yohannes, A. M., & Hanania, N. A. (2008). Anxiety and depression in COPD: Current understanding, unanswered questions, and research needs. *Chest*, 134(4), 43–56.
McGrath, R. E. (2011). Collaboration between pharmacologically trained psychologists and pediatricians: History and professional issues. In G. M. Kapalka (Ed.), *Pediatricians and pharmacologically trained psychologists: Practitioner's guide to collaborative treatment*. New York: Springer.
Moon, P. J. (2015). Anticipatory grief: A mere concept? *American Journal of Hospice and Palliative Medicine*, 33(5), 417–420.
New Jersey Psychological Association. (2016). *New Jersey Psychologist*, 61(1).
Nipp, R. D., El-Jawahri, A., Fishbein, J. N., Eusebio, J., Stagl, J. M., Gaggagher, E. R., . . . Temel, J. S. (2016a). The relationship between coping strategies, quality of life, and mood in patients with incurable cancer. *Cancer*, 1(July), 2110–2116.
Nipp, R. D., El-Jawahri, A., Fishbein, J. N., Gallagher, E. R., Stagl, J. M., Park, E. R., . . . Temel, J. S. (2016b). Factors associated with depression and anxiety symptpoms in family caregivers of patients with incurable cancer. *Annals of Oncology*, 27(8), 1607–1612.
Oliveira Miranda, D., Taís Aparecida Soares de Lima, Azevedo, L. R., Feres, O., Ribeiro da Rocha, J., & Pereira-da-Silva, G. (2014). Proinflammatory cytokines correlate with depression and anxiety in colorectal cancer patients. *BioMed Research International*, http://dx.doi.org/10.1155/2014/739650.
Ornstein, K. A., Aldridge, M. D., Garrido, M. M., Gorges, R., Meier, D. E., & Kelley, A. S. (2015). The association between hospice use and depressive symtpoms. *JAMA Internal Medicine*, 175(7), 1138–1146.
Possel, P., & Knopf, K. (2013). Assessing depression in cancer patients: A longitudinal comparison of three questionnaires. *Annals of Palliative Medicine*, 2(1), 45–47.

Ramos, K., & Fulton, J. J. (2017). Integrating dignity therapy and family therapy in palliative care: A case study of multiple sclerosis, depression, and comorbid cancer. *Journal of Palliative Medicine, 20*(2), 115.

Rasmussen, K. G., & Richardson, J. W. (2011). Elettroconvulsive therapy in palliative care. *American Journal of Hospice and Palliative Care, 28*(5), 375–377.

Romeo, M. J., Parton, B., Russo, R. A., Hays, L. S., & Conboy, L. (2015). Acupuncture to treat the symtpoms of patients in a palliative care setting. *Explore (NY), 11*(5), 357–362.

Rosenfeld, B., Pessin, H., Marziliano, A., Jacobson, C., Sorger, B., Abbey, J., . . . Breitbart, W. (2014). Does desire for hastened death change in terminally ill cancer patients? *Social Science in Medicine, 111*, 35–40.

Rosenstein, D. L. (2011). Depression and end of life care for patients with cancer. *Dialogues in Clinical Neuroscience, 13*(1), 101–108.

Safran, J. D., Muran, J. C., & Eubanks-Carter, C. (2011). Repairing alliance ruptures. *Psychotherapy, 48*(1), 80–87.

Scheffold, K., Philipp, R., Engelmann, D., Schulz-Kindermann, F., Rosenberg, C., Oechsle, K., . . . Mehnert, A. (2015). Efficacy of a brief manualized intervention Managing Cancer and Living Meaningfully (CALM) adapted to German cancer settings: Study protocol for a randomized controlled trial. *BMC Cancer, 15*, 592.

Shaw, C., Chrysikou, V., Davis, S., Gessler, S., Rodin, G., & Lanceley, A. (2017). Inviting end-of-life talk in initial CALM therapy sessions: A conversation analytic study. *Patient Education and Counseling, 100*(2), 259–266.

Solano, J. P., Gomes, B., & Higginson, I. J. (2006). A comparison of symptom prevalence in far advanced cancer, AIDS, heart disease, chronic obstructive pulmonary disease, and renal disease. *Journal of Pain and Symptom Management, 31*(1), 58–69.

Spencer, R., Nilsson, M., Wright, A., Pirl, W., & Prigerson, H. (2010). Anxiety disorders in advanced cancer patients: correlates and predictors of end-of-life outcomes. *Cancer, 116*, 1810–1819.

Stage, K. B., Middelboe, T., Stage, T. B., & Sorensen, C. H. (2006). Depression in COPD: Management and quality of life considerations. *International Journal of Chronic Obstructive Pulmonary Disease, 1*(3), 315–320.

Strada, E. A. (2013a). *Grief and bereavement in the adult palliative care setting.* New York: Oxford University Press.

Strada, E. A. (2013b). *The helping proefessional's guide to end of life care.* Oakland, CA: New Harbinger.

Sulmasy, D. P. (2002). A biopsychosocial-spiritual model for the care of patients at the end of life. *The Gerontologist, 42*(III), 24–33.

Tanco, K., Rhondali, W., Park, M., Liu, D., & Bruera, E. Predictors of trust in the medical profession among cancer patients receiving palliative care: A preliminary study. *Journal of Palliative Medicine, 19*(9), 991–994.

Taraz, M., Taraz, S. & Dashti-Khavidaki, S. (2015). Association between depression and inflammatory/anti-inflammatory cytokines in chronic kidney disease and end-stage renal disease patients: A review of literature. *Hemodialisys International, 19*, 11–22.

Turaga, K. K., Malafa, M. P., Jacobsen, P., B., Schell, M., J., & Sarr, M. G. (2010). Suicide in patients with pancreatic cancer. *Cancer, 117*(3), 642–647.

Watson, M. & Kissane, D. (2011). *Handbook of psychotherapy in cancer care.* Chichester, UK: John Wiley & Sons.

Wilson, K. G., Dalgleish, T. L., Chochinov, H. M., Chary, S., Gagnon, P. R., Macmillan, K., . . . Faisinger, R. L. (2016). Mental disorders and the desire for death in patients receiving palliative care for cancer. *BMJ Supportive Palliative Care, 6*(2), 170–177.

Yohannes, A. M., & Alexopoulos, G. S. (2014). Depression and anxiety in patients with COPD. *European Respiratory Review, 23*, 345–349.

Ziegler, L., Hill, K., Neilly, L., Bennett, M. I., Higginson, I. J., Murray, S. A., & Stark, D. (2012). Identifying psychological distress at key stages of the cancer illness trajectory: A systematic review of validated self-report measures. *Journal of Pain Symptom Management, 41*(3), 619–636.

4

The Fourth Domain of Palliative Care

Social Aspects of Care

> ## Focus Points
>
> - The patient and the family represent the unit of care for the interdisciplinary palliative care team.
> - Attention to the needs of the family includes supporting children and teenagers by promoting coping and providing developmentally appropriate grief and bereavement support.
> - Social stressors (e.g., financial, housing, or transportation issues) need to be readily identified by the team.
> - Family caregivers can experience significant distress associated with caregiving and should be supported in a manner consistent with their cultural values.
> - Palliative psychologists work collaboratively with other palliative care clinicians to promote effective communication between the family, the patient, and the health-care team.
> - Competent bereavement support for family caregivers includes the ability to recognize and manage complications of bereavement (i.e., depression and complicated grief).
> - Family meetings can represent a valuable tool for delivering medical information, facilitating decision making, and providing emotional support to the patient and the family.

Introduction

The fourth domain of palliative care, "social aspects of care," recognizes the patient and the family as the unit of care receiving specialist palliative care. While it is the patient who has been diagnosed with the illness, the entire family system is affected by the experience (Carter & McGoldrich, 2005; Badr & Acitelli, 2017).

To effectively address social needs, it is important to first identify people who are recognized as "family" by the patient and to understand individual roles and responsibilities. This is especially relevant regarding personal care, decision making, and communication with the care team. In addition to family members, caregivers who are considered to be "like family" should also receive care and attention. To illustrate, home health aides represent a vital source of practical and emotional support for patients whose family is either absent or has limited opportunity to participate in caregiving (Aoun, Breen, & Howting, 2014). Often, these relationships are deep and committed. Home health aides may experience significant grief reactions and need emotional support before the patient's death and in bereavement. Recognizing this, hospice bereavement programs frequently extend grief support also to home health aides and invite them to attend memorial services where they can honor the patient's legacy.

When several people are involved in caregiving for the patient, creating a diagram representing the different types of relationships can be helpful. Additionally, it important to note whether each relationship is supportive or challenging for the patient. Family genograms also represent a valuable tool to illustrate different relationships within the family and to assess the quality of support or the presence of conflict that could become problematic in providing care (Hockley, 2000).

Family caregivers experience physical and emotional distress as well as satisfaction in their role. They may face several practical and psychological challenges. Receiving adequate support not only is a comfort to family caregivers, but also helps them to continue performing their roles, facilitating a smoother relationship with the patient and the medical system.

The palliative care team approaches the clinical assessment of the family system from a strength-based approach, validating positive coping, adaptive defense mechanisms, and strategies to manage the challenges involved in living with serious and advanced illness. As social pain is a component of Total Pain, the palliative care team is focused on identifying the presence of distress, risk factors, challenges and needs to address in the plan of care. This comprehensive assessment is complex; it requires that clinicians continually move their assessment and intervention focus between the patient and the family system, depending on the circumstances and needs. The plan of care is developed for the needs of the family system and to ensure that the patient's individual needs are validated and thoroughly addressed (Penrod et al., 2012b).

The core aspects of the social domain can thus be summarized into two main competency areas:

- recognizing, validating, and enhancing the patient and the family's strengths and resources
- recognizing and addressing challenges and sources of social pain.

Competencies for Palliative Psychologists

Social needs can be complex and often overlap with psychological aspects of the patient and family life. Psychologists can provide unique contributions to this comprehensive family work. During graduate training they receive extensive training providing psychological evaluation and assessment to families, including children and older adults. This training extends to the different models of family therapy. Externships, internships, and postdoctoral programs incorporate this focus on the family as the unit of care. Typically, training in family therapy also involves developing a multicultural focus, which is essential in palliative care (see also Chapter 6).

The skills and experience in providing individual, couple, and family therapy uniquely allow palliative psychologists to seamlessly redirect the assessment and intervention focus from the patient's intrapersonal needs (e.g., how the patient as an individual is coping with the illness) to the interpersonal needs of the patient as a member of a family system. The needs and concerns of each family caregiver as well as the needs of the family as a whole are not always aligned and conflict may arise. Effective management of family conflict is essential as it further adds to the psychological suffering that may already be present. Family therapy skills are thus essential to promote communication that is not harmful. A thorough appreciation of the impact of serious illness on family caregivers requires understanding their sociocultural background and developmental stage. Children, teenagers, and older adults are impacted by serious illness in the family in profound yet unique ways. Psychological interventions should match individual needs.

For many, the caregiving role has continued for months or years and represents the core of self-image and personal identity. Caregiver distress may also have been present for variable periods of time and may become exacerbated due to a sudden change in the patient's medical condition. Working with the palliative care team, palliative psychologists need to quickly establish rapport with the family, recognize any long-standing emotional difficulties that must be addressed without delay while also continuing to monitor needs as the patient's condition continues to evolve. Palliative psychologists should recognize the presence of caregiver burden and possible psychiatric complications of caregiving, such as depression and anxiety. Collaboration with other palliative care clinicians is essential. Although overlap exists among disciplines, it is perhaps more evident in the case of psychology and social work. Social workers' clinical focus on improving patients' and families' emotional well-being can promote meaningful and productive collaboration with psychologists and allow for more comprehensive and nuanced treatment plans. The family meeting represents a valuable and frequently used tool in palliative care. It can be a vehicle for safe and compassionate communication between the patient, the family, and the team. Palliative psychologists can lead or co-lead meetings and can use the opportunity for psychological assessment and intervention in the context of interdisciplinary work.

Palliative psychologists should avoid the use of psychological jargon when communicating with other clinicians about the patient and the family. Even though the complex psychological dynamics in a family may call for lengthy and deep explanations, it is important that the psychological plan target specific needs identified during the psychological and interdisciplinary assessment. This approach will maintain a clear focus on the goals of the plan, especially when considering the need to maximize the amount of time available. Box 4.1 summarizes competencies for psychologists in the social domain.

> **Box 4.1 Palliative Psychology Competencies in the Social Domain of Palliative Care**
>
> **KNOWLEDGE**
>
> - understand impact of serious and advanced illness on the family system and on individual family members based on each person's developmental stage
> - recognize impact of sociocultural factors on the way the patient and the family cope with illness
> - understand factors impacting the grieving process in bereavement
> - understand the role and structure of the family meeting in palliative care
> - knowledge of family system work relevant to palliative care
>
> **SKILLS**
>
> - conduct comprehensive assessment of the family needs and develop psychological plan of care
> - facilitate or co-facilitate a family meeting with other providers
> - provide couple therapy and family therapy
> - evaluate family caregivers for caregiver distress, including unmanageable grief reactions and implement an adequate plan of support
> - communicate effectively with other clinicians regarding the needs of family caregivers
>
> **ATTITUDES**
>
> - awareness and appreciation of the importance of the support network for patient
> - nonjudgmental and respectful attitude that honors the family culture, traditions, and rituals
> - multicultural focus that recognizes and values the impact of culture
> - openness toward modifying psychological interventions to match the unique needs of the family
> - recognition of the primacy of social factors and concerns on psychological functioning and behavior

Family Caregivers in Palliative Care: Risk and Protective Factors

Family members frequently assume the role of uncompensated informal caregiver for a family member who is ill and provide most of the care during all phases of illness, including the dying process. According to the National Alliance of Caregiving, about 43.5 million people were caregivers for a family member in 2015 (National Alliance for Caregiving, 2015). Caring for a family member, a loved one, or someone close with serious or advanced illness is a complex process that requires constant mobilization of physical and emotional energy as well as time. Table 4.1 describes common roles of family caregivers and the challenges they may face.

The meaning attributed to caregiving impacts individual responses and adaptation. Depending on the cultural context, caregiving can represent an important opportunity for some; for others it may be primarily the expression of a personal obligation. Family caregivers often experience a multitude of emotions during their activities, and their perception about the meaning may change based on several challenges, including psychological and physical exhaustion, and availability of resources.

Undeniably, caregiving can be rewarding and fulfilling; it can allow for the development of a closer relationship with the patient and increased intimacy during times filled with challenges and vulnerabilities. Many caregivers report feeling proud of their ability to care for the patient, and an increased sense of self-esteem and personal life meaning may result. Relationships that had been strained may be improved by the changes in roles involved in caregiving.

A 43-year-old woman providing care at home for her mother after a diagnosis of advanced lung cancer commented that she felt she could finally make a positive change in her mother's life. She had a history of drug and alcohol abuse and had been estranged

Table 4.1 **Common Roles of Family Caregivers and Associated Challenges**

Role	Practical Function	Possible challenges	Possible negative outcomes
Financial	The caregiver is the main financial provider.	Difficulty managing both roles (primary caregiver and provider)	Guilt, stress, exhaustion, poor physical and mental health
Emotional	The caregiver is the main or only support for the patient during phases of treatment and transitions of care.	The caregiver may disconnect from own emotions and may avoid obtaining support for self.	Loneliness and isolation, depression, anxiety
Direct physical care and nursing tasks	The caregiver provides wound care, medication administration, personal hygiene.	The caregiver may feel inadequately prepared and overwhelmed by the taks.	Irritability and relationship conflict, guilt
Health Care Navigator	The caregiver is in charge of communicating with medical providers and coordinating care.	The caregiver becomes overwhelmed by the complexities of the health care system.	Hopelessness, frustration, dissatisfaction with care, conflict with medical team, guilt

from her mother for years. After completing a drug rehabilitation program, she had maintained her sobriety for five years. Even after reconnecting with her mother, however, she carried a combination of gratitude and guilt. When her mother was diagnosed with advanced lung cancer, her daughter moved in and became her primary caregiver. She attended all medical appointments and became a strong advocate for her mother's care. During a family meeting, the daughter shared that through caregiving she could finally express her gratitude in tangible ways, for the support her mother had provided during the years of her addiction. The challenges of caregiving were significant, however, and increased as the patient's condition worsened. The daughter shared with the team that she felt sleep deprived and exhausted, but she also felt "at peace." The palliative care team assisted the patient's daughter with help from a home health aide who provided respite so that she could attend her AA meetings and psychotherapy. While caregiving was demanding, the meaning attributed to it by the daughter was positive and sustaining. This positive meaning was a protective factor for caregiver distress and it allowed her to cope with the challenges in adaptive ways.

In another example, a 62-year-old woman caring at home for her husband during the advanced stages of COPD and dying process reported that by helping him in practical and emotional ways she began preparing herself for his death. They spent time discussing how she could reorganize her world and continue on with her life. During these conversations, her husband provided her with practical suggestions, as well as emotional support and courage to adjust to his approaching death. He encouraged her to start an informal support group for women caring for spouses who were very ill and insisted that she should continue running the group after his death. He also encouraged her to join a choir, which she had desired to do for years. After his death, she felt a responsibility to continue her life as they had discussed before his death. This provided her with a sense of continuity and purpose and allowed her grieving process to be supported by many positive emotions.

The potential negative impact of caregiving, however, often referred to as caregiver burden can be severe and should not be underestimated. Serving as the primary caregiver for a loved one who is ill and approaching death is emotionally and physically demanding. Family caregivers often lack the emotional and physical energy to engage in meaningful activities, including connecting with acquaintances and friends who are not part of the support around the patient. This may limit their opportunities for receiving support. In addition, family caregivers constantly work to balance their desire to appear strong and positive for the patient with their ongoing grieving process. As a result, they may suppress their grief for fear of distressing the patient (Coelho & Barbosa, 2016).

One spouse commented that, as a result of her full-time caregiving for her husband after his diagnosis of prostate cancer and during his illness, she had stopped returning friends' phone calls because, she "just did not have the energy" to do so. As callers primarily inquired about her husband's condition, she found discussing his condition increasingly difficult and upsetting, especially as he began to decline. She began resenting that no one inquired about her own physical and emotional health. She also realized that her life had become exclusively focused on caregiving and managing her anxiety about her husband's illness. She regretted not having cultivated other personal interests. She felt guilty about how caregiving was impacting her, and she became concerned that she would be considered negatively if she shared her distress. As a result, she became increasingly isolated, which contributed to feelings of hopelessness and depression as her husband's decline continued. She began sharing her distress during psychotherapy after her husband's death. She also expressed sadness and fear about no longer having a caregiver role. Therapy became focused on allowing her to slowly develop an evolving sense of personal identity as part of integrating the pain of loss.

A growing body of literature has focused on the challenging impact of caregiving in several areas of the family caregiver's life. These are briefly described in the following. Palliative psychologists should evaluate whether any of these aspects are relevant to the family caregivers they are supporting.

Physical, emotional, and social aspects. Witnessing a loved one's physical, functional, and cognitive decline may precipitate distress and even anxiety or depression. Sleep can become persistently disrupted and this contributes to physical and emotional exhaustion. Family caregivers often feel they need additional help, especially those with health problems and limited resources. Common stressors are related to housing, insurance and finances, transportation, work, and child care (Clemmer et al., 2008; Penrod et al., 2012a; Schulz & Sherwood, 2008). Caregivers who are overwhelmed and do not receive adequate support are at increased risk for depression and overall reduction in quality of life. They often need to balance their caregiving role with the need to maintain a full-time job. Or they may need to reduce their work hours, which may cause financial difficulties and additional stress. Months or years of intense caregiving do not necessarily facilitate anticipating the death of the loved one or feeling emotionally prepared at the time of death (Breen, 2012). A Danish nationwide population-based cohort indicated that one third of family caregivers of patients with advanced cancer experienced severe pre-death grief and depressive symptoms. While caregivers who were partners experienced the highest levels of depression, adult children caregivers experienced the highest level of caregiver burden (Nielsen, 2016a, 2016b).

Caregivers' personality traits have also been associated with the impact of caregiving. A study of 227 patient-family caregiver dyads showed that extroversion was a protective factor in caregiver burden. Depressive symptoms and neuroticism were positively correlated with caregiver burden; however, neuroticism was not a significant factor when there was an adjustment for depressive symptoms (Kim et al., 2016). In a sample of 304 patient-caregiver dyads, presence of a hopeful attitude in caregivers was determined by less depressive symptoms, active coping strategy, and lower burden (Kim et al., 2014).

Caregiving styles are associated with risk and protective factors. To illustrate, a qualitative study of patient-caregiver dyads in an oncology setting and a hospice setting identified and described four types of caregiving styles: the Manager caregiver, the Carrier caregiver, the Partner caregiver, and the Lone caregiver (Wittenberg-Lyles et al., 2012; Goldsmith et al., 2016). Manager caregivers tend to make decisions independently and may become the self-appointed spokesperson for the family. Carrier caregivers are focused on ensuring they meet every patient's needs, but seek constant reassurance and validation for their performance from the care team. Partner caregivers approach caregiving in collaboration with family and the care team. Lone caregivers tend to be isolated in caregiving and focus on one aspect of care (e.g., physical symtpoms). Subsequently, a model of family caregiver communication was developed and validated to understand the impact of each communication style on levels of psychological distress, skill preparedness, family inventory of needs, and quality-of-life domains (Wittenberg et al., 2017). Results indicated that while Partner and Lone caregivers reported the lowest levels of psychological distress, Carrier caregivers reported lowest levels of preparedness, and Manager caregivers reported the lowest level of physical quality of life.

The patient's type of disease also affects the burden on family caregivers. This is because different diseases create different challenges for both patient and caregiver. For instance, in patients with gliomas, symptoms may interfere with end-of-life decisions, creating additional stress for family caregivers (Koekkoek, Chang & Taphoorn, 2016). Further, a qualitative study of the experience of family caregivers of patients with motor neuron disease identified three main themes in the caregiver's experience. These were described by the authors as the Thief, the Labyrinth, and Defying Fate (Anderson et al., 2016). The first theme identified the illness (the Thief) as responsible for the progressive losses and grief experienced by the patient and the caregivers during the disease trajectory. The second theme (the Labyrinth) illustrated the complex process of identifying and using strategies to manage the ongoing challenges. The third theme highlighted the importance of resilience and hope in the caregiver's life (Defying Fate).

Training and preparation for caregiving. Ensuring adequate preparation for the practical and emotional tasks involved in caregiving is essential. These tasks vary based on the type of disease, symptom burden experienced by the patient, and response to treatment. It is important to ensure physical, emotional, social, and functional home care safety (Lang et al., 2015). Adequate training to provide care to the patient is a critical aspect of safety. *Physical safety* includes specific criteria for the home environment that ensure safety of both the patient and the caregiver as the unit of care. *Emotional safety* addresses the emotional impact of caregiving on family members and patients, as well as on their relationship. *Social safety* considers potential risk factors in the social environment, such as ensuring adequate transportation and access to medical care and needed social services. All these components should be addressed. Family caregivers' perceived preparedness should be assessed during every hospitalization. Hospice clinicians are routinely involved in training family members to perform various tasks. They should consider that grief and stress may affect family caregivers' ability to process and retain information. Thus, it is important to regularly assess the adequacy of training provided to them.

The use of validated assessment tools can be considered. A study explored the reliability and validity of a hospice survey developed to assess the quality of training received by 262 primary caregivers. Most caregivers were females and non-Hispanic white (DiBiasio et al., 2016). Survey questions focused on pain management, medication side effects, management of agitation, safely moving the patient, and addressing symptoms such as difficulty swallowing and difficulty breathing. Additionally, the overall quality of information provided about what to expect during the dying process was also assessed. Results highlighted the importance of exploring family caregivers' competence, level of comfort, and feelings of adequacy in performing tasks directly related to the patient's medical care. Exploring these areas can be an important component of the work of palliative psychologists.

Stress related to performing nursing tasks. Family caregivers are often required to perform nursing tasks, such as giving injections, managing IVs and medication, and providing wound care and hygiene. This causes a change in family roles. Although some caregivers may appreciate being able to assist loved ones with medical needs, others may feel anxious, scared, inadequately trained, or even repulsed by the task. Spouses may grieve the loss of their role and the way the illness has changed the relationship. Adult children may have difficulty relating to their parents' physical and emotional vulnerability, especially when the parent has always valued a sense of personal agency and control.

During bereavement therapy, one spouse shared that she had dreaded using the suctioning device for her husband during his illness. Even though the hospice nurse had showed her how to perform the procedure correctly and had reassured her about her skills, she felt anxious and admitted trying to avoid the task at the risk of causing more discomfort for her husband. She also felt uncomfortable administering medication, especially for pain. Even though she followed the nurse's instructions correctly, she worried when her husband fell asleep, and was afraid that the medication would hasten his death. The most troublesome aspect of caregiving for her was the complete attention required by "nursing" tasks. She felt she missed the opportunity to truly connect emotionally with her husband because of her primary focus on his personal care and hygiene. After her husband died, she began wondering if she had somehow hastened his death by administering the pain medication. Reassurance by the nurse that she had correctly followed instructions did not relieve her concern and instead caused great emotional distress, which complicated her bereavement process. In this case, receiving adequate training for performing nursing tasks did not mitigate this spouse's distress because she felt these tasks kept her from being emotionally present for her spouse. Therefore, it is important not only to ensure that caregivers can perform a task correctly; it is also necessary to assess their psychological readiness and need for support.

Symptom control. Adequate symptom management is critical not only for the patient but also for family caregivers. Witnessing poorly controlled pain, hyperactive delirium, and other physical symptoms in the patient is traumatic and can complicate the bereavement process (see also Chapter 7). In one study, while patients who experienced dyspnea were likely to become distressed, their family caregivers were also more likely to experience distress. (Freeman, Hirdes, Stolee, & Garcia, 2016).

Perceived preparedness for caregiving and satisfaction with EOL care. Family caregivers' perception of being prepared for the practical tasks of caregiving also directly impacts their level of satisfaction with hospice services and their willingness to remain in a hospice program. Pain management is an important risk area. A systematic review indicated that many family caregivers report inadequate knowledge and skills in pain management, poor communication with the treatment team about pain, and misunderstanding of the use of pain medication (Chi and Demiris, 2017). Notably, poorly managed symptoms and caregiver distress are among the main reasons for choosing hospitalization and discontinuation of hospice services.

A qualitative study of hospice disenrollment and hospital admission indicated additional causes: lack of clarity about prognosis, confusion about hospice services, caregiver burden, difficulty managing symptoms at home, caregiver reluctance to administer morphine, faster response time from 911 than from hospice, desire to continue receiving care from the primary physicians at the hospital, and families' difficulty accepting the patient's impending death (Phongtankuel et al., 2016).

Live discharges from hospice because the patient no longer meets criteria can also create confusion and distress for family caregivers. Caregivers of patients with dementia represent a particularly vulnerable group in this regard. A qualitative study focused on 24 family caregivers whose family members with advanced dementia were discharged from hospice (Wladkowski, 2016). For these family caregivers, the ongoing grief was compounded by the difficulty reconciling that a terminal illness no longer met hospice criteria and the stress of losing the important practical and emotional support from hospice. A study examining differences in frailty between spousal caregivers showed that those caring for a spouse with dementia had over 40% higher likelihood of experiencing increased frailty by the time the patient died. Additionally, they had over 90% higher chance of developing frailty in the two years following the patient's death compared with non-dementia caregivers (Dassel & Carr, 2016). Caregiving for a spouse who has dementia has been also associated with greater cognitive decline (Dassel, Carr, & Vitaliano, 2017).

Although caregiving and caregiver burden have received increasing attention, more research is needed. Kent et al. (2016) provided the following recommendations for research:

- prevalence and burden of family caregivers for patients with cancer
- interventions targeting patients, caregivers, and the patient-caregiver dyad
- ways of integrating caregivers into the health care system
- role of technology in supporting caregivers.

Kent et al. (2016) identified the need to increase research focused on vulnerable caregivers, such as minorities, isolated caregivers, and older caregivers. The authors also advocated for increasing diversity participation in research. Regarding technology, they emphasized the importance of identifying groups of caregivers more likely to benefit from use of technology, including virtual support. Risks associated with online support were noted, including the potential for spreading inaccurate information.

ASSESSING THE NEEDS OF FAMILY CAREGIVERS

Responses to the stress of caregiving are modulated by personal history, personal strengths, history of loss, financial resources, and availability of practical and emotional support. According to family system theory, a family is an emotional unit, and the members cannot be understood in isolation from one another. Rather, their behavior often occurs in response to changes in the family that cause anxiety, in an attempt to preserve the family identify by reducing that anxiety. The behavior of the patient and the family observed by the palliative care team is the result of years of complex history and dynamics intended to generate and maintain homeostasis. Thus, symptoms and dysfunctional patterns may develop in response to situations that threaten the perceived family integrity (Kerr & Bowen, 1988).

Caregiving is characterized by interdependence of roles and responsibilities. Serious illness and end of life are intensely stressful situations for a family and can cause the unraveling of coping skills and defense mechanisms. Because there is a mutual association between the quality of life of patient and caregiver (Krug et al., 2016), family caregivers should receive regular and ongoing assessment of their burden and its impact (Table 4.2).

Table 4.2 **Areas of Need for Family Caregivers**

Caregiver Need	What the Palliative Psychologist Should Assess the Caregiver for	How the Palliative Psychologist Can Help the Caregiver
Information	Does the caregiver feel that he or she is receiving adequate information from the medical team? Does he or she feel comfortable asking questions?	Help caregivers prepare list of questions for medical providers, help them rehearse asking questions and expressing concerns
Grief	How is the caregiver expressing grief?	Provide psychoeducation about the grieving process; psychotherapy
Navigating the medical system	Does the caregiver recognize when he or she needs help with the various tasks? Does the caregiver need resources?	Help the caregiver identify his or her caregiving style. Facilitate access to additional resources for older patients, disable patients or caregivers, veterans, Holocaust survivors.
Psychological/Psychiatric	Does the caregiver have untreated depression, anxiety, exacerbation of preexisting mental illness?	Depending on the circumstances, provide psychotherapy or referrals to community mental health, referrals to primary care providers. Ensure caregiver is able to follow up on referrals.
Relationship with the patient	Is the caregiver experiencing abuse from the patient or perpetrating abuse?	Explore any concerning behaviors by the patient or the caregiver and implement plan for safety and support.
Physical health	Is the caregiver maintaining personal health (e.g., making or keeping medical appointments, taking medications as prescribed)?	Provide referrals to primary care physicians; assist caregiver in understanding importance of caring for self while caregiving for patient; coordinate with social work to facilitate respite for caregiver (e.g., by providing home health care assistance, case managing services, etc.).

The assessment process should also be expanded and focus on understanding the structure and function of the family system as a whole. It is also important to identify strengths and protective factors, as well as risk factors, and to understand how the family has coped with loss in the past (Table 4.3). The psychologist should constantly

Table 4.3 **Assessment of the Family System**

Family structure and values	What are the expectations and roles defined within the family? What are the family stories that make the family unique? How does the family adapt to change? How does the family define its identity? What are the alliances in the family? What is the nature of attachments? How are emotions expressed within the family?
Communication style	What is the primary communication style in the family? Direct or indirect? Does everyone have the ability to express his or her thoughts and needs? Are there rules about how communication should occur?
Decision-making style	How are medical decisions discussed and achieved in the family?
Cultural practices	What is the meaning of the illness for the family, and what cultural practices are necessary to preserve a sense of meaning and purpose within the family?
Developmental aspects	How is the illness affecting each family member's developmental stage?
History of loss and trauma	Has the family experienced losses/trauma in the past? How has the family coped? What are the strategies that have been successful, and what are behaviors that may have threatened cohesiveness?

maintain awareness of the purpose of the assessment, which goes beyond the general desire to join and support the family. Rather, it should help understand how the different aspects of the family functioning are affected by the experience of illness and caregiving (Tinetti, Esterson, Ferris, Posner, & Blaum, 2016; Turan et al., 2011).

To illustrate, hope is an important source of support that can promote coping. The assessment should explore how hope is conceptualized, experienced, and expressed by the patient and family caregivers. A study of female caregivers of patients with advanced cancer living in rural areas explored their relationship with hope (Williams et al., 2013). The narratives provided by the caregivers offered insight into the different types of hope they held. For the family caregivers in the study, hope can be specific and concrete and focused on the immediate future. Hope can also be held despite evidence that the patient's condition is worsening. This type of hope, described as "hope against hope," highlights the ongoing intrapsychic strategies used by caregivers to maintain a sense of purpose in the face of challenges. Additionally, hope and emotion-oriented coping have been identified as relevant in limiting development of anxiety and depression in family caregivers after diagnosis (Rumpold et al., 2016).

A skillful assessment should also identify the presence of sensitive issues that caregivers may not voluntarily disclose due to shame or concerns about harming the patients. For instance, family caregivers of patients with advanced Parkinson's disease reported high rates of physical and sexual aggression by the patient (Bruno et al., 2016). In the study, two questions asking about physical and sexual aggression were added to the Zarit Caregiver Burden Interview and were endorsed by most caregivers during the initial palliative care interview. This early detection of the problem enabled the palliative care team to implement strategies to support caregivers. As part of the interventions, caregivers received psychoeducation about the causes of aggression and counseling. They were taught techniques to deescalate the patient's behavior and received additional education about medication management. Results showed that instances of aggression were significantly reduced at the second palliative care visit.

Potentially abusive behaviors by family caregivers should also be promptly identified. Instances of using a harsh tone of voice, yelling at the patient, or calling them names can escalate to abuse (Lafferty, Fealy, Downes, & Drennan, 2016). Additionally, if it appears that family caregivers are pressuring the patient to make decisions contrary to their expressed wishes, clinicians should assess and intervene to safeguard the patient (see also Chapter 8). Many factors can contribute to this development, including caregiver distress. Early identification can allow the implementation of strategies that can promote safety and support relationships.

As mentioned previously, screening and assessment tools can be used in conjunction with the clinical interview, provided they are culturally relevant and not burdensome. Palliative psychologists can assist the palliative care team by identifying appropriate tools to facilitate routine assessment of family caregivers' needs. A systematic review indicated the existence of validated assessment tools with good psychometric qualities both for caregivers of adult and pediatric patients (Tanco et al., 2017). As an example, the Carer Support Needs Assessment Tool (CSNAT) is a helpful tool for assessing support needs in caregivers of patients with primary brain cancer (Aoun, Deas, Howting & Lee, 2015). Assessment tools can also be modified to address specific diseases where caregiver needs are not routinely assessed, as in progressive interstitial lung disease. In this case, an adaptation of the Progressive Disease-Cancer Needs Assessment Tool demonstrated face and content validity and allowed for the inclusion of family caregivers as additional sources of information (Boland et al., 2016).

Interventions for Supporting Family Caregivers

The range of psychological support for family caregivers can range from information and psychoeducation, to general supportive strategies (e.g., empathic listening and reassuring), to family therapy. While there is general agreement that family caregivers need support, it is also necessary to identify family caregivers who are more likely to benefit from interventions and determine how to provide caregivers with the appropriate intervention. Assessment of baseline vulnerability can help match interventions with specific caregiver needs. To illustrate, caregivers who did not report significant benefit from receiving a psychosocial intervention in one study were found to have higher levels of preparedness and competence before the interventions (Holm et al., 2017).

A systematic review (Chi, Demiris, Lewis, Walker, & Langer, 2015) concluded that educational and cognitive-behavioral interventions had a positive impact on measures of quality of life in family caregivers. Cognitive-behavioral interventions aimed at identifying challenges and modifying behaviors showed more robust outcome. The authors of the review, however, describe family caregivers as woefully underrepresented in palliative care research and call for additional studies.

The impact of grief-focused family therapy for families identified to be at risk due to dysfunctional relationships was studied in families identified as either low communicating, low involvement, or high conflict. They were randomly assigned to standard care or to receiving 6 or 10 sessions of a manualized family therapy intervention during palliative care and continued into bereavement. Results indicated that grief-focused therapy significantly reduced the risk of complicated grief for these families (Kissane et al., 2016).

In most non-academic palliative care settings, the clinicians providing psychological intervention need to determine which approaches are appropriate each time they meet with family caregivers. The sessions often blend assessment, pragmatic education, and deeper family therapy intervention that can address recent or long-standing conflict. The family meeting, described in the following, can be considered a valuable tool for providing psychosocial interventions to family caregivers.

THE FAMILY MEETING

The family meeting, also known as "family conference" and "patient-family conference," is commonly used in the health-care system to review and discuss the patient's illness, the medical treatment, and overall care (Fineberg, Kawashima & Asch, 2011). It also offers the opportunity to explore preferences and cultural values impacting on decision-making, to engage in collaborative planning, and to provide emotional support (Joshi, 2013). For these reasons, the family meeting can be considered an intervention for supporting family caregivers.

A family meeting can take place in the hospital, in an outpatient setting, or in the patient's home if home-based palliative care or hospice care is being provided. It usually includes the family, or other caregivers who have legal rights to make decisions for health care. The patient's participation depends on their physical and cognitive condition. One of the key elements is ensuring participation of clinicians who are directly involved in the care of the patient so their input and insight can help the conversation evolve in productive ways. The number of clinicians present at the meeting should not be overwhelming for the family, however, as this may be intimidating.

Palliative psychologists with training in family therapy will appreciate the value and complexity of bringing people together for delineating a coherent and reasonable plan that not only makes sense from a medical standpoint but also respects patients and families' preferences. This is particularly challenging when there are different goals and expectations (Lum & Sudore, 2016).

The family meeting has several functions, which are often intertwined (Table 4.4). A family meeting has a *pragmatic function* when medical information is communicated and options are described (e.g., test results, updates on treatment, treatment options). It also has an *emotional function*, because it allows the patient and the

Table 4.4 **Functions of the Family Meeting in Palliative Care**

Pragmatic Function	Emotional Function	Process-Oriented Function	Assessment Function
Share information about diagnosis and prognosis; discuss treatment options; discuss treatment updates	Facilitate expression of emotions; safely contain affect; normalize and support; manage conflict within the family and between the family and treating team	Discuss advance care planning; explore ethical issues; facilitate communication; redirect focus on plan	Assess coping skills; assess family communication and decision-making process; assess severity of grief reactions

family to safely express distressing emotions and receive support from the team (e.g., when receiving serious or bad news). The meeting allows for a longer exchange with the family, which enables clinicians to assess coping skills and immediate needs, the *assessment function*. The meeting can also have a *process-oriented function* when complex decisions and plans must be addressed and finalized. As an example, advanced care planning discussions, safe discharge planning, or ethical discussions involve not only the delivery of information and expression of emotions, but also the development of a plan based on complex information. And, it may be necessary to address difficult family dynamics with conflict among family members about the care the patient is receiving.

The family meeting can involve an important opportunity for assessment of the patient and family coping skills, communication style, and grieving style. While the family meeting is not family therapy, the framework of single-session therapy has been used as a helpful tool in the development of guidelines for successful family meetings (Hudson et al., 2008; Hudson et al., 2009). In summary, the family meeting can accomplish the complex task of facilitating communication between the medical team, the family, and patient. It can help strengthen the alliance between the medical team and the family by providing an opportunity to discuss the patient's medical condition, developing a plan of care, and facilitating decision making. It is important to note that while the value of family meetings is generally recognized to improve psychological distress in family caregivers by providing them with needed information and support (Reed & Harding, 2015; Sullivan, da Rosa Silva, & Meeker, 2015), the evidence of benefit is limited by the small number of quality studies. Additionally, the evidence of benefit in intensive care unit (ICU) populations is inconsistent, with most studies indicating evidence of benefits, and one study indicating no benefit and perhaps even worsening of distress in family members (Carson et al., 2016). Future research should focus on identifying specific models and approaches to family meetings that can meet the needs of different populations. Nonetheless, family meetings are a common intervention in palliative care, and palliative psychologists can be instrumental in improving their clinical effectiveness.

Structure of the Family Meeting

Family meetings are considered structured interventions, and guidelines for their effective planning and execution have been developed (Hudson et al., 2008; Gritti, 2015). The main components are pre-meeting, meeting, and follow-up (Table 4.5). Respecting the structure and preparing for the meeting is important; however, it may be challenging if rapid changes in the patient's condition require urgent conversations with family members.

The *pre-meeting* allows clinicians to prepare context and strategy before meeting with the patients and the family. Depending on the purpose of the meeting, preparation may include reviewing the necessary medical and psychosocial information, reviewing the information to be shared with the family, and identifying the facilitator and the agenda for the meeting. The type of information that will be shared and the agenda may

Table 4.5 **Structure of the Family Meeting**

Before the Meeting	During the Meeting	Follow-Up
Identify the purpose of the meeting (e.g., discussing test results)	Allow participants to introduce themselves	Plan individual or family meetings for support if needed
Be aware of any family conflict or complex dynamics that may complicate outcome of the meeting	Sit in circle if possible and avoid seating arrangements that may convey a family versus team message	Debrief meeting with team members
Review relevant medical and psychosocial information about the case	Discuss purpose and goal of the meeting and check for agreement from participants	Maintain ongoing communication with family members about the plan
Determine what is the main goal of the meeting (e.g., come to an agreement about treatment)	Convey information using clear and simple language	Communicate with other team members about plan
Determine who will lead the meeting	Check for understanding from family members	Identify and address any indication that family caregivers may no longer be in agreement with the plan
Resolve any disagreements among clincians about patient care before the meeting	Allow for expression of emotions and affect and attend to nonverbal communication	
	Close the meeting with agreed-upon plan and clarify steps going forward	

determine who should facilitate a meeting. If the goal of the meeting is to review medical information about diagnosis and treatment, a physician or a nurse will generally lead the meeting. If the nature of the meeting is psychological or psychosocial, the facilitator can be a social worker, a psychologist, or a chaplain. However, if the family feels particularly comfortable with the psychologist or the social worker, he or she may facilitate the meeting, even though the agenda may be primarily medical. It is important that family caregivers feel as comfortable as possible during the meeting; a facilitator who has good rapport with the family can help communication and de-escalate emotions if conflict arises.

It is important to have obtained an interdisciplinary perspective on the patient and the family. Knowledge of a family-preferred communication style can allow clinicians to promote a smoother meeting. Additionally, any information about psychiatric illness in any of the family caregivers or the patient should be reviewed and considered for possible impact on the meeting's outcome.

Any disagreement among medical providers about the patient's prognosis or about the appropriate treatment options and medical plan should be clarified during the preparation phase, avoiding confusion for the family. The goals identified for the meeting need to be realistic and accomplishable within the amount of time allocated for the meeting, which is generally not more than one hour. If the goal of the meeting is communicating information that is likely to generate distress (e.g., that disease has continued to worsen despite treatment), it is important to recognize that allowing the patient and the family to absorb and process the information may be the only goal accomplished. If the patient is an adult able to make decisions and his or her level of function allows, he or she will be present at the meeting and may decide which family members should participate. Family members who have legal rights to make decisions as health-care proxy agents or surrogates should also attend.

The meeting. At the beginning of the actual meeting, the facilitator will introduce the purpose of the meeting and introduce participants. The agenda for the meeting should be stated clearly and in simple language, and the facilitator should ensure that the participants are all in agreement with the purpose. For example, the facilitator may say, "We are meeting today to discuss the results of the recent scan. Does everyone agree this is the purpose of this meeting?" The tone should convey respect, but the language used should be simple and convey that the clinicians are approachable and empathetic. The clinicians should also speak slowly and ensure that everyone can hear well and understand. It is important to avoid medical jargon and avoid overloading the patient and the family with information.

Delivering serious or bad news (e.g., cancer diagnosis, recurrence of disease, lack of effectiveness of treatment) is recognized as one of the most challenging tasks for health-care professionals. The acronym SPIKES (Baile et al., 2000; Kaplan, 2010) is a communication protocol for facilitating these difficult discussions. Initially developed for the oncology setting, it is applicable to any clinical situation requiring communication of medical facts that are likely to cause distress for the patient and the family. Briefly, S stands for *Setting up the interview*; P stands for *Perception*; I stands for *Invitation*; K stands for *Knowledge*; E stands for *Empathy*; and S stands for *Summarize*. These step-wise recommendations have been developed specifically for physicians and other providers who do not routinely receive training in psychotherapy.

Setting up the interview involves ensuring that the meeting will be conducted in a private area, with chairs, and availability of tissues for family members. Additionally, the physician is encouraged to silence his or her phones and pagers or switch them to a vibrate mode. *Perception* involves starting the meeting by asking the patient and/or the family what is their current understanding of the medical situation overall, including diagnosis and prognosis. *Invitation* involves asking the patient how much information he or she would like to receive about the results of the test. *Knowledge* involves providing the information to the patient simply and directly, avoiding complex medical jargon. This is followed by *empathy*, allowing the patient and family to react to the difficult news. During *summary*, the physician can discuss available options and strategies moving forward.

Managing a family meeting is a complex task requiring excellent communication skills from the palliative care team. It involves not only the ability to convey medical information and discuss medical options but also the management of expectations, affect, worldview, fears, all in the context of the need to develop a care plan and facilitate decisions regarding next steps. Even after all the necessary planning has taken place, the family meeting contains several elements of unpredictability. Family caregivers may react negatively to the sharing of bad news and refuse to discuss any options. Family conflict previously latent may be activated by the stress elicited by the information shared.

Psychologists' training and expertise conducting therapy with individuals and families will allow them to offer unique contributions to planning and conducting a family meeting. Their expertise managing complex communication in challenging clinical scenarios can be especially helpful in supporting patients and/or family caregivers who have become overwhelmed during the meeting. Receiving bad news or discussing difficult topics (e.g., advanced directives) can trigger severe grief reactions ranging from disengagement and numbness to anger, despair, or overt antagonism toward the team or to the complete inability to process the information. To illustrate, after receiving news that treatment is not effective and should be discontinued (e.g., "I am very sorry to have to tell you this, but the MRI showed that the chemotherapy does not seem to be working as we had hoped"), the family may react with distress and may doubt the validity of the medical conclusions and recommendations. A failure to recognize these reactions and the grief that often underlies anger may generate stress and resentment in the medical provider and promote antagonism towards the family.

Palliative psychologists can have an important role in educating staff about grief reactions and recognizing grief when it is not expressed through sadness but through anger. This is vital to preserving a critical alliance between the patient, the team, and all clinicians, at a time when the patient and the family are most vulnerable and in need of support.

A *follow-up* plan about what will be the next step should end the meeting. This could be a simple statement: for example, "We recognize that what we discussed today was very difficult. It takes some time to adjust and for all of you to process as a family. Would it be ok to meet again tomorrow discuss any questions you may have?" If the patient is hospitalized and the family distressed, it may be appropriate to offer a meeting the same day with the psychologist, the clinical social worker, or chaplain to facilitate processing of information and emotions.

CASE VIGNETTE 4.1

Malcolm is a 69-year-old man with advanced COPD, admitted to the hospital with severe shortness of breath. The patient also suffers from recurrent depression, and symptoms have been managed on medication. He has been living independently and has been able to manage his daily routines receiving four hours of home care three days a week. He is divorced, currently single, and has two adult children who live in the area. The patient assumed he would be able to return home after receiving care at the hospital. Unfortunately, his condition begins to quickly deteriorate after admission, changing discharge plans. A family meeting is called with the attending hospitalist, the consulting pulmonologist, the palliative care physician and psychologist, the patient, and the patient's family. The medical team shares the bad news of the worsening condition and explains that the patient's needs for home care have increased significantly. The patient comments that he understands his condition and asks his son to help him receive more hours of home care. The children explain they have full-time jobs and cannot assist him, and they are concerned about their father returning to his apartment. One of the children mentions that his father could be transferred to a skilled nursing facility near his home so that it would be easier for them to visit regularly. Malcolm remains silent for most of the meeting but becomes agitated when the nursing home is mentioned. He begins crying, saying he just wants to die. He accuses his children of not caring about him and the doctors of just wanting to "discard" him "like a bag of garbage." The team reassures the patient that he is the only one in charge of making decisions about his life and his future. The psychologist reflects that the change in the patient's condition is difficult news, and it is normal that it will generate anxiety and even distress. She comments that it is understandable for the children to suggest solutions that can ensure safety for the patient. She adds that it is important to slow things down and fully understand what Malcolm thinks and wants. The meeting continues and the skilled nursing facility is not mentioned again. The patient's son feels mortified about causing distress for his father. The psychologist asks him to express these feelings directly to his father. For about ten minutes the meeting focuses on repairing the fracture between father and son. The patient is then invited to explain what living independently means to him and what he values most. At the end of the meeting, the psychologist summarizes that three important aspects have emerged from the meeting. First, and most important, is the medical information about the patient's health. Though distressing, this information cannot be ignored. Second, it is important to preserve the patient's independence and his decision-making ability. Third, she acknowledges the commitment and love of the children. She also comments that the situation would be challenging for any family and that the team is committed to supporting them.

Despite the challenges, the meeting ended on a positive note. It was decided that the social worker and psychologist would work together to ensure the discharge plan home was physically and emotionally safe for the patient. Additionally, the children agreed to create a schedule so their visits would not overlap and they could maximize the time each of them spent with their father. Developing and implementing the plan required significant interdisciplinary work, but ensured that the patient's preferences were respected and his well-being preserved.

As illustrated in this case, patients used to living independently with some assistance can become distressed by the transition to a different living situation. A transfer to a facility may trigger profound grief reactions, fear of abandonment, and anger at family members and medical providers. Thus, the family meeting can represent an important opportunity to explore the options that are available, in the best interest of the patient.

Bereavement Care for Family Caregivers

As the different aspects of grief—cultural, psychological, social, and spiritual—are interconnected, attention to the grieving process is relevant in all eight domains of palliative care. This section continues the discussion about grief (see chapter 3) by focusing on family caregivers' grieving process *after* the death of the patient, known as bereavement.

For many family caregivers, grieving is a process that begins at the time of diagnosis and continues, with variations and fluctuations, throughout treatment, transitions of care, during the dying process, and in bereavement. Providing continuity of care by ensuring access to competent psychological support is critical, because bereavement carries a high risk for long-term distress and morbidity.

The understanding and conceptualization of bereavement has evolved significantly. From an early emphasis on identifying and promoting conventional, or "healthy" grieving, the focus of current models has shifted toward an appreciation of the grieving process as uniquely personal for each individual and thus also unpredictable with regards to "symptoms" and duration (see also Strada, 2013, for a review) For many, the normal grieving process also involves a fluctuation between moments of engagement in life-enhancing activities and moments characterized by great distress. After the patient's death, the importance of maintaining an emotional connection with the memory and sense of presence of the deceased has also been recognized as supportive. Thus, bereavement care should support the individual's unique and personal grieving process, ensuring safety, but without a preconceived notion of how that process should present or develop.

With this new appreciation of the personal, unique, and unpredictable nature of grief reactions palliative psychologists should focus on identifying risk factors for developing bereavement complications, such as bereavement-related depression and complicated grief. This is particularly relevant for palliative care and hospice programs, because early identification of risk factors can facilitate access to psychological support and community referrals.

CLINICAL FEATURES AND OUTCOMES OF NORMAL BEREAVEMENT

Normal bereavement involves a grieving process of variable duration and intensity. Even in its normal presentation, it can be associated with severe physical, psychological, and spiritual distress and negative health outcomes. Physical manifestations of loss may include shortness of breath, feelings of emptiness and heaviness, physical numbness, headaches, dizziness, nausea, gastrointestinal problems, and heart palpitations. There can be an increased risk for hypertension, atrial fibrillation, acute cardiovascular events, and overall reduction in quality of life (Carey et al., 2014; Graff et al., 2016). The risk of death following partner bereavement also increases, especially within three months of the death (King, Lodwick, Jones, Whitaker & Petersen, 2017).

Several manifestations of bereavement can resemble depression, panic attack, or generalized anxiety disorder. There may be crying spells, fatigue, disturbances in sleeping and eating patterns, anorexia and weight loss, or weight gain. Spouses who were also the patient's primary caregiver represent a vulnerable population in bereavement. While bereavement can increase the risk of major depression, studies have indicated that depressive symptoms are common after spousal bereavement and can negatively affect quality of life even if their severity does not meet criteria for major depression (Grassi, 2007).

Normal bereavement can also include transient visual and auditory hallucinations, impaired short-term memory, constant worry, slowed and disorganized thinking, and passive suicidal ideation, and constantly thinking about the deceased. The content of visual or auditory hallucination may be focused on difficult circumstances surrounding the death, or on unresolved relationship issues that may elicit guilt, anger, or shame. While bereavement may deepen one's connection with a faith or spiritual community, it may also trigger conflicts in faith beliefs or loss of meaning and purpose.

In normal bereavement, the severity of distress fluctuates and subsides over time allowing for adjustment. With adequate psychosocial and spiritual support most bereaved caregivers can slowly integrate the pain of loss, maintain or regain ability to function adequately for their life demands, and maintain acceptable physical and emotional health. Adaptation is an ongoing process involving a variable and unpredictable amount of time. Some family caregivers experience severe distress immediately after the death. Others become focused on practical tasks necessary for continuation of family routines. This is often the case for parents of children or teenagers who have lost a spouse. They may suppress the intensity of their grief in order to return to work and continue supporting their children. And yet, the daily demands of work and parenting can become overwhelming, especially when social and practical support is lacking.

COMPLICATIONS OF BEREAVEMENT

Complicated Grief

Even though most bereaved caregivers can slowly adjust to the death of a loved one after a variable period of time, 15%–25% continue experiencing persistent reactions and psychiatric symptoms that are disabling and non-adaptive, causing unremitting suffering and a significant impairment in their level of functioning. Based on a large body of research, complicated grief and prolonged grief disorder were both proposed for inclusion as formal diagnoses in the *Diagnostic and Statistical Manual of Mental Disorders* (5th edition). The DSM Task Force concluded that insufficient evidence exists to support inclusion. Instead, Persistent Complex Bereavement Disorder (PCBD) was included as a condition warranting further study. The criteria of PCBD include features of complicated grief and prolonged grief disorder that should be used for research purposes. *Complicated grief* and, less frequently, *prolonged grief disorder* remain terms that are commonly used in the palliative care and hospice setting.

Complicated grief indicates a pathological process that can occur in adults and also children, caused by grief that is not effectively processed and integrated by the bereaved (Bryant, 2013; Melhem et al., 2013; Shear, Ghesquiere, & Glickman, 2013). As a result, the distressing symptoms continue to cause severe and disabling impairment long after the loss has occurred. For instance, grief-related panic symtpoms are prevalent (Bui et al., 2015). Additionally, the presence of maladaptive cognitions about the loss and the grieving process continue to interfere with the griever's ability to integrate the loss (Skritskaya et al., 2017). Furthermore, complicated grief is also associated with a significant increase in suicidal ideation and behavior (Baker et al., 2016).

Psychological interventions that include exposure to the memories of the death have shown to be more effective than modalities that do not incorporate exposure (Bryant et al., 2017). Complicated grief therapy (CGT) is an individual and group, evidence-based psychological treatment for complicated grief, supported by several trials and adapted for different patient populations, including bereaved caregivers of patients with dementia (Glickman, Shear & Wall, 2016; Shear, 2015; Supiano, Haynes, & Pond, 2017). This intervention includes psychoeducation, imaginal, and in-vivo exposure, Gestalt techniques, and homework assignments to target traumatic memories and negative cognitions while also promoting development of positive life goals. A randomized controlled study has indicated that antidepressants can be used in conjunction with CGT to address comorbid depression, with overall improved outcome (Bui, Nadal-Vicens & Simon, 2012; Shah et al., 2013; Shear et al., 2016).

Research is now beginning to compare the effectiveness of the three sets of diagnostic criteria (complicated grief, prolonged grief disorder, and persistent complex bereavement disorder) in clinical and community settings to identify which performs best (Friedman, 2016). It has been argued that while PCBD is essentially the same as prolonged grief disorder (Maciejewski et al., 2016), the name PCBD should be changed because it does not reference a clinical entity (grief), but only an event (bereavement). Additionally, while PCBD criteria are effective in excluding normal grief, there may be indications that they do not perform as well in identifying clinical cases, where criteria for complicated grief are superior (Cozza et al., 2016). Even though complicated grief continues to be used by most clinicians in palliative care and hospice, the issue of criteria and identification of risk factors will continue to be relevant. Palliative psychologists should be familiar with this literature and developments in the field.

Bereavement-Related Depression

Major depression can become a complication of bereavement, but it may also predate it. Family caregivers who develop depression during the period of caregiving often do not seek support, and thus remain undiagnosed. In bereavement, they may continue experiencing preexisting depression in addition to acute grief. Others may develop depression in the context of bereavement. Considering the similarity between bereavement-related depression and depression developing in the context of other stressors, the DSM-5 has eliminated the bereavement exclusion criterion from the diagnostic criteria of the major depressive episode. This change implies that an individual who is recently bereaved can also be diagnosed with major depression without the need to wait two months (Pies, 2014). Some have objected to this change, arguing that it may lead to over-diagnosing depression and the medicalization of grief, resulting in over-prescribing psychotropic medication.

Differentiating depression from bereavement in acute grief can indeed be challenging because of symptom overlap. In normal bereavement, the individual generally maintains some ability to emotionally connect with others and receive support; suicidal ideation is rare and, when present, it is focused on joining the loved one; the pain of loss is generally mixed with good memories about the relationship; grief is often experienced as moments of profound distress, alternating with the ability to feel connection to others. While normal grief is characterized by mood fluctuation with ability to experience positive emotions, clinical depression often presents with nearly constantly depressed mood that often does not respond to emotional support. Additionally, while basic self-esteem is generally maintained in grief, clinical depression is often characterized by a sense of profound worthlessness and guilt (Table 4.6).

Table 4.6 **Difference Between Grief in Normal Bereavement and Depression**

Clinical Presentation	Grief	Depression
Predominant affect	Feelings of emptiness and loss	Persistent depressed mood; inability to anticipate happiness or pleasure
Nature of distress	Likely to decrease in intensity over the weeks and months; occurs in waves (pangs of grief); associated with thoughts or reminders of the deceased	More persistent; not tied to specific thoughts or preoccupations
Duration	Fluctuates; decreases in intensity over time	More persistent
Presence of positive emotions	Positive emotions and humor can be present.	Unhappiness and misery are pervasive.
Thought content	Preoccupation with thoughts and memories of the deceased	Self-critical or pessimistic rumination
Self-esteem	Generally preserved	Feelings of worthlessness and self-loathing are common.
Self-derogatory ideation	Feelings of having failed the deceased by not visiting frequently enough, or by not expressing enough love to the deceased	Pervasive feelings of worthlessness, or excessive, or inappropriate guilt
Thoughts of death and dying	Perceived as a way of joining the deceased or escaping the pain of loss	Death is wished as a result of feeling worthless, undeserving, or unable to cope.

The focus on avoiding a medicalization of grief should not prevent the recognition and treatment of depression, a psychiatric disorder. Normalizing a pathological process that creates suffering for the bereaved and even increases risk of suicide would indicate substandard care. Furthermore, the fear of medicalization is grounded in concerns that a diagnosis of depression will result in over-prescription of antidepressants. The key issue appears to be the clinician's competence in recognizing the difference between grief and depression and determining the most effective and least burdensome treatment approach.

RISK AND PROTECTIVE FACTORS FOR COMPLICATIONS OF BEREAVEMENT

A family caregiver's grieving process during bereavement is facilitated or hindered by several factors. Facilitating *self-perceived preparedness for the death* of a family member can have an important protective factor. A study that investigated bereavement outcomes among family caregivers indicated that those who perceived being more prepared for the death showed better adjustment to the bereavement process (Kim et al., 2017). Overall however, many family members continued to display high levels of bereavement-related distress several years after the death of the patient.

The *patient's age and developmental stage* will also impact on the grieving process. A study exploring the relationship between caregiving, the age of the patient, and bereavement indicated that family caregivers who cared for middle-aged patients ages 40–59 were at increased risk for severe grief reactions and depression. On the other hand, family caregivers of patients between the ages of 60 and 79 more often appeared to experience relief (Francis et al., 2016).

Traumatic distress, separation distress, and severe emotional grief symptoms before the death were significantly associated with the presence of complicated grief in a group of Italian family caregivers of terminally ill patients admitted to hospice (Nanni, Biancospino & Grassi, 2014). Traumatic distress may be present also in the absence of complicated grief. To illustrate, bereaved caregivers who have experienced traumatic events during the loved one's death may experience intrusive memories, presenting a clinical picture that has been described as the "shocked caregiver" (Sanderson et al., 2013).

Acting as a surrogate decision-maker for a patient at the end of life has an impact on caregivers' bereavement (Tinetti et al., 2016; Turan et al., 2011). In one study, caregivers who made end-of-life decisions that focused on prolonging the patient's survival, rather than comfort, experienced significantly higher levels of guilt and complicated grief (Lovell, Smith, & Kannis-Dymand, 2015).

Pessimistic attitudes and *stressful life events*, in addition to the illness of a loved one, were significantly associated with complicated grief. Additionally, *lack of social support* and *current of history of depression* were also significantly associated with complicated grief (Tomarken et al., 2008). In a longitudinal study of 301 family caregivers, measures of their psychological distress were collected at initial contact with the palliative care team and were then collected again six months after the death of the patient and at 13 months (Thomas et al., 2014). Despite attrition (end $n = 143$), results indicated that symptoms of prolonged grief at initial contact with palliative care were strong predictors of prolonged grief after the loss. In particular, *poor family functioning, low levels of optimism, being a spouse to the patient,* and *strong impact of caregiving* on their life activities were strong predictors of complicated grief.

The presence of depressive symptoms in family caregivers before the death of the patient and after 1 month, 3 months, 6 months, and 13 months was explored in 186 family caregivers in Taiwan (Ling et al., 2013). Results indicated that depressive symptoms were more significant 1 month after the death and became less prominent in the course of the first 13 months after the death. Additionally, higher levels of depressive symptoms were present in caregivers who had cared for a spouse, had more health problems, and had experienced *more depressive symptoms prior to the patient's death*. Conversely, patients who had cared for older patients and had more social support prior to the patient's death reported lower levels of depressive symptoms.

Four trajectories of depressive symptoms were described in a study of 447 caregivers. Symptoms were explored at four different points in time before the patient's death and later than 180 days after the death (Tang et al., 2013). The four trajectories were

- endurance
- resilience
- moderately symptomatic
- chronically distressed.

Weaker psychological resources characterized caregivers in the moderately symptomatic and chronically distressed trajectory. The endurance trajectory included caregivers who had less education and provided care to older patients with higher symptom distress; however, they had adequate financial support and adequate psychological resources to cope with their caregiving role. Those in the resilience trajectory faced more challenges in terms of caring for a younger patient, had fewer psychological resources, and they were more likely to be the patient's spouse. However, they were older and perceived less distress in their role.

The prevalence of complicated grief symptoms was also studied in a group of 152 spouses and adult children caring for a patient with lung cancer (Kramer et al., 2010). Caregivers with lower education levels who cared for a patient with higher fear of death and difficulty accepting the illness, as well as higher levels of family conflicts near the end of life, were associated with higher levels of complicated grief. In this study, hospice care had a positive impact on caregivers' bereavement process.

Other studies have indicated that receiving hospice care may be a protective factor for caregivers and is associated with a modest reduction of depressive symptoms (Ornstein et al., 2015). A study of family caregivers of patients who died with advanced colorectal cancer explored their perception about quality of end-of-life care comparing those who enrolled in hospice and those who did not. Family caregivers enrolled in hospice reported higher quality of end-of-life care, better symptom control, and more respect for patients' wishes (Kumar et al., 2016).

In summary, the quality of support family caregivers receive during the patient's illness and in end of life can improve their experience not only during caregiving but also in bereavement, thus mitigating the likelihood of complications (Box 4.2).

> *Box 4.2* **Protective Factors in Bereavement for Family Caregivers**
> - perception of being prepared for the death of the patient
> - receiving adequate training, information, and psychoeducation during caregiving
> - receiving hospice care
> - optimism and positive emotions
> - social support

The Spectrum of Bereavement Support

Bereavement care through hospice. Hospice provides specialist palliative care to patients with advanced illness whose life expectancy is about six months or less. It also provides bereavement care for family caregivers and others who were closely involved in caring for the patient. According to Medicare regulations, hospice programs are required to provide bereavement care to any family member or relative of a patient who died on the hospice program. This bereavement support is required to be continued for up to 13 months after the death of the patient.

Continuity of support can allow hospice clinicians to identify family members who subsequently develop depression or complicated grief. Predicting the course of bereavement for a family caregiver is challenging because grieving is unique and the intensity of distress may be unexpected or surprising. For this reason, it is important to screen family caregivers for caregiver burden, depression, and severe anxiety at initial contact with the palliative care team or hospice team. Screening should be repeated regularly and especially after specific stressors. A cross-sectional survey explored psychosocial services provided by 591 hospice programs. The goal of this study was to gather information about whether hospice program screened for depression or complicated grief at the time of death or provided access to bereavement therapy for depression and complicated grief. Results indicated that only 55% of hospice programs screened for complicated grief and depression and provided access to bereavement grief therapy (Ghesquiere et al., 2015).

There is significant variability among hospice programs in terms of quality, intensity, and availability of bereavement support. The Medicare requirement of 13 months of bereavement support is often accomplished by a combination of short-term counseling, phone support, support groups, memorial services, and workshops and lectures designed to provide general psychoeducation and support related to the grieving process. Some hospice programs provide both individual counseling and support groups. Others only provide support groups tailored to different types of loss (e.g., spousal, parental, and child loss). Some programs use primarily licensed mental health and spiritual professionals such as clinical psychologists, licensed clinical social workers, and board certified chaplains. Others may rely primarily on volunteers who have previously been recipients of hospice care for a family member and are now committed to helping others during the grieving process. Thus, the ability to recognize risk factors or presence of psychopathology and the ability to provide adequate psychological interventions depends on the training and skill level of hospice bereavement counselors and psychosocial clinicians. For this reason, bereaved family caregivers with major depression or symptoms of complicated grief are often referred to mental health professionals in the community for long-term treatment. The key is ensuring that hospice clinicians have the skills to recognize the development of a pathological grieving process and to ensure appropriate care. This identifies a clear role for palliative psychologists as educators and clinical supervisors, as well as providers of treatment when indicated.

Bereavement care through palliative care services. Bereavement care coordination is especially important if the patient received palliative care and died in the hospital but was not enrolled in a hospice program. In this case, family caregivers will not automatically receive bereavement outreach from hospice. It may also not be feasible for them to receive bereavement care from the palliative care team. To address these limitations, palliative care programs can prepare a list of community resources for grief and bereavement support and make it available to bereaved family caregivers. Palliative care programs can also partner with hospice programs that offer bereavement support to members of the community (Table 4.7).

DEVELOPING A BEREAVEMENT PLAN OF CARE FOR FAMILY CAREGIVERS

Palliative psychologists can have important roles in providing bereavement care in palliative care and hospice settings. Psychological interventions for supporting the grieving process are on a continuum based on intensity and severity of the distress. These interventions include supportive psychoeducation, counseling, and psychotherapy. The ability to provide the bereaved with the level of support that is adequate for their needs is an important competence.

Normalizing the grieving process by clarifying misconceptions and unsupportive beliefs about the grieving process can help family caregivers understand their own

Table 4.7 **Bereavement Care for Family Caregivers**

Patient Enrolled in Hospice	Patient Not Enrolled in Hospice
Hospice provides up to 13 months of individualized bereavement support.	The palliative care team should provide referrals to community resources for bereavement support.
Each family member receives a comprehensive bereavement assessment and a plan of care is formulated.	Family members in need of support should be referred before the death of the patient to facilitate coordination of care.
There is great variability among hospice programs in terms of quality, intensity, and availability of bereavement support.	The palliative care team should conduct ongoing assessment of grief reactions to identify needs and risk factors for complications of bereavement.

grieving process. Even in normal grief, some wonder if they are "grieving the right way," "the healthy way," whether the distress they are experiencing is normal, or whether their apparent lack of distress is normal. These bereaved caregivers need to be reassured their reactions are not pathological or dysfunctional. Many who rely on family members and their social network for support may not need to receive deeper psychological support in addition to psychoeducation.

As an example, a 45-year-old man working in the military began experiencing memory loss, difficulty concentrating, difficulty making decisions and recurrent gastrointestinal problems after the death of his wife, who died only five months after being diagnosed with metastatic lung cancer. For the first time in his life, he was experiencing a loss of control that felt confusing and threatening. After being reassured by his physician that there were no medical problems causing his symptoms, he contacted the palliative psychologist who had provided therapy to his wife in the last months of illness. Two sessions of psychoeducation two weeks apart provided normalization and a context for his "symptoms," as well as a general "road map" about the grieving process. He returned monthly for a check-in session to discuss his adaptation process. Describing himself as a pragmatic man focused on completing tasks assigned to him, he was concerned about "completing this grief work the right way" and felt the sessions helped him to be "less strict." Accepting the fluctuations and unpredictability of the grieving process allowed integration of the loss to occur naturally over time. This approach proved important in the relationship with his teenage son, who had started exhibiting disruptive behavior in school and benefited from receiving psychoeducation about grief from his father. The adequate amount and type of supportive education allowed this grieving widower to feel supported and to become more effective as a parent.

The following treatment aspects should be taken into consideration when working with a bereaved family member in any setting.

Meeting the bereaved caregivers where they are emotionally. It is important to suspend any preconceived notions about how people will navigate the grieving process and be prepared for a variety of different presentations, behaviors, and goals. A bereaved family caregiver may grieve openly with crying spells and anxiety and may wish to talk about the patient's death directly. Another may present with lack of overt affect, focused on practical tasks that need to be completed. They may discuss the circumstances of the death in a factual manner and wonder out loud why they reached out to the therapist in the first place. When supporting normal grief, it is important to follow the family caregiver's lead and adapt to his or her style. Some caregivers will benefit from delineating a plan after the first session; others would feel uncomfortable with the idea of "goals" and prefer a free-flowing session.

Providing supportive psycho-education as needed. When bereaved caregivers explain feeling overwhelmed, it is helpful to note that the grieving process can affect every thought and emotion; it may sometimes seem as if their mind does not have space for anything other than the pain of grief. It is also beneficial to discuss the range and uniqueness of grief reactions and clarify unsupportive beliefs (e.g., I am not grieving the right way, I should not be feeling these emotions, I should not be thinking these thoughts, etc.). By listening carefully to the caregiver's experience, normalizing and explaining that many experience similar distress when grieving, the therapist can help diffuse the sense of isolation. It can also be helpful to acknowledge that although grief is normal, it does not feel normal, and it is only natural to have concerns about what one is experiencing. Importantly, psychoeducation about the range of expected responses in grieving should focus on the areas described as significant by the caregiver to avoid overwhelming with information with long descriptions of all the possible manifestations.

For instance, if a bereaved caregiver reports difficulty with short-term memory, it is useful to clarify that this can be, though unwelcome, a normal component of bereavement. It may be important to explain that tasks performed without any difficulty previously, such as reading a book, may now require special effort and make it necessary to read the same page several times. If the bereaved is feeling distressed by losing objects more frequently or having difficulty remembering appointments, it can be helpful to suggest practical strategies for managing the daily demands, including creating lists and setting reminders. At the core of bereavement support for normal grief is helping the bereaved cope with the emotional and practical demands imposed by the loss of a loved one.

Identifying co-morbid medical and psychiatric conditions. The psychologist's assessment of the caregivers' resources, coping skills, severity of distress and risk level for complications of bereavement should be ongoing, even if the grieving process appears normal. This is especially important when bereaved caregivers are older, socially isolated, or have a history of psychiatric illness. Every assessment is valid at the point in time when it is performed, and there is no guarantee that it will not change. Thus, sudden health crises or unexpected psychosocial stressors may intensify grief reactions and cause the distress to become unmanageable. Family caregivers described by the palliative care or hospice team as "prepared for the death" may begin experiencing significant distress several months after the loss and become overwhelmed by it.

In case of complicated grief or bereavement-related depression an integrative treatment approach should be followed to maximize outcome. For moderate to severe depression, it may appropriate to refer the patient for a medication evaluation in addition to psychotherapy treatment. Developing a collaborative approach with primary care physicians involved in the care will ensure that needs are addressed in a comprehensive manner. If the bereaved caregiver reports that sleep is persistently disrupted, it is important to explain that adequate rest is necessary to support the grieving process. Teaching relaxation and self-hypnosis techniques can lead to improvement, but the bereaved should also be encouraged to visit a primary care physician. Similarly, if they report using maladaptive strategies to disconnect from the pain of grief, such as binging on alcohol, using drugs, or taking more of certain prescribed medication such as opioids or benzodiazepines, the primary care physician or the specialist prescribing medication should be involved in the bereavement care plan. After referring a bereaved caregiver to a primary care physician, the therapist should follow up to ensure coordination of care. Bereaved caregivers often resist the suggestion to visit their physician due to lack of physical and emotional energy, lack of motivation, and fear that their emotional pain will not be understood.

Identifying protective factors and sources of strength. The grieving process is best approached from a strength-based perspective. It is important to focus on identifying individual and family strengths that can support adjustment and promote healing. Because of the intense pain of grief, family caregivers may temporarily lose their connection with the unique strengths and resources they have developed and have normally accessed. Therefore, an important function of grief support is helping the bereaved "remember" and reconnect with these important sources of support. For instance, a family may have developed a style of communication that is particularly supportive of each member, optimism, a good sense of humor, or the capacity to allow family members to be vulnerable without negative judgment. These qualities can support the family during bereavement and can facilitate normal grieving.

Importantly, the presence of strengths can promote hope, but it certainly does not reduce the pain of grief. Highlighting individual and family strengths should be done tactfully to avoid conveying the impression that the challenges and distress in the grieving process are being minimized.

Helping the caregiver identify needs and personal style in grieving. Grief support needs to be consistent with the caregiver's culture, values, and belief system. At the same time, it should help the caregiver recognize their needs and developing strategies accordingly. When personal needs and cultural expectations clash, most caregivers appreciate help finding a balance without alienating their community.

CASE VIGNETTE 4.2

Rose and Jim were referred for psychological support during Jim's admission to an inpatient palliative care unit for pain from metastatic colorectal cancer. They were both in their early sixties and had been married for 12 years. When the psychologist approached the couple in their hospital room, they both greeted her politely but stated that they were focused on spending every moment together and did not need additional support. Jim died two weeks after admission, and Rose began seeing the psychologist weekly for bereavement support.

Immediately after his death she experienced several physical manifestations of grief: anxiety, pains and aches throughout her body, memory impairment, and severe GI distress. She received psychoeducation about grief, and the psychologist also recommended making an appointment with her primary care physician for a physical examination. The physician ruled out any physical concerns and prescribed a short-acting benzodiazepine for symptomatic relief. However, Rose felt that simply knowing her symtpoms were the result of anxiety and grief would help her cope. Additionally, she was a strong believer in complementary approaches and chose to not take the medication. The therapy sessions became focused on practicing self-hypnosis to decrease anxiety, which Rose found beneficial. Specific strategies for managing exacerbations of anxiety were discussed and practiced. An art therapy approach was used to facilitate the creation of a "healing journal" that comprised all the psychological techniques and practices that Rose was learning. She also began drawing mandalas to express the different emotions of her grieving process.

As Rose's symptoms of acute grief subsided, she started talking about Jim and reviewing the positive aspects of the relationship. Her memories were all positive, and she emphatically described her life with Jim as "a movie." At every session she became focused on emphasizing her husband had been her "soulmate" and "the perfect husband." Rose also made frequent positive remarks about the therapist and offered her constant reinforcement by repeating, "you are a healer" and "no one can help me like you do." It was clear she had idealized the therapist. The therapy sessions felt somewhat contrived to the psychologist; she felt that Rose was working hard to build the image of the psychologist as powerful, protective, and all-knowing.

A major shift in the therapy occurred one day, when the psychologist was 30 minutes late for the session due to traffic, and having left her cell phone at home, she could not call Rose to alert her. The psychologist apologized profusely, and Rose reassured her that everything was fine, expressing worry about the stress of being stuck in traffic.

During the session a guided imagery exercise was used to encourage Rose to identify her own needs during the grieving process. In the exercise, Rose saw herself being shut down like a jack-in-the-box and feeling intensely angry. During processing of the exercise, it became clear that the disappointment caused by the psychologist's apparently careless behavior—not calling to inform she would be late—created a fracture in the idealized image of the therapist and resulted in an impossible situation for Rose. While Rose did not feel she could express her anger safely, she also could no longer continue therapy as if nothing had happened. Integrating the image of the psychologist as a healer with the image of a human being with flaws created anxiety for Rose. She also became aware of feeling disempowered during most of her life, unable to express her wishes or anger for fear of damaging relationships. She realized that the difficulties developing a more complex but realistic image of the therapist paralleled her difficulty reconciling negative feelings about her husband.

After this breakthrough, Rose began sharing aspects of her marriage that had troubled her during Jim's illness. She shared that he had started behaving abruptly after being diagnosed with cancer, perhaps as a result of his distress. She also felt annoyed that his many friends would visit Jim for several hours at a time, both at home and at the hospital. She felt as if she was being "robbed" of intimacy with Jim and had resented his lack of boundaries. She regretted not sharing these feelings with Jim prior to his death. Recalling these memories was particularly painful for Rose and the frequency of sessions was temporarily increased to twice a week. She grieved remembering that Jim had felt conflicted at the beginning of their relationship and had expressed ambivalence about committing to one woman because "he loved women." Rose had experienced unsafe boundaries in the relationship with her mother and her siblings and had quietly resented Jim for not providing a safer emotional environment for her.

She also began exploring her relationship with her own support network more deeply. On the one hand, she admitted feeling resentment that other friends and family members seemed to be doing "just fine" after Jim's death. On the other hand, she became annoyed when they overtly expressed distress and grief.

She felt that somehow they "did not have the right" to grieve openly as she did. As layers of memories and awareness unfolded, Rose began appreciating the complexity of her own emotional life and grieving process and became progressively comfortable allowing contrasting emotions to exist, without suppressing them. She commented, "When you are in the midst of chaos you can't just tie a nice big bow."

The evolution of bereavement therapy allowed Rose to slowly develop a richer and more authentic narrative about her life and her marriage. As she became increasingly able to tolerate the complexity of the grieving process, she developed more tolerance and compassion for Jim's own challenges dealing with illness and death. This process allowed her to fully reconnect with the positive legacy of her marriage. During a body relaxation exercise, she described feeling surrounded by a clear and smooth gel-like substance that made her feel safe and protected. However, when she brought her attention to her back, she described feeling cold and noticing that her back was not covered by the substance. As a result, she described feeling cold, exposed, and somewhat unsafe.

In debriefing the exercise and exploring the meaning of the image, she commented "I know what it is. No matter what, Jim had my back. Now my back is exposed." Realizing the strong support she had received from her husband allowed for additional healing.

CASE VIGNETTE 4.3

Mindy had been the primary caregiver for her husband John during his brief illness. Diagnosed with metastatic pancreatic cancer, he died seven months after the initial diagnosis. Both in their early forties, they had two young children and worked full-time. Even though John had been told quite bluntly by his oncologist that the prognosis was poor, he refused to consider that he was dying. John had managed the household finances, and before he became ill he had often commented that Mindy should learn the skills because she would feel lost if something happened to him. After chemotherapy and radiation proved ineffective, Mindy began to realize that John would die soon. Heartbroken, she attempted to discuss this with him, planning to use the time left also for becoming knowledgeable about running the household. She was surprised at John's reaction. He became visibly upset, accusing her of being insensitive and already used to the idea that he would die. He continued to pay bills and manage finance until a week before his death. She was mortified by his reaction and did not raise the topic again. After his death, she immediately focused on the finances and became consumed with contacting all the financial institutions while working full-time and ensuring that her children were cared for. Mindy was not receptive to receiving emotional support from family and friends, stating she was too busy to focus on her grief. She declined bereavement support from a local hospice that partnered with the hospital where John died, but kept the bereavement counselor's phone number. Eight months later she contacted the bereavement counselor. During the initial session she explained feeling increasingly angry at her husband for being unwilling to help her get control of practical financial matters before he died. She resented him for his accusations when she raised the topic and admitted the fracture created that day was not healed before his death. She felt emotionally shut down and constantly fluctuated between guilt and anger. Moreover, she felt unable to unable to think about her marriage because she would become flooded with anxiety about the negative interaction with her husband. By avoiding thinking about her marriage, however, she was also prevented from experiencing support from the positive memories and legacy. Mindy's grieving process appeared centered around re-experiencing painful memories and emotions. This created anxiety and amplified her sense of loss, which perpetuated her avoidance. Mindy did not experience symptoms of major depression; however, her grieving process appeared complicated. Psychotherapy allowed Mindy to slowly integrate traumatic memories about the last months of her husband's illness and to reframe the meaning of the conflict. Trauma-focused modalities, including Eye Movement Desensitization and Reprocessing (EMDR), were used to process difficult events (her husband's diagnosis, the rapid decline, his reaction to her requests), to process intrusive images of his reaction that she interpreted as angry and accusatory, and to change the negative cognitions she had developed.

This approach allowed Mindy to begin understanding her husband's reaction in the context of his personal grief about imminent death. During a session she mentioned that when her son was two years old and she got him out of bed to brush his teeth, he told her he hated her and she was a bad mom. She remembered feeling empathy and compassion for her son, and even a mild sense of amusement. She then commented that her husband's grief had prevented him from helping her with finances. By avoiding the topic, he somehow avoided acknowledging his impending death. Like her son, her husband had become angry because she was asking him to do something that was difficult. Helping Mindy take control of finances would mean that he would not be alive to continue doing it. She then felt great compassion for her husband's suffering and was able to release anger. This facilitated her grieving process and her emotional adjustment and allowed her to feel supported by the many positive memories of her marriage.

References

Anderson, N. H., Gluyas, C., Mathers, S. Hudson, P., & Ugalde, A. (2016). "A monster that lives in our lives": Experiences of caregivers of people with moto neuron disease and identifying avenues for support. *BMJ Supportive & Palliative Care*. doi: 10.1136/bmjspcare-2015-001057.

Aoun, S. M., Breen, L. J., & Howting, D. (2014). The support needs of terminally ill people living alone at home: A narrative review. *Health Psychology and Behavioral Medicine*, 2(1), 951–969.

Aoun, S. M., Deas, K., Howting, D., & Lee, G. (2015). Exploring the support nees of family caregivers of patients with brain cancer using the CSNAT: A comparative study with other cancer groups. *PLoS One*, 10(12). doi: 10.1371/journal.pone.0148074.

Badr, H., & Acitelli, L. K. (2017). Re-thinking dyadic coping in the context of chronic illness. *Current Opinions in Psychology*, 13, 44–48.

Baile, W. F., Buckman, R., Lenzi, R., Glober, G., Beale, E. & Kudelka, P. (2000). SPIKES—A six-step protocol for delivering bad news: application to the patient with cancer. *The Oncologist*, 5, 302–311.

Baker, A. W., Goetter, E. M., Bui, E., Shah, R., Charney, M. E., Mauro, C., ... Simon, N. M. (2016). The influence of anxiety sensitivity on a wish to die in complicated grief. *Journal of Nervous and Mental Disease*, 204(4), 314–316.

Blackler, L. (2016). When families pressure patients to change their wishes. *Journal of Hospice and Palliative Nursing*, 18(4), 184–191.

Boland, J. W., Reigada, C., Yorke, J., Hart, S. P., Bajwah, S., Ross, Y., ... Johnson, M. J. (2016). The adaptation, face, and content validation of a needs assessment tool: progressive disease for people with interstitial lung disease. *Journal of Palliative Medicine*, 19(5), 549–555.

Breen, L. (2012). The effect of caring on post-bereavement outcome: Research gaps and practice priorities. *Progress in Palliative Care*, 20(1), 27–30.

Bruno, V., Mancini, D., Ghoche, R., Arshinoff, R. & Miyasaki, J. M. (2016). High prevalence of physical and sexual aggression to caregivers in advanced Parkinson's disease: Experience in the palliative care program. *Parkinsonism & Related Disorders*, 24, 141–142.

Bryant, R. A. (2013). Is pathological grief lasting more than 12 months grief or depression? *Current Opinion in Psychiatry*, 26(1), 41–46.

Bryant, R. A., Kenny, L., Joscelyne, A., Rawson, N., Maccallum, F., Cahill, C., ... Nickerson, A. (2017). Treating prolonged grief disorder: A 2-year follow-up of a randomized controlled trial. *Journal of Clinical Psychiatry*. doi: 10.4088/JCP.16m10729.

Bui, E., Horenstein, A., Shah, R., Skritskaya, N. A., Mauro, C., Wang, Y., ... Simon, N. M. (2015). Grief-related panic symptoms in complicated grief. *Journal of Affective Disorders*, 170, 213–216.

Bui, E., Nadal-Vicens, M., & Simon, N. M. (2012). Pharmacological approaches to the treatment of complicated grief: rationale and a brief review of the literature. *Dialogues in Clinical Neuroscience*, 14(2), 149–157.

Carey, I. M., Shah, S. M., DeWilde, S., Harris, T., Victor, C. R., & Cook, D. G. (2014). Increased risk of acute cardiovascular events after partner bereavement: a matched cohort study. *JAMA Internal Medicine, 174*(4), 598–605.
Carson, S. S., Cox, C. E., Wallenstein, S., Hanson, L. C., Danis, M., Tulsky, J. A., . . . & Nelson, J. E. (2016). Effect of palliative care-led- meetings for families of patients with chronic critical illness: A randomized clinical trial. *JAMA, 316*(1), 51–62.
Carter, B., & McGoldrick, M. (2005). The expanded family cycle. In B. Carter & M. McGoldrick (Eds.), *The expanded family cycle: Individual, family, and social perspectives.* Boston, MA: Allyn & Bacon.
Chi, N. C., & Demiris, G. (Family caregivers' pain management in end of life care: a systematic review. *American Journal of Hospice and Palliative Medicine, 34*(5), 470–485.
Chi, N. C., Demiris, G., Lewis, F. M., Walker, A. J., & Langer, S. L. (2016). Behavioral and educational interventions to support family caregivers to support family caregivers. *American Journal of Hospice and Palliative Medicine, 33*(9), 894–908.
Clemmer, S. J., Ward-Griffin, C., & Forbes, D. (2008). Family memebrs providing home-based palliative care to older adults: The enactment of multiple roles. *Canadian Journal on Aging, 27*(3), 267–283.
Coelho, A., & Barbosa, A. (2016). Family anticipatory grief: An integrative literature review. *American Journal of Hospice & Palliative Medicine, 1*, 12. doi: 10.1177/1049909116647960.
Cozza, S. J., Fisher, J. E., Mauro, C., Zhou, J., Ortiz, C. D., Skritskaya, N., . . .& Shear, M. K. (2016). Performance of DSM-5 persistent complex bereavement disorder criteria in a community sample of bereaved military family members. The *Amedican Journal of Psychiatry, 173*(9), 919–929.
Dassel, K. B., & Carr, D. C. (2016). Does dementia caregiving accelerate frailty? Findings from the health and retirement study. *Gerontologist, 56*(3), 444–450.
Dassel, K. B., Carr, D. C., & Vitaliano, P. (2017). Does caring for a spouse with dementia accelerate cognitive decline? Findings from the health and retirement study. *Gerontologist, 57*(2), 319–328.
DiBello, K. K. (2015). Grief and depression at the end of life. *Nurse Practitioner, 40*(5), 22–28.
DiBiasio, E. L, Teno, J. M., Clark, M. A., Spence, C., & Casarett, D. (2016). Development of an assessment to examine training of the hospice primary caregiver. *Journal of Palliative Medicine, 19*(6), 639–645.
Fineberg, I. C., Kawashima, M., & Asch, S. M. (2011). Communication with families facing life-threatening illness: A research-based model for family conferences. *Journal of Palliative Medicine, 14*(4), 421–427.
Francis, L. E., Kypriotakis, G., O'Toole, E. E., & Rose, J. H. (2016). Cancer patient age and family caregiver bereavment outcomes. *Supportive Care in Cancer, 24*(9), 3987–3996.
Freeman, S., Hirdes, J. P., Stolee, P., & Garcia, J. (2016). A cross-sectional examination of the association between dyspnea and distress as experienced by palliative home care clients and their informal caregivers. *Journal of Social Work in End of Life & Palliative Care, 12*(1–2), 82–103.
Friedman, M. (2016). Seeking the best bereavment-related diagnostic criteria. *The American Journal of Psychiatry, 173*(9), 864–865.
Ghesquiere, A. R., Aldridge, M. D., Johnson-Hurzeler, R., Kaplan, D., Bruce, M. L., & Bradley, E. (2015). Hospice services for complicated grief and depression: Results from a national survey. *Journal of the American Geriatric Society, 63*(10), 2173–2180.
Glickman, K., Shear, M. K., & Wall, M. (2016). Exploring outcomes related to anxiety and depression in completers of a randomized controlled trial of complicated grief treatment. *Clinical Psychology & Psychotherapy, 23*(2), 118–124.
Goldsmith, J., Wittenberg, E., Platt, C. S., Iannarino, N., & Reno, J. (2016). Family caregiver communication in oncology: Advancing a typology. *Psychooncology, 25*(4), 463–470.
Graff, S., Fenger-Gron, M., Christensen, B., Pedersen, H. S., Christensen, J., Li, J., & Vestergaard, M. (2016). Long-term risk of atrial fibrillation after the death of a partner. *Open Heart, 3*(1). doi: 10.1136/openhrt-2015-000367

Grassi, L. (2007). Bereavement in families with relatives dying of cancer. *Current Opinions in Supportive Palliative Care, 1*(1), 43–49.

Gritti, P. (2015). The family meetings in oncology: Some practical guidelines. *Frontiers in Psychology.* https://doi.org/10.3389/fpsyg.2014.01552.

Hockley, J. (2000). Psychosocial aspects of palliative care: Communicating with the patient and the family. *Acta Oncologica, 39*(8), 905–910.

Holm, M., Arestedt, K., Carlander, I., Wengstrom, Y., Ohlen, J., & Alvariza, A. (2017). Characteristics of the family caregivers who did not benefit from a successful psychoeducational group intervention during palliative cancer care: A prospective correlational study. *Cancer Nursing, 40*(1), 76–83.

Hudson, P., Quinn, K., O'Hanlon, B., & Aranda, S. (2008). Family meetings in palliative care: Multidisciplinary clinical practice guidelines. *BMC Palliative Care, 7,* 12.

Hudson, P., Thomas, T., Quinn, K., & Aranda, S. (2009). Family meetings in palliative care: Are they effective? *Palliative Medicine, 23*(2), 150–157.

Iglewicz, A., Seay, K., Zetumer, S. D., & Zisook, S. (2013). The removal of the bereavement exclusion in the DSM-5: Exploring the evidence. *Current Psychiatry Reports, 15*(11), 413.

Joshi, R. (2013). Family meetings: An essential component of comprehensive palliative care. *Canadian Family Physician, 59*(6), 637–639.

Kaplan, M. (2010). SPIKES: a framework for breaking bad news to patients with cancer. *Clinical Journal of Oncology Nursing, 14*(4), 514–516.

Kent, E. E., Rowland, J. H., Northouse, L., Litzelman, K., Chou, W. Y., Shelburne, N., ... Huss, K. (2016). Caring for caregivers and patients: Research and clinical priorities for informal cancer caregiving. *Cancer, 122*(13), 1987–1995.

Kentish-Barnes N., Chaize M., Seegers V., Legriel, S., Cariou, A., Jaber S., . . . Azoulay, E. (2015). Complicated grief after death of a relative in the intensive care unit. *European Respiratory Journal, 45*(5):1341–1352.

Kentish-Barnes, N., Chevret, S., Champigneulle, B., Thirion, M., Souppart, V., Gilbert, M., ... Azoulay, E. (2017). Effect of a condolence letter on grief and symptoms among relatives of patients who died in the ICU: A randomized clinical trial. *Intensive Care Medicine, 43*(4), 473–484.

Kerr, M. E., & Bowen, M. (1988). *Family evaluation: An approach based on Bowen theory.* New York: W. W. Norton & Company.

Kim, Y., Carver, C. S., Spiegel, D., Mitchell, H. R., & Cannady, R. S. (2017). Role of family caregivers' self-perceived preparedness for the death of the cancer patient in long term adjustment to bereavement. *Psychooncology, 26*(4), 484–492.

Kim, H. H., Kim, S. Y., Kim, J. M., Kim, S. W., Shin, I. S., Shim, H. J., ... Yoon, J. S. (2016). Influence of caregiver personality on the burden of family caregivers of terminally ill cancer patients. *Palliative and Supportive Care, 14*(1), 5–12.

Kim, S. Y., Kim, J. M., Kim, S. W., Kang, H. J., Shin, I. S., Shim, H. J., . . . Yoon, J. S. (2014). Determinants of a hopeful attitude among family caregivers in a palliative care setting. *General Hospital Psychiatry, 36*(2), 165–171.

Kim, Y., Shaffer, K. M., Carver, C. S., & Cannady, R. S. (2016). Quality of life of family caregivers 8 years after a relative's cancer diagnosis: Follow-up of the national quality of life survey for caregivers. *Psychooncology, 25*(3), 266–274.

King, M., Lodwick, R., Jones, R., Whitaker, H., & Petersen, I. (2017). Death following partner bereavement: A self-controlled case series analysis. *PloS ONE, 12*(3). doi: org/10.137/journal.pone.0173870.

Kissane, D. W., Zaider, T. I., Li, Y., Hichenberg, S., Schuler, T., Lederberg, M., Lavelle, L., Loeb, R., & Del Gaudio, F. (2016). Randomized controlled trial of family therapy in advanced cancer continued into bereavement. *Journal of Clinical Oncology, 34*(16), 1921–1927.

Koekkoek, J. A., Chang, S., & Taphoorn, M. J. (2016). Palliative care at the end-of-life in glioma patients. *Handbook of Clinical Neurology, 134,* 315–326.

Kramer, B. J., Boelk, A. Z., & Auer, C. (2006). Family conflict at the end of life: Lessons learned in a model program for vulnerable adults. *Journal of Palliative Medicine, 9*(3), 791–801.

Kramer, B. J., Kavanaugh, M., Trentham-Dietz, A., Walsh, M., & Yonker, J. A. (2010). Complicated grief symtpoms in caregivers of persons dwith lung cancer: The role of family conflict, intrapsychic strains, and hospice utilization. *Omega (Westport)*, 62(3), 201–220.

Krug, K., Miksch, A., Peters-Klimm, F., Engeser, P., & Szecsenyi, J. (2016). Correlation between patient quality of life in palliative care and burden of their family caregivers: A prospective observational cohort study. *BMC Palliative Care*, 15, 4. doi: 10.1186/s12904-016-0082-y.

Kumar, P., Wright, A. A., Hatfield, L. A., Temel, J. S., & Keating, N. L. (2016). Family perspectives on hospice care experiences of patients with cancer. *Journal of Clinical Oncology*, 35(4), 432–439.

Lafferty, A., Fealy, G., Downes, C., & Drennan, J. (2016). The prevalence of potentially abusive behaviours in family caregiving: Findings from a national survey of family carers of older people. *Age and Ageing*, 45(5), 703–707.

Lang, A., Toon, L., Cohen, S. R., Stajduhar, K., Griffin, M., Fleiszer, A. R., . . . Williams, A. (2015). Client, caregiver, and provider perspective of safety in palliative home care: A mixed method design. *Safety in Health*, 1, 3. doi: 10.1186/2056-5917-1-3.

Ling, S. F., Chen, M. L., Li, C. Y., Chang, W. C., Shen, W. C., & Tang, S. T. (2013). Trajectory and influencing factors of depressive symptoms in family caregivers before and after the death of terminally ill patients with cancer. *Oncology Nursing Forum*, 40(1), 32–40.

Lovell, G. P., Smith, T., & Kannis-Dymand, L. (2015). Surrogates end of life care decision makers' postbereavement grief and guilt responses. *Death Studies*, 39(10), 647–653.

Lum, H. D., & Sudore, R. L. (2016). Advanced care planning and goals of care communication in older adults with cardiovascular disease and multi-morbidity. *Clinics in Geriatric Medicine*, 32, 247–260.

Maciejewski, P. K., Maercker, A., Boelen, P. A., & Prigerson, H. G. (2016). Prolonged grief disorder and persistent complex bereavement disorder, but not complicated grief, are one and the same diagnostic entity: An analysis of data from the Yale Bereavement Study. *World Psychiatry*, 15, 266–275.

Melhem, N. M., Porta, G., Walker Payne, M., & Brent, D. A. (2013). Identifying prolonged grief reactions in children: Dimensional and diagnostic approaches. *Journal of the American Academy of Child & Adolescent Psychiatry*, 52(6), 599–607.

Nanni, M. G., Biancospino, B., & Grassi, L. (2014). Pre-loss symptoms related to risk of complicated grief in caregivers of terminally ill cancer patients. *Journal of Affective Disorders*, 160, 87–91.

National Alliance for Caregiving (2015). Caregiving in the U.S. http://www.aarp.org/content/dam/aarp/ppi/2015/caregiving-in-the-united-states-2015-report-revised.pdf. Retrieved on May 15, 2016.

Nielsen, M. K., Neergaard, M. A., Jensen, A. B., Vedsted, P., Bro, F., & Guldin, M. B. (2016a). Predictors of complicated grief and depression in bereaved caregivers: a national prospective cohort study. *Journal of Pain and Symptom Management*, 53(3), 540–550.

Nielsen, M. K., Neergaard, M. A., Jensen, A. B., Bro, F., & Guldin, M. B. (2016b). Do we need to change our understanding of anticipatory grief in caregivers? A systematic review of caregiver studies during end of life caregiving and bereavement. *Clinical Psychology Review*, 44, 75–93.

Ornstein, K. A., Aldridge, M. D., Garrido, M. M., Gorges, R., Meier, D. E., & Kelley, A. S. (2015). Association between hospice use and depressive symtpoms in surviving spouses. *JAMA Internal Medicine*, 175(7), 1138–1146.

Penrod, J., Baney, B., Loeb, S. J. McGhan, G., & Shipley, P. Z. (2012a). The influence of the culture of care on informal caregivers' experiences. *Advances in Nursing Science*, 35(1), 64–76.

Penrod, J., Hupcey, J. E., Shipley, P. Z., Loeb, S. J., & Baney, B. (2012b). A model of caregiving through the end of life: Seeking normal. *Western Journal of Nursing Research*, 34(2), 174–193.

Phongtankuel, V., Scherban, B. A., Reid, M. C., Finley, A., Martin, A., Dennis, J., & Adelman, R. D. (2016). Why do hospice patients return to the hospital? A study of hospice providers perspectives. *Journal of Palliative Medicine*, 19(1), 51–56.

Pies, R. W. (2014). The bereavement excusion and DSM-5: An update and commentary. *Innovations in Clinical Neuroscience*, 11(7–8), 19–22.

Reed, M., & Harding, K. E. (2015). Do family meetings improve measurable outcomes for patients, carers, or health care system? A systematic review. *Australian Social Work, 68*(2), 244–258.

Rumpold, T., Schur, S., Amering, M., Ebert-Vogel, A., Kirchheiner, K., Masel, E., . . . Schrank, B. (2016). Hope as determinant for psychiatric morbidity in family caregivers of advanced cancer patients. *Psychooncology, 26*(5), 672–678. doi:10.1002/pon.4205.

Sanderson, C., Lobb, E. A., Mowll, J., Butow, P. N., McGowan, N., & Price, M. A. (2013). Signs of post-traumatic stress disorder in caregivers following an expected death; a qualitative study. *Palliative Medicine, 27*(7), 625–631.

Schulz, R., & Sherwood, P. R. (2008). Physical and mental health effects of family caregiving. *American Journal of Nursing, 108*(9 Suppl), 23–27.

Shah, S. M., Carey, I. M., Harris, T., DeWilde, S., Victor, C. R., & Cook, D. G. (2013). Initiation of psychotropic medication after partner bereavement: a matched cohort study. *PLoS One, 8*(11).

Shear, M. K., Ghesquiere, A., & Glickman, K. (2013). Bereavement and complicated grief. *Current Psychiatry Reports, 15*(11), 406.

Shear, M. K. (2015). Clinical practice: Complicated grief. *New England Journal of Medicine, 372*(2), 153–160.

Shear, M. K., Reynolds, C. F., Simon, N. M., Zisook, S., Wang, Y., Mauro, C., . . . & Skritskaya, N. (2016). Optimizing treatment of complicated grief: A randomized clinical trial. *JAMA Psychiatry, 73*(7), 685–694.

Skritskaya, N. A., Mauro, C., Olonoff, M., Qiu, X., Duncan, S., Wang, Y., . . . Shear, M. K. (2017). Measuring maladaptive cognitions in complicated grief: Introducing the typical beliefs questionnaire. *American Journal of Geriatric Psychiatry, 25*(5), 541–550.

Strada, E. A. (2013). *Grief and bereavement in the adult palliative care setting*. New York: Oxford University Press.

Sullivan, S. S., Ferreira da Rosa Silva, C., & Meeker, M. A. (2015). Family meetings at end of life: A systematic review. *Journal of Hospice and Palliative Nursing, 17*(3), 196–205.

Supiano, K. P., Haynes, L. B., & Pond, V. (2017). The process of change in complicated group therapy for bereaved dementia caregivers: An evaluation using the Meaning of Loss Codebook. *Journal of Gerontology & Social Work, 60*(2), 155–169.

Tanco, K., Park, J. C., Cerana, A., Sisson, A., Sobti, N., & Bruera, E. (2017). A systematic review of instruments assessing dimensions of distress among caregivers of adult and pediatric cancer patients. *Palliative and Supportive Care, 15*(1), 110–124.

Tang, S. T., Huang, G. H., Wei, Y. C., Chang, W. C., Chen, J. S., & Chou, W. C. (2013). Trajectories of caregiver depressive symptoms while providing end-of-life care. *Psychooncology, 22*(12), 2702–2710.

Thomas, K., Hudson, P., Trauer, T., Remedios, C., & Clarke, D. (2014). Risk factors for developing prolonged grief during bereavement in family carers of cancer patients in palliative care: A longitudinal study. *Journal of Pain and Symptom Management, 47*(3), 531–541.

Tinetti, M. E., Esterson, J., Ferris, R., Posner, P., & Blaum, C. S. (2016). Patient priority-directed decision making and care for older adults with multiple chronic conditions. *Clinics in Geriatric Medicine, 32*(2), 261–275.

Tomarken, A., Holland, J., Schachter, S., Vanderwerker, L., Zuckerman, E., Nelson, C. . . . Prigerson, H. (2008). Factors of complicated grief pre-death in caregivers of cancer patients. *Psychooncology, 17*(2), 105–111.

Turan, B., Goldstein, M. K., Garber, A. M., & Carstensen, L. L. (2011). Knowing loved ones' end of life health care wishes: Attachment security predicts caregiver's accuracy. *Health Psychology, 30*(6), 814–818.

Waller, A., Turon, H., Mansfield, E., Clark, K., Hobden, B., & Sanson-Fisher, R. (2016). Assisting the bereaved: A systematic review of the evidence for grief counseling. *Palliative Medicine, 30*(2), 132–148.

Williams, A., Duggleby, W., Eby, J., Cooper, D., Hallstrom, L. K., Holtslander, L., & Thomas, R. (2013). Hope against hope: exploring the hopes and challenges of rural female caregivers of persons with advanced cancer. *BMC Palliative Care, 12,* 44. doi:10.1186/1472-684X-12-44.

Wittenberg, E., Kravits, K., Goldsmith, J., Ferrel, B., & Fujinami, R. (2017). Validation of a model of family caregiver communication types and related caregiver outcomes. *Palliative and Supportive Care, 15*(1), 3–11.

Wittenberg-Lyles, E., Goldsmith, J., Parker Oliver, D., Demiris, G., & Rankin, A. (2012). Targeting communication interventions to decrease oncology family caregiver burden. *Seminars in Oncology Nursing, 28*(4), 262–270.

Wladkowski, S. P. (2016). Live discharge from hospice and the grief experience of dementia caregivers. *Journal of Social Work in End of Life & Palliat Care, 12*(1–2), 47–62.

5

The Fifth Domain of Palliative Care

Spiritual, Religious, and Existential Aspects of Care

Focus Points

- The palliative care team is committed to facilitating the expression of spiritual and religious beliefs and practices throughout the disease trajectory and after the patient's death.
- Every member of the palliative care team has a responsibility to explore and support patients' spiritual and religious values.
- Spiritual screening, spiritual history, and spiritual assessment are important tools for recognizing spiritual needs
- Palliative psychologists should include a spiritual screening and spiritual history in their comprehensive evaluation of the patient and family caregivers.
- Palliative psychologists are open to exploring spiritual and religious values in the therapy session and ensure appropriate referrals to spiritual care providers.

Introduction

The fifth domain, which consists of spiritual, existential, and religious aspects of care, emphasizes the focus of palliative care as an integrated system. Comprehensive care in this domain is multidimensional, recognizing and honoring patients and family caregivers' spiritual and religious needs as well as facilitating their individual and unique expression (Speck, 2016). Additionally, it includes the ability to recognize the presence of spiritual and religious suffering, assess its sources, and provide competent interventions that can relieve distress. Accordingly, the *Clinical Practice Guidelines* also recommend that spiritual care providers be included on the palliative care team to provide assessments and diagnosis of spiritual distress and to offer adequate interventions to relieve spiritual suffering. Spiritual, religious, and existential care begins at the initial contact with the palliative care team; it continues during the dying process and involves facilitating and honoring rituals and practices related to the time surrounding death. Bereavement care of family caregivers after the patient's death must continue to honor and support what is important to them from a religious, spiritual, and existential perspective.

Spiritual suffering is a component of Total Pain that can severely compromise patients' well-being. Therefore, spiritual care is an expression not only of competent care but also of compassionate care (Johnson-Bogaerts, 2015; Sinclair et al., 2016). As the patient and family caregivers represent the unit of care, all should receive assessment and intervention in this area (Sun et al., 2016).

It has been increasingly recognized that spiritual and religious values may represent an important resource for individuals and groups across the life span and especially when facing challenges (Richardson, 2014). This is evidenced by a growing body of literature identifying the central role of spiritual and religious beliefs in the quality of life of patients with advanced illness (Bussing et al., 2014; Peteet & Balboni, 2013).These beliefs are centered around faith for many, but also around such constructs as dignity and community (Dobratz, 2013). Religion and spirituality can improve quality of life and can have a significant impact on medical decisions at the end of life. Additionally, they are especially relevant for how some ethnic groups understand and cope with illness (Balboni et al., 2013; El Nawawi, Balboni & Balboni, 2012).

A study of patients with advanced cancer showed that those who perceived themselves as less religious and leading a less spiritual life reported higher levels of spiritual pain and reported more physical and emotional symptoms (Delgado-Guay et al., 2011). In another group of patients with advanced cancer, "being at peace with God" was the most common wish at end of life. Also considered important by patients were prayer, having family present, being free from pain, not being a burden to family, trusting the doctor, keeping a sense of humor, saying good-bye to the important people, having family prepared for death, and being able to help others (Delgado-Guay et al., 2016). The importance of spiritual and religious beliefs was also found in patients with advanced cancer receiving palliative radiation (Vallurupalli et al., 2012). Furthermore, studies have increasingly indicated religion and spirituality to be important quality-of-life elements also in patients with advanced heart and lung disease, heart failure, and end-stage renal disease (Bekelman et al., 2007; Elliott et al., 2012; Strada et al., 2013).

The role of religion and spirituality appears to be important in studies investigating patients' and families' perception of what represents a "good death." However, it is noteworthy that spirituality and religion may be given different levels of importance by the patient and the family. For example, a review of studies investigating patients' perspectives and preferences for end-of-life care found that religiosity and spirituality were described as important more frequently by patients than by family caregivers (Meier et al., 2016). This indicates the importance of promoting effective communication between patients, caregivers, and the medical team to ensure patients' preferences are correctly identified and supported. Patients and caregivers may share many goals and values, but clinicians also need to recognize individual differences and discrepancies within the family system. Furthermore, the patient's relationship with spirituality, religious beliefs, or organized religion may evolve or change during the illness, warranting changes to the psychospritual care plan.

Studies have also consistently indicated that patients would like their health-care providers to inquire about their spiritual and religious beliefs, and that health-care providers recognize the importance of exploring these issues with patients (Sulmasy, 2006, 2009). For many, this becomes particularly important when discussing a life-threatening illness or after the death of a loved one (McCord et al., 2004).

The constructs "spirituality" and "religion" have often been used interchangeably in the literature. Although there are overlaps, it is important to be aware of the unique aspects of each. Additionally, "existential distress" indicates a separate, but related construct.

Religion has been defined as "an individual's beliefs, values, behaviors, and experiences related to ultimate meaning, often involving deities and dogma, formulated by faith groups or institutions over time" (Sinclair & Chochinov, 2012, p. 260). For some religious patients, the term "religion" subsumes also spiritual and existential aspects. Others may consider their religious affiliation primarily an expression of their cultural and family history, but not necessarily the ultimate source of meaning in life.

Spirituality is currently understood as a broad construct that is directly related to how people make meaning of their lives. Spirituality involves a dynamic process that continues to develop throughout life, and it is an important expression of patients' culture (Delgado-Guay, 2014). Spirituality is not only used to indicate a quest or search for meaning but often indicates a framework that supports the individual through specific beliefs and practices. As such, the construct can be used in both religious and secular contexts.

Many definitions of spirituality exist, each focusing on certain aspects of the human experience. The definition of spirituality adopted by the *Clinical Practice Guidelines for Quality Palliative Care* is as follows: "Spirituality is the aspect of humanity that refers to the way individuals seek and express meaning and purpose, and the way they experience their connectedness to the moment, to self, to others, to nature, and to the significant or sacred" (Puchalski et al., 2014, p. 643). In a more recent rewording the focus is expanded: "Spirituality is a dynamic and intrinsic aspect of humanity through which persons seek ultimate meaning, purpose, and transcendence, and experience relationship to self, family, others, community, society, nature, and the significant or sacred. Spirituality is expressed through beliefs, values, traditions, and practice" (Puchalski et al., 2014, p. 648). This definition identifies meaning and purpose as the focus of the experience of spirituality. And, it recognizes the existence of several modalities, secular or religious, to seek, experience, and express this meaning and purpose in life.

Existential distress is increasingly being recognized as one of the main sources of suffering in patients with advanced illness (Milstein, 2008). Although the term "existential" has been widely used in the palliative care literature, there is lack of agreement on definition, theoretical frameworks, and clinical applications, limiting the development of targeted interventions. In the literature, it appears that "existential" is more often used in conjunction with distress, pain, questions, and concerns. It seems to point to the struggle of the individual who is experiencing the anguish derived from a lack of answers or comfort. Furthermore, "spiritual" and "existential" are often used interchangeably, or as expressions of an individual's psychological functioning (Boston, Bruce & Schreiber, 2011).

Existential concepts are rooted in existential philosophy, which focused on the exploration of life's limitations and possible ways of overcoming them. Believing that life lacks inherent meaning, early existential philosophers pondered constructs such as authenticity, freedom, death, and aloneness. Existential psychology developed from efforts to create meaning in life and in suffering, to establish authentic and deep connections, and to live fully in the absence of obvious meaning. Existential psychotherapy also focuses on the main questions of existence: How can one live fully and with authenticity? How does one find the strength to live with the awareness of death? How does one relate to existential loneliness? What is the meaning of freedom, given the constraints of human existence? (Yalom, 1998).

Based on these premises, existential questions or concerns can become especially relevant for patients with serious and advanced illness, regardless of religious affiliation or spiritual orientation, affecting patients who are religious, and those who are atheist or agnostic (Ettema et al., 2010; Steger et al., 2008). Demoralization has emerged as a manifestation of existential distress caused by loss of meaning and purpose (Robinson et al., 2016). The patient and family caregivers may reflect on the meaning of hope and how they can maintain hope in the face of imminent death. The struggle to maintain some element of control and personal freedom in the context of advanced disease is common. And maintaining a sense of dignity and belonging to avoid alienation often takes a prominent focus. Every member of the palliative care team has a responsibility to provide basic elements of spiritual screening and support. A *spiritual screening* allows clinicians to recognize symptoms of spiritual and religious distress that need prompt attention. Additionally, a more thorough understanding of the spiritual and religious beliefs of the patient and the family is facilitated by obtaining a complete *spiritual history*. Tools have been developed for this purpose, and they will be described in this chapter. A *spiritual assessment* is different from a spiritual history and a screening. It is an in-depth process that allows diagnosis of religious, spiritual, and existential distress and development of a care plan. Although any member of the interdisciplinary team can administer a spiritual screening or obtain a spiritual history, it is recommended that a formal spiritual assessment be performed by a licensed spiritual care provider who can diagnose different manifestations of distress in this domain (Puchalski, 2010).

Competencies for Palliative Psychologists

Competencies in this domain involve the ability to explore, recognize, and support religious, spiritual, and existential needs in patients and family caregivers. In settings other than palliative care, exploration of spiritual needs may not be routinely included in a psychological assessment. For this reason, palliative psychologists will benefit from developing skills in administering a spiritual screening and obtaining a spiritual history tool as part of the exploration of values and needs.

The focus on addressing spiritual needs should not, however, encourage generalizations on the part of clinicians such as "everyone has a spirituality" or "everyone has spiritual needs" or "every human being has a spiritual dimension." It is essential that clinicians do not make assumptions based on personal values and preconceived ideas. As the term "spiritual" may not be secular enough to represent a patient's worldview, the language used with the patient and the family should be carefully chosen to open channels of communication. Psychologists working in medical settings are also aware of the necessity to balance the sharing of information relevant to the care plan with other team members and referral sources, with the need to protect patient confidentiality.

Interventions specifically targeting spiritual and existential distress, such as existential and meaning-centered approaches, offer an important addition to psychotherapy approaches designed to provide broad psychological well-being, such as supportive psychotherapy (Strada & Sourkes, 2015). Familiarity and clinical comfort with different psychological modalities can allow the psychologist to adapt them to meet the patient's needs in different circumstances. While palliative psychologists are certainly not required to have a spiritual or religious orientation, it is important that their professional development include an ongoing exploration of their own relationship with spirituality and existential values. This will help ensure that, regardless of what their personal beliefs may be, they are able to convey to patients and families a sense of welcoming respect, relating to them in a nonjudgmental manner that honors their journey. Awareness of their own beliefs and biases in the area of spirituality and religion also will allow them to lay their personal agenda aside and be able to effectively work with patients and families, better recognizing their unique way of experiencing the world (Williams et al., 2011). Box 5.1 summarizes competencies for psychologists in this domain.

Psychospiritual Care of the Patient and the Family

While the relationship between psychology and spirituality has increasingly become more integrated, it has a complex history. Psychology and psychiatry were initially developed as disciplines dedicated to the cure of mental illness as an expression of pathology. This focus on the medical model was evident in initial psychoanalytic work, focusing on the patient, the illness, the cure (psychotherapy as the talking cure), and the doctor as the authority during this curative process. Freud wrote extensively about religion as "comparable to a childhood neurosis" (Freud, 1927), characterizing religious beliefs as pathological. However, for some a rigorous separation between religious or spiritual domains and psychological functioning may also be considered forced and detrimental to well-being.

In the last two decades there have been significant development and growth in the disciplined and scientific study of religion and spirituality. The development of more sophisticated research tools has now allowed researchers to study in depth the impact of religious and spiritual variables on many areas of human experience (Loetz et al., 2013). With a growing number of scientific journals dedicated to the study of spirituality and religion, understanding of these domains has been deepened. The Society for the Psychology of Religion and Spirituality is a division within the American Psychological Association that promotes research and clinical application of different forms of religion and spirituality.

Exploration of the spiritual domain with patients who are seriously ill can be conceptualized as an intrinsic aspect of psychological work (Patton, 2006). Spirituality as a construct related to searching, finding, and maintaining a sense of meaning and purpose in life is an area well within the realm of psychology. Meaning is a central construct of psychology and is being increasingly explored in numerous empirical studies and clinical applications. For example, the Meaning-Making model describes the components of meaning. It distinguishes between *global meaning*, as the totality of global values and goals determining how individuals perceive themselves and the world, and *situational meaning*, which can be impacted by stressful events, such as a diagnosis of serious illness.

> **Box 5.1 Palliative Psychology Competencies in the Spiritual, Religious, and Existential Domain of Care**
>
> **KNOWLEDGE**
>
> - knowledge of the existing literature on importance of spirituality and religion in palliative care
> - understanding of the role of spiritual care providers on the interdisciplinary team
> - knowledge of common manifestations of spiritual, religious, and existential distress in advanced illness and end of life
> - knowledge of the difference between spiritual screening, spiritual history, and spiritual assessment
> - knowledge of commonly used screening and spiritual history tools
> - understanding of different ways of integrating spirituality in the therapy session
>
> **SKILLS**
>
> - ablity to administer a spiritual screening and a spiritual history to the patient and the family
> - ability to recognize and address psychological aspects of spiritual distress
> - ability to develop and demonstrate comfort and ease exploring patients' spiritual and religious beliefs and preferences
> - ability to integrate spiritual perspective in psychotherapy, as appropriate
> - ability to address existential needs in patients who do not define themselves as spiritual or religious
> - ability to coordinate care with interdisciplinary team and work collaboratively with spiritual care providers.
>
> **ATTITUDES**
>
> - maintain ongoing awareness of personal beliefs in spirituality and religion
> - demonstrate openness and receptivity toward patient and family
> - exhibit a nonjudgmental attitude toward practices and beliefs that may be in contrast with one's own
> - maintin a willingness to engage in ongoing personal inquiry regarding the meaning of life and death

In the model, stress results from a discrepancy between global and situational meaning. (Markman, Proulx, & Lindberg, 2013; Park, 2013).

Frankl (1959), also discussed meaning as a central psychospiritual construct. He distinguished *ultimate meaning*, the ultimate belief that life has inherent meaning, from *meaning of the moment*, which indicates a practical, day-to- day determination of meaning based on individuals' choices given their circumstances. In this sense, he conceptualized a meaningful life as a trajectory composed of an infinite number of points of meaning while realizing the unique meaning of each moment. In his words, "For the meaning of life differs from man to man, from day to day, and from hour to hour. What matters therefore, is not the meaning of life in general but rather the specific meaning of a person's life at a given moment" (p. 106).

Helping patients maintain a sense of meaning is often central to psychological treatment even with patients who are not medically ill. For example, major depression and severe anxiety can threaten and erode a personal sense of meaning and purpose. Additionally, major life transitions, such as deaths of loved ones, divorce, or loss of job can also threaten the fabric of personal and societal meanings. Questions such as, "How can I continue on," or "What is the point of going on given what has happened to me?" can therefore be conceptualized as psychospiritual questions centered around meaning. They frequently become a focus of psychotherapy.

It is necessary to understand not only what makes a person's life meaningful, but also what can threaten that sense of meaning. The feeling that life is meaningful depends on the ability to continually attribute meaning to it, in a constant flow (Warmenhoven et al., 2016). Stressors can interrupt the person's connection from that flow. For instance, patients with serious illnesses may begin to feel their life has become defined by medical appointments and challenging treatments without guarantees about their survival. For some, death represents the ultimate threat to a sense of integrity and meaning.

CASE VIGNETTE 5.1

Dorothy was 45 years old when she received a diagnosis of pancreatic cancer after experiencing two months of fatigue, sense of bloating, and weight loss. Subsequent scans showed the cancer had metastasized to several areas of the liver. A yoga instructor who was married with two young children, Dorothy had followed a vegetarian diet for the past thirteen years, did not smoke, meditated regularly, and drank only a glass of wine occasionally. She felt she had done all she could to support a healthy lifestyle and minimize risk factors. She experienced a profound loss of meaning immediately after receiving the diagnosis and asked her doctor what had been the point of trying to eat healthy and take care of herself. At that meeting, Dorothy received psychoeducation about cancer and began to accept that she had chosen the right path by following a healthy lifestyle; that cancer, however, is a complex issue and diet is not the only factor involved. The oncologist recommended chemotherapy to slow the spread of disease in the hope that it would prolong her life. He told Dorothy he would use a combination of drugs to increase effectiveness and was confident she could tolerate the side effects. Dorothy felt an upsurge of meaning; she identified herself as a fighter and chose to pursue all the available treatment. She decided not to entertain the thought that treatment may not be successful and focused on remaining positive. However, Dorothy felt very ill for several days after each treatment and her quality of life was poor. She regretted not being able to spend quality time with her children and her husband, but she found meaning in thinking that after treatment was over she would be able to feel better. She was aware she could not be cured of the disease, but her oncologist had expressed optimism about the treatment, so she felt encouraged. Unfortunately, five months of chemotherapy was minimally effective in reducing the size of the cancer. Additionally, Dorothy felt weak and exhausted. During a family meeting, the oncologist told her and her family that it was unlikely that continuing treatment would help and recommended against it. The medical team recommended a referral to palliative care for quality of life.

Dorothy experienced a new, profound loss of meaning, with sadness and moments of hopelessness. During psychotherapy sessions with the palliative psychologist, she articulated that she had tolerated treatment expecting it would be effective. She now felt it had been "meaningless." She felt she had "wasted" the previous five months postponing living and waiting for an improvement in her condition that would never occur. Dorothy was not religious and did not consider herself particularly spiritual. However, she strongly resonated with the idea of meaning, which she described as the life force that allowed her to engage in the world. She now felt cut off from that source of life energy.

Psychotherapy treatment with Dorothy involved helping her reconnect with a sense of meaning in life. She believed she could not allow the disease to erase her life legacy. The idea of a global sense of meaning did not resonate with her. Rather, she strongly related to the concept of "infusing" every moment of her remaining life with meaning. Because of her meditation and mindfulness practice, she was aware that by giving full attention to each experience and each interaction, she was keeping anxiety, disappointment, and fear away from her awareness. She begin thinking about her life as an ongoing meditation practice. She joked that the psychotherapy approach should be named "living with cancer as a spiritual practice." In psychotherapy, Dorothy developed a keen awareness of the impact of her focus of attention on her mood. She noticed that when she felt fully present, she noticed smells, colors, background noises, nuances in temperature, and the rhythm of her breathing. In these moments, she felt fully alive and connected to a sense of meaning. When she allowed fear and resentment to be prominent, she felt her ability to perceive the world around her became restricted. She practiced these different ways of existing within the safe psychotherapy space and felt empowered to apply these skills to her relationship with her children and her spouse.

There is great variability in how practicing psychologists approach their patients' existential, spiritual, or religious concerns. Training background, professional setting, patient population, and preferred theoretical framework are relevant factors. Some therapists may believe that spiritual or religious beliefs do not belong in the therapy session. Others may have incorporated a spiritual or religious focus in their approach to psychotherapy and identify these aspects as central to their work. For instance, psychologists trained in the Transpersonal Psychology model typically value and encourage all forms of spiritual and transcendent experience and approach all human experience, including psychopathology, from a psychospiritual perspective. Additionally, psychologists with a specific religious orientation generally describe themselves through that lens (e.g., a Christian clinical psychologist). Spiritually oriented psychotherapy has received increasing attention in the last decade, resulting in the development of models and approaches integrating psychological and spiritual constructs. Most psychotherapy frameworks can effectively incorporate attention to the spiritual domain. Psychologists with training and experience incorporating spirituality in clinical practice are certainly supported by a growing body of literature indicating that, for many, this integration represents an important step toward healing.

Historically, cognitive behavioral therapy has included limited exploration of the patient's spiritual or religious beliefs. This may be especially true in behavioral health and primary care settings when psychological interventions are typically aimed at improving specific health outcomes, such as treatment adherence in diabetes or lower-back pain.

However, the recognition of spiritual and religious aspects as central to many patient's lives has facilitated adaptation of therapy models to include these themes (Waller, Trepka, Collerton, & Hawkins, 2010). For instance, several therapy models have integrated a broad understanding of spirituality, which is often conceptualized as mindfulness. Dialectical Behavioral Therapy, Acceptance and Commitment Therapy, and Mindfulness-Based Cognitive Therapy for Depression are examples of this approach. Additionally, Religiously Integrated Cognitive-Behavioral Therapy is a manualized intervention for the treatment of major depression in patients with chronic medical illness. A patient's religious beliefs are specifically incorporated in each of the therapy sessions, and the manuals have been developed for Christianity, Judaism, Islam, Budddhism, and Hinduism (Pearce et al., 2015).

The *Clinical Practice Guidelines for Quality Palliative Care* used as a framework for this book define the ability to recognize and address patients' and families' spiritual needs as a core competency for all specialist palliative care clinicians. In particular, palliative psychologists should provide a therapeutic space where religious, spiritual, and existential concerns can be safely explored, without judgment or stigma. This will indicate that they are not primarily focused on detecting signs of psychopathology, but on identifying what are important sources of meaning and purpose for the patient and the family (Sperry & Shafranske, 2005; Sperry, 2012).

Avoiding exploration of the spiritual domain would represent a disservice to the patient because it ignores central aspects of their experience. Of course, psychologists and others must offer services within their scope of practice and within the boundaries of their competence. They are not expected to function as spiritual care professionals and should not improvise spiritual or religious interventions. Rather, their openness about spiritual and religious needs will allow them to work collaboratively with spiritual care providers in the best interest of the patient.

Spiritual Screening, Spiritual History, and Spiritual Assessment

The importance of assessing the spiritual/religious domain is recognized in medicine, nursing, and psychiatry. For instance, spiritual distress is included in the spiritual diagnosis taxonomy for nursing, evaluating the patient's suffering in several categories, including connections to self; connections with others; connections with arts, music, literature, nature; and connections with power greater than self. Additionally, the fourth edition of the *Diagnostic and Statistical Manual of Mental Disorders* (DSM-IV-TR) included, for the first time, a new category called "Religious and Spiritual Problems." This category was maintained in the DSM-5. Categories and problem lists in this section (V codes or Z codes) are not considered mental disorders, but they are listed in the DSM because of their potential impact on the patient. In describing religious or spiritual problems, the DSM notes, "This category can be used when the focus of clinical attention is a religious or spiritual problem. Examples include distressing experiences that involve loss or questioning of faith, problems associated with conversion to a new faith, or questioning of spiritual values that may not necessarily be related to an organized church or religious institution" (p. 725).

Similarly, palliative care clinicians should incorporate spiritual screening, spiritual history, and spiritual assessment in the care of the patient and the family (Puchalski, 2010). This will ensure the prompt recognition of needs in the spiritual domain, as well as spiritual and existential suffering. In the literature, spiritual screening, history, and assessment are often used interchangeably, creating confusion regarding professional roles and responsibilities.

Every palliative care clinician should be able to screen a patient for spiritual distress or obtain a spiritual history. However, because licensed spiritual care professionals are the experts in assessing the spiritual and religious domain, they are uniquely qualified for administering formal spiritual assessments, formulating spiritual diagnoses, and developing treatment plans.

A *spiritual screening* is a procedure designed to quickly determine the patient's spiritual or religious orientation and affiliation, and whether the patient and the family are experiencing spiritual distress warranting an immediate referral to a spiritual care provider. The screening also enables identification of any cultural or religious practices that are relevant to the patient's hospital stay and medical care (LaRocca-Pitts, 2012). A screening generally contains one or two questions and it is a static procedure, not designed for further exploration at the moment of administration.

In the hospital setting, a nurse typically administers the screening upon admission to identify any urgent spiritual needs that would prompt a referral to a spiritual care professional. Due to low chaplain availability and the need to use resources efficiently, it is important that the screening procedure identify those patients who are more likely to benefit from an assessment by a spiritual care provider. At the same time, the screening should not automatically eliminate patients solely because they do not admit having spiritual or religious beliefs that are important to them. An example of screening algorithm developed for the hospital setting (Fitchett & Risk, 2009) begins with the question, "Is religion or spirituality important to you as you cope with your illness? If the patient answers "yes," the follow-up question asks, "How much strength/comfort do you get from your religion/spirituality now?" If the answer to the initial question is "no," the follow-up question asks, "Was there a time in the past when it was helpful?"

Screening tools can be modified to meet the specific cultural needs of the patient population in a particular setting. For example, the tool described above was modified in another study (Blanchard, Dunlap & Fitchett, 2012) by asking the patient upon admission, "Our team is committed to the whole person. Do you have a belief, spiritual or otherwise, that is important to you?" If the patient responds "yes," the follow up question asks, "Is that helping you now?" Based on the patient's answer, the clinician can determine the best course of action. For example, if the patient acknowledges any difficulties with their spiritual beliefs, they should be asked if they would like to share their concerns with a spiritual care provider. If they deny any interest in spiritual or religious aspects, they can be gently reminded that the health-care team remains available for any conversation in the future.

Spiritual screenings have limitations. For example, they can sometimes become focused on obtaining a quick "yes" or "no" answer from the patient. Additionally, the questions on a screening tool presuppose a shared understanding of the terms. To illustrate, a patient who is an atheist or an agnostic may respond "no" to the screening question because she may not want to be associated with religion, and the term "spiritual" may also seem too close to religion for her. However, she may have "spiritual" needs in the area related to the process of meaning-making, connectedness, and hope. And, some may actually welcome a "secular" conversation with a chaplain or another clinician who is able to explore these areas (Mais, 2010).

In a hospital setting, palliative psychologists are generally not the primary clinicians administering the screening to patients. They typically become involved after the patient's admission and after the patient has already received an assessment from nursing and medicine. However, they need to be aware of the results of these screening procedures as they are shared with team members. Additionally, they can incorporate basic spiritual screening questions as part of their clinical interview.

A *spiritual history* represents a lengthier, in-depth, and dynamic process that allows the clinician to interview the patient about spiritual or religious beliefs, practices, and values. It focuses on identifying the sources of strength, meaning, and purpose that are supporting them during their illness. It allows exploring the evolution of those resources in the patient's life and how their function may have changed. It has been recommended that a spiritual history be performed more than once during the hospitalization, especially if there is a change in the patient's medical condition that can impact personal coping and resources (LaRocca-Pitts, 2012).

When working in teams with other psychosocial-spiritual professionals, coordination of care is essential to avoid replication of services. The patient and the family should not be burdened by several clinicians asking the same questions or repeatedly exploring the same issues. On the other hand, a patient can certainly be followed by different psychosocial providers, even if there are overlaps. For instance, a patient may receive care from the psychologist, the chaplain, and the social worker for different needs. During interdisciplinary discussion the clinicians should clarify the general target of their intervention to facilitate collaboration and coordination of care.

Several spiritual history tools have been developed. Some of the available tools were initially developed to facilitate physicians' ability to explore spiritual beliefs with their patients. The questions/items on the spiritual history tools can be followed as a template or can be used as a general guide for discussion that will cover many aspects of the patient's values and worldview, including how their spiritual or religious resources and practices are supporting them as they are dealing with illness.

For a palliative psychologist, the process of spiritual history taking could be described as conducting a psychospiritual interview, where the patient is not only asked to describe events and situations, but also and foremost what type of meaning they attributed to the event, and what sources of strength are continuing to support them. Psychologists who are new to palliative care can benefit from becoming familiar with one tool and using it consistently. This will then allow them to expand on that tool and integrate other questions that may be relevant. The process of spiritual history taking can become a therapeutic and creative intervention because it gathers important information relevant to the care plan and also deepens the relationship with the patient and the family. For a detailed discussion of spiritual models and tools applicable to the palliative care setting, see Puchalski and Ferrell (2010). Those who do not feel comfortable exploring spiritual or existential needs should seek training and supervision opportunities to enhance their knowledge and skills. Making joined patient visits with spiritual care providers and shadowing them when possible can facilitate clinical comfort with spiritual issues and enhance competence.

The following examples of spiritual history tools are commonly used in the palliative care setting.

The FICA spiritual tool (Puchalski & Romer, 2000; Borneman, Ferrell, & Puchalski, 2010) explores the following dimensions:

- *Faith and beliefs*: Spiritual, religious, or otherwise
- *Importance*: Are these beliefs important in the context of the present illness?
- *Community*: Is there a community—religious, spiritual, or otherwise—that is supportive for the patient?
- *Address*: The clinician asks patients how spiritual or religious issues important to them can be incorporated into their care.

The HOPE spiritual history tool (Anandarajah & Hight, 2001) explores the following dimensions:

- *Hope*: What are the patient's sources of hope, meaning, comfort, and peace during difficult times?
- *Organized*: Is the patient part of organized religion or a spiritual community and how is the community supporting the patient at this time?
- *Personal spirituality/practice*: Does the patient have spiritual practices that are supportive at this time?
- *Effects on medical care and end of life issues*: Has the illness and the medical care affected the patient's ability to practice and connect with sources of meaning, faith, or spirituality?

The OPEN-INVITE tool (Saguil & Phelps, 2012) is a patient-centered tool developed for physicians and focuses on gently "opening the door" to spiritual dialogue by asking the patient if they have a religious or spiritual background. Additionally, clinicians can ask what has helped the patient cope during difficulty times. If the patient is willing to engage in the dialogue, there can be more focused questions by "inviting" further exploration. For example, it would be helpful to can ask how the patient's spirituality or religion affects medical care and their medical decision making.

A *spiritual assessment* is an in-depth process allowing the spiritual care provider to build a spiritual profile (LaRocca-Pitts, 2012) and identify spiritual concerns and sources of spiritual distress. In the palliative care setting, formal spiritual assessments include diagnostic considerations and treatment plan that should be completed by a licensed spiritual care professional (Puchalski & Ferrell, 2010). The treatment plan includes recommendations for relieving the patient's spiritual pain or for allowing sources of support to remain present and active in the patient's life during the hospitalization and afterward.

CLINICAL CONSIDERATIONS

The process of obtaining a spiritual history can identify the interplay of psychological, religious, and spiritual issues in the manifestations of a patient's worldview and personal sense of meaning. It can help the clinician appreciate how the patient understands and defines his or her image of God, or a higher power. To illustrate, there are differences between patients who believe in God as a personal and defined entity, patients who have a more undefined belief in a divine presence, and those patients who do not believe in a personal God or a divine presence but may value experiencing a sense of connectedness with something larger than themselves.

The constructs of "God image" and "God concept" have been used to explore the nature of these relationships in patients who believe in a personal God or a higher power. Ana-Maria Rizzuto (1979) differentiated between the God Concept and the God Image. According to her conceptualization, while the God Concept is an intellectual definition, the God Image is an internal psychological model resulting from memories and associations developed from various sources, which allows the individual to develop and internalize a sense of who God is in a personal relationship. It is a relevant construct, as individuals' God Image impacts on psychological functioning. To illustrate, a study exploring the relationship between God images among adolescents, showed that those who held the God image of a merciful and compassionate God had higher scores on empathy compared to those who held a God image based on justice (Francis, Croft, & Pike, 2012). The God Image Inventory is an eight-scale instrument with 156 items to measure the individual's image of God. The scales explore issues of belonging (as presence and challenge) goodness (as acceptance and benevolence) and control (as influence and providence). Due to its length, the God Image Inventory has limited application in the palliative care setting. However, the key aspect for palliative psychologists exploring spirituality is the importance of understanding how patients relate to the concept, image, and identity of God, and the importance of recognizing how this impacts on the patient's overall coping, adaptation, and well-being (Lawrence, 1997).

Exploring the patient's image of God, whether it is the result of the teachings of a defined religious group or the expression of personal spirituality, can help shed light on the patient's current relationship with sources of meaning and support. This can be especially valuable when there is psychological or spiritual distress.

For example, a patient who is experiencing depression may report that his understanding of God as a personal entity has changed. While a patient experiencing depression may rely even more closely on God's help to feel better emotionally, another may instead begin feeling more distant from God and become convinced that she is being judged or punished. What used to be an image of God as merciful and supportive may become, in the context of depression or unrelieved grief, an image of an unforgiving, judgmental, and uncaring presence. This change can cause profound spiritual pain and alienation, with fear of being abandoned by God and becoming separated from a main source of meaning and strength in the patient's life.

Because of the overlap between psychological and spiritual constructs, the presence of spiritual or existential distress, such as sense of meaninglessness, alienation, or despair should be carefully understood. Although these can also be present in the context of clinical depression due to the overlap between depression and spiritual distress, research is indicating that they represent two different dimensions of human experience. A study of 185 older patients compared their depression scores on the 15-item Geriatric Depression Scale (GDS-15) and spiritual distress on the Spiritual Distress Assessment Tool (SDAT). Results indicated that depression symptoms and spiritual distress represented two different dimensions. Although high depression scores were associated with spiritual distress, the study found that patients with low depression scores were associated with great variability of spiritual distress scores (Bornet et al., 2016).

Recognizing Spiritual and Existential Needs in Understudied Populations

Palliative care clinicians should ensure that spiritual and existential needs are adequately addressed in patients who are not religious and those who hold belief systems that are incompatible with conventional ideas of religion or spirituality (Thiel & Robinson, 2015).

ATHEISTS

Patients who described themselves as atheists represent a group that has been understudied in palliative and end-of-life care. According to the American Atheists website (2017), Atheism is not an affirmative belief that there is no god nor does it answer any other question about what a person believes. It is simply a rejection of the assertion that there are gods. Atheism is too often defined incorrectly as a belief system. There are over 1.6 million self-defined atheists in the United States, and they represent a growing minority. According to statistics released by the Pew Foundation, in 2015, nearly one-fourth of Americans described themselves as non-religious (Pew Foundation). Atheism is not a belief system or a religion, but it can be described as a lack of belief in God, or supernatural beings, and atheists generally advocate for complete separation of church and state.

Importantly, atheists do not share a common belief system and assumptions cannot be made about what values and practices are important. The lack of belief in God can be described as the only common denominator among atheists. Atheism can be expressed in different ways—thus, the importance for clinicians of understanding the unique worldview of each patient without assumptions. Allowing the patient and the family to educate the clinician about their beliefs and values facilitates communication and promotes understanding.

A study conducted with 88 participants, involving members of two national atheist organizations, explored end-of-life preferences and assessed potential interventions based on a model of spiritual care (Smith-Stoner, 2007). This model defined spirituality as the integration of the following needs:

- to find meaning in life (intrapersonal dimension)
- intimacy in relationships (interpersonal dimension)
- connection to nature and the environment (natural dimension).

A 26-question survey was developed to explore participants' needs and perceptions in the three dimensions of the model. Results allowed identification of five areas that were important for participants: comfort, decision making, autonomy, spirituality, and natural.

In the area of *comfort*, participants' responses indicated that they valued evidence-based medical care and considered pain management and symptom relief important components of a "good death." In the area of *decision making*, participants indicated that being part of this process was important, and they did not advocate for futile care. Additionally, they regarded physician-assisted suicide as a way of achieving a dignified death and reducing suffering for family caregivers. In the area of *autonomy*, participants considered it important that health-care providers respect their wishes not to receive prayers or judgment about their lack of belief in God. In the area of *spirituality*, they valued intrapersonal experience and identified ways of honoring it by finding time to relax and to review their life. In the *interpersonal* dimension, participants expressed the desire that family members should organize memorial services as an opportunity to receive grief and bereavement support. In the *natural* dimension, some participants chose cremation as a way of disposing of the body and stated valuing time in the outdoors and time spent with animals.

This information points to the importance of adopting a broad framework when discussing spiritual needs with palliative care patients. Because of the strong associations between spirituality and religion, some patients who do not believe in God or disapprove of organized religion may have strong negative reactions when asked specific questions about their spirituality. Additionally, some may react negatively when hearing the term "spirituality" because they may associate it with spiritualism, which is characterized by a belief in God and especially the belief that spirits can communicate with the living (Mais, 2010). Therefore, while asking screening questions about spiritual beliefs can be perfectly appropriate for some patients, it may be counterproductive when used with patients who have strong negative associations to the words spiritual and religious. Perhaps, asking patients what gives their life meaning and purpose and what they consider important in life can be a better opening for exploring their values and beliefs. This approach will allow clinicians to establish rapport, without eliciting negative responses.

The ability to respect non-religious values and attitudes is also particularly important for providing competent and sensitive care during bereavement.

PAGANS AND WICCANS

Members of paganism and Wicca are also a growing minority in the United States. Paganism is often described as an earth religion, a religion that is not based on specific dogma but on following and respecting natural laws and cycles of nature and the cosmos. Activities are guided by the cycles of nature and the seasons. Depending on the particular coven, Wiccans may worship a male god and a female goddess, or only one. For example, covens of feminist activists may decide to only welcome feminine energy in their activities, rituals, and worship. Many pagan worshippers have rejected the patriarchal roots of organized religion and advocate for supremacy of the feminine. The use of magic is fully integrated into the lives of Wiccans. Magic is regarded as a way of focusing intention and energy to bring about a desired change. During their magic rituals, Wiccans may utilize the energy of herbs, rocks, or any other natural resource. Symbols are commonly used to represents the elements: fire, water, earth, and metal. There is great variation within the pagan community, with some following a number of gods and goddesses and others focusing on a specific symbol of life force (Hollins, 2009).

Members of pagan and Wiccan religions may be reluctant to disclose their spirituality to health-care professionals, especially in a hospital setting. The various biases and misconceptions about this religion have created significant stigma around its members. Wiccans are often incorrectly associated with worship of Satan and negative forces. However, Wicca prohibits use of magic ritual to create damage. Many Wiccans may be solitary practitioners, because they may not live in an area where covens are available.

If asked about their spiritual beliefs during a hospitalization, pagans and Wiccans may remain vague and choose not to disclose their faith for fear that they will be judged negatively. They may also be concerned that the quality of the medical care they receive will be affected by how they are perceived by the medical staff. However incorrect and unfounded these concerns may be, they ultimately contribute to a sense of isolation in the patient. Patients may, however, feel more comfortable disclosing their faith during a general psychospiritual interview. It is important to exhibit sincere interest in further understanding the patient's worldview, with the goal of improving the ability to meet the patient's needs.

Smith-Stoner and Young (2007) applied Steinhauser's framework for defining a good death as a guide to describe Wiccans' end-of-life needs and surveyed 2,607 individuals who defined themselves as Wiccan, pagan, or nature spiritualists about their preferences and practices. Most respondents expressed a preference for a death at home, cremation, and organ donation. Additionally, while many participants valued pharmacological treatment of pain, they also valued autonomy and clear decision-making, as well as the importance of ritual and connectedness.

Exploring Manifestations of Religious, Spiritual, and Existential Distress

In clinical practice, spiritual distress, existential distress, and psychological distress often overlap, and the patient's experience may include a combination of different sources of suffering (Kissane, 2012). Understanding the core of the patient's experience may be helpful to tailor the intervention and develop a treatment plan.

Some patients ask "why" the illness is happening to them, and what it means. The lack of a meaningful or acceptable answer may trigger spiritual pain. A religious patient may begin to feel abandoned by God. Another patient struggling to find meaning in the worsening of illness may believe there is a lesson he needs to learn and understand in order to heal. This struggle to make meaning of the illness may create distress, and spiritual pain may result. A patient may become convinced that the illness is the result of maladaptive psychological patterns that if successfully addressed, would directly and positively impact the course of the disease. When the focus on finding meaning in illness creates spiritual pain, it is important to explore with the patient what strategies she is using to conduct this meaning-making inquiry and whether these are supportive, or have the potential to create more distress.

CASE VIGNETTE 5.2

Mary Jane was a 65-year-old woman with advanced ovarian cancer. The referral questions for the palliative care consultation team were pain, anxiety, and need to discuss goals of care. After the initial diagnosis 14 months prior, followed by surgery and chemotherapy, the patient was told the cancer was in remission. Six months later she developed a bowel obstruction, which caused severe pain and required hospitalization. After a scan showed extensive spread of disease to the bowels, she was told that active treatment was no longer indicated or helpful and the focus of the care should be symptom management. The news that the cancer had spread so quickly and aggressively felt like the ultimate betrayal to Mary Jane. The palliative care team offered psychological support, but Mary Jane declined because she was already seeing a therapist and felt supported by her. However, she offered to describe her therapy to the palliative psychologist. Mary Jane explained that soon after diagnosis she had used several complementary approaches to manage the distress caused by the disease and by the side effects of treatment. During treatment she saw her therapist twice a week and focused on processing and expressing her emotions through writing, painting, and singing. She made meaning of the diagnosis by believing that it was primarily caused by her difficulty expressing anger in relationships, especially toward her husband. She believed that years of suppressed anger had created fertile ground for the cancer to grow. And she was convinced that by removing what she described as "emotional blocks" she could enhance the effectiveness of chemotherapy and radiation. According to Mary Jane, her therapist had encouraged her belief system and approach. After being told the cancer had metastasized, her initial reaction was that she needed to work harder to develop a relatively peaceful coexistence with her cancer. She was willing to allow the cancer to stay in her body, provided it did not kill her.

Her therapist encouraged Mary Jane to use past-lives regression therapy. Mary Jane believed that if she was willing to explore in depth her feelings, thoughts, and emotions about the cancer, she could limit its aggressiveness. She intensified her personal therapeutic work, connecting with several holistic therapists. The message she consistently received from the different therapists was that if she really worked hard to remove her emotional and mental blocks, she could control the cancer. However, this concept began to cause her distress, as she could not identify any significant blocks that could be responsible for the cancer spread. She decided to work even harder, in therapy and with her group of healers. Despite all her efforts, the cancer not only continued to spread, but also started causing significant pain. Overwhelmed by the rapid progression of her illness and her inability to stop it, she became highly anxious and distressed. Her emotional pain escalated with the increase of physical pain. The palliative care team recommended opioid therapy to control the pain; however, Mary Jane was reluctant to take the medication regularly because she thought it would cause an altered state of mind that would prevent her from using effective cancer-fighting strategies. Her physical pain continued to increase, as did her emotional distress and spiritual pain. In the last 10 days of her life she accepted more pain medication, and her overall distress subsided. While she continued to carefully monitor how much morphine she was being given, she acknowledged that adequate pain management had a positive impact on her emotional state.

Discussion

In Case Vignette 5.2, Mary Jane had developed the belief that the worsening of the disease was caused by her inability to release "emotional blocks." She could not entertain the possibility of alternative explanations and continued seeking answers from her community of healers. During a palliative care team meeting, some of the clinicians questioned whether Mary Jane was being manipulated by the group of healers and therapists, and questions were raised about whether she was being hurt emotionally by them. During the following visit at the palliative care clinic, the psychologist and the social worker met with Mary Jane and her husband and gently but directly shared the team's concerns. The psychologist and social worker also wondered out loud if there was something they could do to alleviate Mary Jane's suffering.

Mary Jane and her husband thanked the clinicians for being concerned about her and for being direct about it. They explained that they felt supported by their community and that Mary Jane felt in control at all times. She stated that her main therapist knew the family had financial difficulties and did not charge her for the work they did together. Her friends would take turns spending time with her so that her husband could have respite; they were attentive, offering to massage her feet and prepare food. Mary Jane said that at this point she needed to continue on her path because, in addition to being with her family, seeking to heal herself was all that gave her life meaning and purpose. It was clear from the interview that Mary Jane had decisional capacity, and there was no evidence that she was being abused emotionally.

While the palliative care clinicians admitted after the interview that they experienced countertransference, they also recognized that as Mary Jane had articulated, this was "her path," and their responsibility was to support her while ensuring that she was safe in this process. Unfortunately, Mary Jane did not obtain the answers she was looking for, or the outcome she wished for, before she died. She did not develop any new insights about what caused her cancer and why she had not succeeded in controlling its activity, in spite of all the personal work she engaged in. During the psychological evaluations with the palliative care psychologist, she did not meet criteria for depression or for an anxiety disorder. One can speculate that the abrupt news of a recurrence, compounded by the quick progression of disease, may have seriously compromised Mary Jane's coping skills and ability to process the change in disease stage and rapid deterioration. Mary Jane deeply valued being in control of her life and felt she could affect the disease the way she had been able to control other events and situations in her life.

The communication of a terminal diagnosis created such a profound rupture in her personal narrative that she could no longer continue to create meaning in a way that was supportive of her well-being. The news created a spiritual and existential crisis, with profound suffering. Additionally, the rapid worsening of disease and deterioration did not allow her enough time to fully consider different explanations and ways of thinking about the disease, other than a self-blaming focus on emotional "blocks." Paradoxically, it appears that her meaning-making process became detrimental. And yet it was her "journey," and the palliative care team respected her wishes and continued to bear witness to her story. According to her belief system, the ability to successfully eliminate psychological blocks would result in the cancer becoming controlled and no longer threatening her life. While Mary Jane's beliefs and expectations appeared to support her sense of meaning and connection to her community, the inflexibility of her belief, which involved only one possible outcome, created a challenging situation and magnified her spiritual and existential suffering.

As suggested by Niemeyer, "human beings are inveterate meaning makers p. 184." The process of making meaning can lead patients on a path of self-discovery, possibilities, growth, and emotional healing. However, it can also lead them on an increasingly narrow path, devoid of possibilities. Still, the task for palliative psychologists is to always "be with" the patient, regardless of the path he or she chooses, witnessing the unfolding of his or her story, respecting boundaries, while attempting to expand opportunities for emotional and existential healing.

Palliative psychologists may gently challenge what appear to be unsupportive beliefs and practices, but ultimately they have a responsibility to accompany the patient, without judgment, without a desire to fix, without a preconceived notion of what type of spiritually evolved death they should have. In essence, patients may experience spiritual distress not only when they lose the ability to make meaning of the events in their lives, but also when the strategies and processes utilized to make meaning deprive them of opportunities rather than expanding them.

ALIENATION

Religious patients may experience spiritual alienation as a sense that God is distant and unreachable. Spiritual alienation may cause patients to feel abandoned, alone, and undeserving of support and comfort. The therapist could explore with patients what it was like when they felt spiritually connected to either God, a divine presence, their deepest sense of self, or any other representation of a sense of connectedness. The therapist could also explore what factors or stressors may have contributed to the feeling of alienation.

Spiritual alienation in patients who have a secular approach may present as a feeling of being disconnected from loved ones and from values they once deemed important. This condition may present in a manner similar to depression and demoralization in symptomatology. In essence, patients may experience a sense of feeling abandoned, with loss of a sense of connection and purpose.

LOSS OF FAITH OR SPIRITUAL BELIEFS

Religious patients may feel they have lost God's love, or they may fear they no longer have a personal relationship with God. This sense of loss can trigger a profound grief reaction, which can be as intense and devastating as bereavement. Patients who describe themselves as spiritual and not religious may report they have lost the relationship with their sense of self. Spiritual loss is deeply connected to the sense of spiritual alienation, which can turn their image of the universe into something distant, detached, uncaring, or even hostile.

In the midst of challenging circumstances that test the patient's and the family's coping skills, some may experience doubt or conflict in their faith. Some may find it challenging to reconcile their image of a loving divine presence with the reality that they have been "allowed" to develop the disease. Thus, a patient may believe the disease is evidence that God is punishing them or no longer protecting them. Patients who do not believe in a personal God may still blame "life itself" for being unfair.

Worsening disease and approaching death can test a patient's spiritual, religious, or secular beliefs. The therapist should not assume that the beliefs that have supported patients during their lives will automatically offer the same level of support as they approach death.

SPIRITUAL COMPONENTS OF ANXIETY AND DEPRESSION

From a psychospirtual perspective, depression and anxiety in patients with serious and advanced illness are not merely behavioral manifestations of a biological disorder. They also affect patients' sense of meaning and purpose and their relationship with themselves and others. Accordingly, they could be conceptualized as manifestations of spiritual distress related to loss of meaning and purpose. For this reason, depression has also been described as "the dark night of the soul," to indicate the spiritual counterpart of the diagnosis.

Anxiety and fear also have profound spiritual implications. Patients who constantly worry about the future and envision worst-case scenarios may also become disconnected, both cognitively and emotionally, from sources of spiritual strength and support. Fear of dying is common when patients experience spiritual anxiety. It is important to explore the sources of this fear. Is the patient afraid of suffering from unmanaged pain and other physical symptoms? Is there fear of losing control by becoming dependent on others and losing one's dignity? Is there fear about what will happen after their death? Patients who are not religious may begin wondering about the concept of an afterlife, even if they have never believed in it. Some may become anxious about lacking a clear belief to support them during the dying process. They may also feel terrified at the idea of nonexistence after death, and contemplating that possibility may trigger profound anxiety and even terror.

A palliative psychologist following an integrative approach in diagnosis and treatment will always try to understand the spiritual implications of any manifestation of psychological distress or psychiatric disorder. While palliative psychology actively addresses psychopathology, it also explores how psychological distress develops, how it affects the individuals belief system and values, and how it is in turn affected by those values.

GUILT

While not all patients will engage in a review of their lives and evaluation of their actions, some may become focused on past actions and experiences that have hurt others and damaged relationships. As a result, some may feel a variety of emotions, ranging from regret to profound guilt and remorse. The underlying spiritual or religious question they may struggle with is whether they will be able to receive forgiveness, and if God will welcome them after their death. Patients who do not believe in a personal God may still fear some form of undefined retribution after their death. Or, the guilt about their past actions may develop into profound sense of demoralization and meaninglessness. Exploring the concept of forgiveness with these patients can help clinicians understand whether patients are wishing for forgiveness from someone specifically, or if they are hoping for a more general sense of acceptance and understanding.

Patients may disclose to therapists past actions that may challenge the clinician's ability to convey a sense of openness, safety, and complete acceptance. The issue of confidentiality in therapy may become relevant in this context. For example, patients may reveal having physically or sexually abused their children in the past. There may be graphic descriptions of the abuse and expressions of profound remorse. Or a patient may disclose that he has killed someone as a result of an altercation or drunk driving. He may reveal that he fled the scene and never told anyone. Yet now that his life is coming to an end, he may feel that the emotional burden is unbearable and that he needs to share his actions with someone in the hope of some reconciliation and acceptance.

Any communication offered during therapy is protected by confidentiality. There are exceptions if there is reason to believe that the abuse of a child, older person, or vulnerable adult is ongoing or there is potential for new or further abuse. Although reporting responsibilities need to be carefully considered and followed by all clinicians, it is important to note that patients who report past harmful or criminal behavior in therapy may wish to "confess" and receive symbolic "forgiveness" from the therapist. Applying Roger's principle of unconditional positive regard for the patient during therapy will help clinicians convey a sense of acceptance. While the psychologist cannot actually "forgive" or "absolve" past crimes, it is possible to convey a sense of deep human understanding. Close collaboration between spiritual care providers and psychologists can prove extremely beneficial and facilitate the experience of healing and peace for the patient and for the family. Psychological and spiritual interventions focused on legacy building can also help facilitate the experience of positive, healing emotions.

A palliative psychologist can embody the ability to understand, hold, and embrace complexity and ambiguity. They can do so by witnessing a patient's humanity with respect, wisdom, and even tenderness. If the patient expresses the desire to receive formal "absolution" for past or current actions, a referral should be promptly made to a spiritual care provider, who will evaluate the appropriateness of a spiritual or religious ritual to relieve suffering.

ANGER

There are multiple reasons why religious patients may develop anger toward their religion and, consequently, at God. They may have experienced abuse at the hand of a religious leader and they may have never reported it. Anger is a strong emotion that can be manifested in different ways based on the unique psychological makeup of each person. Nonetheless, it is often associated with high levels of energy and it highlights the interplay of the spiritual and psychological domain. It certainly can create significant distress for the patient and the family witnessing the patient's suffering.

Integrating Spirituality in the Palliative Psychology Session

Addressing the etymology of the word "psychology" as blending the roots of *psyche* and *logos*, Hillman (1983, location 251, kindle edition) described it as "reason or speech or intelligible account of soul." Interestingly, the term "psychotherapy" comes from the Greek *therapeia*, which means support and caring. Psychotherapy can then be understood as a process of serving the patient's soul. For this reason, Jungian psychology refers to psychotherapy as "soul making."

The therapeutic space created by the palliative psychologist needs to be welcoming, safe, and ready to accommodate the patient and the family to the full extent of human experience, including spirituality and religion. In the therapeutic space patients reveal their suffering, their hopes and fears and they can explore healing and sources of healing. Here, they can explore what infuses their life of meaning and what annihilates a sense of meaning and purpose. The therapist witnesses, welcomes, and symbolically holds the pain, helping the patient work through or process the content and source of the suffering. In this way the patient can "make sense" of the suffering, understanding its personal and universal significance. Thus, the meaning-making process of suffering is not only a cognitive and emotional process but it can also be a spiritual one.

In this sense, facilitating a deeply personal connection to a sense of meaning helping the patient reclaim their personal narrative is a spiritual process. This allows the patient to identify and maintain a sense of continuity and congruence in the midst of medical crises and ongoing challenges that threaten their most meaningful connections. The quality of connection or presence provided by the therapist can be described as "an attitude of palpable, immediate, kinesthetic, effective, and profound attention" (Schneider, 2008, p. 60). For some, the quality of this experience has a felt sense of the spiritual.

In addition to incorporating screening questions, palliative psychologists can also integrate a spiritual history as a component of the clinical interview. Elements of spiritual history can then continue to be fluidly incorporated in each subsequent meeting with the patient and addressed based on their relevance. Because of its focus on therapeutic alliance, relationship building, and respectful and supportive exploration, the process of obtaining a spiritual history can provide immediate benefits to the patient and the family. It can create a space where they feel understood and where their core beliefs are valued.

The process of obtaining a spiritual history in the course of a therapy session can include exploration of the following areas:

- patient's understanding of the meaning of life and the meaning of his or her *own* life
- any religious beliefs and practices and their evolution over time
- importance of prayer in the patient's life
- beliefs about life after death
- use of contemplative practices, such as meditation, mystical poetry, and others
- any past experiences that had spiritual impact, such as near-death experiences, or traumatic experiences that triggered a spiritual journey
- importance of the religious or spiritual community as a source of support.

When there is significant overlap of spiritual and psychological components of distress, it may be beneficial if a psychologist and spiritual care provider can visit a patient jointly, in addition to individually. This can allow each clinician to provide expertise in unique aspects of his or her discipline, while honoring the overlaps, with the goal of providing maximal support for patients in distress.

In the course of a therapy session, a psychologist may develop the impression that the patient's beliefs and practices in the area of religion or spirituality that used to be sustaining for the patient are no longer supporting her, but are actually causing distress. For example, patients may describe that since they became ill they think of God as angry, impossible to please, and punishing. Or they may develop severe anxiety about the future of family members who do not follow the same religion and "will not be saved." A patient may believe that the illness is the result of divine retribution for bad past behavior, and the pain is punishment. As a result, they may refuse pain medication or other interventions intended to relieve suffering. They may even articulate that "dying in pain" is the only way to make up for the past wrong. Patients in abusive relationships may have received or interpreted the teachings from their spiritual leaders as condoning of the abuse. Thus, they may believe that they have to continue tolerating the abuse. Patients with depression may feel that their psychological difficulties are the result of their lack of spirituality or inability to follow religious practices as they should. As a result, they may not be willing to accept treatment, be it structured psychotherapy or pharmacological interventions. They may have developed the belief that only God can help them feel better and that if help is not provided, it means they do not deserve it.

Upon discovering these sources of distress, the psychologist may believe that psychological intervention should be used to modify a belief system that does not appear to be supportive of the individual. There may be a combination of strong countertransference reactions together with a true desire to relieve the patient's suffering. The pull for "fixing" can be particularly strong in clinicians who are new to the field. Additionally, there may be a perception of urgency due to the patient's poor prognosis and the transferential wish to allow for "a good death." Self-awareness of personal beliefs, biases, and agenda becomes critical in these scenarios. The clinician must develop the ability to truly "be with" before even contemplating "change" especially if the patient had not expressed any desire to modify their belief systems.

Patients' autonomy remains important even in the midst of medical crises, psychosocial distress, and the clinician's desire to "fix" is sometimes based on his or her own anxiety or countertransference—or prior experiences with death and dying. It is important to keep in mind that religious and spiritual beliefs systems are generally deeply rooted in the patient's life and that challenging them may be perceived as offensive and disrespectful, as well as being outside the competency of a psychologist. Certainly, not all the patients' concerns may be addressed by using a psychological framework, however broad, inclusive, holistic, or integrative. If religious and spiritual beliefs appear to cause significant distress to patients, it is important to involve a spiritual care professional in the care.

CASE VIGNETTE 5.3

Roy was a 49-year-old African American man with metastatic appendiceal carcinoma, admitted to the hospital for severe pain and anxiety. He had received multiple chemotherapy treatments. With progression of the disease, causing extension of the cancer through the abdominal wall and small bowel obstruction, he walked with difficulty and was uncomfortable most of the time. The medical team thought that the prognosis was in order of a few months. Roy was also a veteran who had been in active combat. He had a history of alcohol abuse but had been sober for 10 years. He was raised Baptist but had disconnected from organized religion. The medical team requested a palliative care consult to address the patient's unwillingness to accept pain medication even in the presence of severe pain and his unwillingness to allow nursing staff to provide support with daily hygiene. The medical team was also concerned about Roy's severe anxiety and overall emotional distress and what they described as a profound distrust of the medical system. They were also concerned about Roy's comments that he wished he could die in his sleep.

In the course of the comprehensive assessment conducted jointly by the psychologist and the chaplain, several sources of suffering were identified:

Presence of untreated PTSD due to having experienced sexual assault in the military. Roy shared that three men in his platoon had accused him of being homosexual and had sexually assaulted him. He reported the assault but stated he was encouraged not to pursue the matter. Roy tried to forget the assault but began experiencing flashbacks of the assault, recurrent nightmares, and hyper-vigilance. When the male nurses approached him for the daily hygiene, he felt as if he was in danger and became anxious. Yet, a sense of shame and embarrassment prevented him from openly discussing the reasons for his reaction.

Suicidal ideation. Roy felt that the memory of the assault and the physical pain he was currently experiencing made life unbearable for him. The psychological assessment revealed that Roy had passive suicidal ideation without a plan or means. However, he said that thinking about dying was the only thing that comforted him. While he did not appear to be in imminent danger, it was obvious that Roy was suffering. During the suicide assessment, Roy shared that his girlfriend had left him because she could not cope with the idea that he had been sexually assaulted. Roy felt isolated, neglected, and unworthy. These feelings created ongoing pain, and he thought about suicide as a way of stopping the suffering.

Low social support. Roy had an older brother who occasionally visited him at the hospital. He felt very anxious about social interactions and was convinced that people could "see" from his demeanor that he had been sexually assaulted. He had attended a support group for veterans after his discharge but felt there was a barrier between him and other people. He felt trapped by these feelings and unable to reach out for emotional support.

Guilt and need for forgiveness. Roy felt extremely guilty for having caused human deaths during combat. He stated that he was unable to forgive himself and felt no one else could. He felt God would never forgive him and this was the main reason he had stopped connecting with his church community.

Pervasive loss of meaning and legacy. Roy commented that he was facing the end of his life "with nothing to show for." He felt that overall he had made bad decisions in his life and did not have anything meaningful to leave behind. He thought of his life as a negative narrative but wished he could identify a positive legacy to leave behind.

Undertreated pain and unsupportive belief system related to the use of medication. Roy was suffering with severe pain, but did not take pain medication as prescribed. He was concerned that taking opioid medication regularly meant he was sliding back into a pattern of addiction. His AA sponsor had related stories about people in recovery who had started using again after "trying opioids." Hence, Roy was convinced he should be able to cope with the pain without medication. He was suffering deeply and felt "trapped" by his own rules.

Negative self-concept. Roy had developed negative cognitions about himself. As a result, he had a negative self-concept, which appeared to undermine any attempt to establish a connection with a sense of meaning. Core negative cognitions were (1) I failed to protect myself from the assault; I am unable to take care of myself, and I cannot be safe in social interactions; (2) I do not deserve forgiveness; (3) I am unlovable as a human being; and (4) my life was a waste, and I cannot leave a meaningful legacy behind.

Roy was clearly experiencing high levels of distress on multiple levels. He also met criteria for depression. The chaplain and the psychologists coordinated a psychological/spiritual plan with the rest of the team to address Roy's needs. Because it was not clear how long he would be in the hospital, it was important to prioritize interventions to ensure goals would be realistic and could be met.

It appeared that addressing the active PTSD symptoms, physical pain, and profound guilt needed to be targeted first. With Roy's consent, the psychologist provided Eye Movement Desensitization and Reprocessing (EMDR) to address PTSD from the sexual trauma. In the course of three sessions, some of the core negative cognitions were targeted, specifically "I am unsafe" and "I am unlovable." The metaphor of safely observing a traumatic scene from a moving train was used when explaining this treatment to Roy. EMDR treatment was effective for Roy. His level of anxiety drastically decreased, and he reported he could still remember the assault but felt as if he was watching the scene from a moving train—so he was no longer present at the scene.

The palliative care chaplain worked with Roy to address his spiritual guilt and need for forgiveness. Together, they read scriptures from the Christian tradition, prayed, and meditated on the scriptures' emphasis on forgiveness. Roy felt great emotional relief and healing from the spiritual counseling sessions and began to re-establish a relationship with God. His God image became merciful and forgiving. The chaplain and the psychologist both met with Roy for a joint session to discuss pain management, which was still under-managed. Jointly, the psychologist and the chaplain discussed with Roy the difference between addiction and adequate pain management.

The psychologist guided Roy in an imagery exercise asking him to imagine God in front of him receiving all of Roy's fears, anxieties, and hopelessness and sending back love, acceptance, and forgiveness. He was asked to continue focusing on that exchange as pain management was discussed. Both the psychologist and the chaplain told Roy that it was clear to them that he wanted to maintain a sober lifestyle and did not want to use medication inappropriately. The chaplain mentioned that he believed God also knew this to be the truth. Roy cried during most of the session but remained oriented and grounded, so both clinicians felt the intervention was safe. At the end of the session, Roy said he was willing to start taking his medication as prescribed, so he would feel less distressed and better able to actively engage in reading the scriptures. This important reframing of the purpose and role of pain medication was facilitated by Roy's engagement in a meaning-making process that allowed him to reconnect with his beliefs in God.

The psychologist and the music therapist engaged Roy in a legacy project to address his distress about failing to lead a meaningful life. The first step consisted in identifying the recipient of the project. Roy was not close to his brother and had no close friends. He did not feel his brother would value receiving his legacy project. After considering various options, Roy chose a local organization supporting victims of sexual assault. His legacy project consisted in the creation of a video interview and a journal, both of which were created with the palliative care team during his hospitalization. The director of the organization was contacted, and she expressed a strong interest in using Roy's legacy project to empower and help other survivors. In the video, Roy told his story about the assault and described how the trauma and shame had negatively affected his life. He spoke about how reconnecting with his faith had brought new meaning into his life. He provided encouragement for victims of sexual assault not only to report the assault, but also to seek support. The journal contained poems and thoughts that illustrated Roy's healing process, and he wrote in it daily.

Roy remained at the hospital for two weeks. His pain became better controlled, and he felt the traumatic sexual assault no longer defined him. He was now defined by the transformative experience of forgiveness and reconciliation with God. He reconnected with an important source of meaning, his relationship with God, and found peace. He had found a home for a positive legacy of resilience, hope, and healing. He was transferred to a nursing home, where he received supportive counseling from the chaplain and social worker on staff until his death, three months later. According to the nursing home social worker who contacted the palliative care team after Roy's death, he continued writing in his book every day, with the last entry being two days before he died.

CASE VIGNETTE 5.4

Connie was a 55-year-old woman with advanced congestive heart failure. She had severe edema of the lower extremities and could no longer lie down. She spent her days sitting in an upright chair and a hospital bed at night. Her physician was direct about her prognosis, which he believed to be about six months. He recommended hospice, but Connie said she needed some time to make the decision. Diagnosed with cardiomyopathy in her twenties, she had experienced a progressive worsening of the disease. She worked from home as a technical writer and lived with her elderly mother, a retired school teacher. She avoided romantic relationships most of her life, because she did not feel she had enough energy for them. Connie's cardiologist thought she was depressed and consulted the hospital-based palliative psychologist. The physician thought that Connie appeared too calm and he was concerned she was not allowing herself to grieve her approaching death to avoid upsetting her mother, who was her primary caregiver.

During the meeting with the psychologist, Connie explained that she had been an atheist for over thirty years. She felt that the idea of the existence of a personal God did not make any sense to her. She believed she had been able to maintain a good quality of life precisely because she did not believe in God. Had she not been an atheist, she would have asked questions about her illness that could not be answered, such as "why me." She was glad she was not "burdened" with the need to find a reason why God would not allow her to have a better life. She reacted with slight irritation when the psychologist inquired about her sources of meaning and purpose in life, commenting "The issue of meaning has no meaning for me." She added that people reacted negatively when she explained she did not believe in God and in the past she had felt discriminated against for being an atheist.

She explained that the only things that mattered to her was whether the psychologist would be able to "show up" for her and be with her through her different emotions, including despair, without trying to change it or "fix" it somehow. Connie stated that what she wanted from people was "absolute presence." The therapy session became focused on exploring what Connie meant by absolute presence and how people around her could offer that quality of experience. She was also invited to explain how that quality of presence in people had been supportive during her life. Connie found comfort in focusing on what she was doing without letting her mind wander or ruminate. She could spend several moments simply observing a flower in all its details, and described feeling a sense of balance during those activities. Connie had never been trained in mindfulness or other mediation practice. When asked how she had developed such a rich way of approaching life, she related that her illness "pushed" her to do the best she could with her human capabilities because she did not believe in the existence of a reality outside of immediate experience. During her explanation, Connie appeared engaged and smiled while holding the psychologist's hand.

During the second therapy session, Connie shared that she had recurring nightmares where she felt she was drowning and admitted being afraid that her actual dying process would feel like drowning. The psychologist offered to explore hypnosis as a tool for improving Connie's sleep, and she responded to the intervention, commenting that it brought her "equilibrium." She did not like using words such as "peace" or any words that could possibly have a spiritual connotation. Hospice services were discussed during the session, and Connie felt she was ready to accept these services, as long as no one tried to discuss spiritual issues with her. The psychologist explained that hospice would actively manage any symptoms and its main goal was to prevent suffering, especially during the dying process. With Connie's permission the psychologist discussed her concerns about the dying process with her cardiologist.

Connie's story highlights patients' uniqueness and the need for palliative care clinicians to constantly adjust their perceptions, assessments, and interventions to meet the needs of a particular patient. The ability to be present and explore spiritual and existential aspects of the patient's life should not prevent accurate assessment and active intervention. Connie's nightmares and fear about dying in distress had to be addressed in the care plan. An important element in the palliative care psychology session is the therapist's ability to switch to different modes depending on the evolution of the session and patient's needs.

While the psychologist used in her assessment the word "meaning," which is generally considered neutral, the patient did not feel it applied to her. Most patients would probably not feel triggered by the word "meaning," and it is possible that Connie's response was also impacted by her experience of discrimination for her belief system. However, Connie willingly shared quite a sophisticated approach to life, which could be described as a mindfulness practice. The particular quality of presence that Connie pursued in her life and she expected from others could be conceptualized as her main source of meaning and purpose, although she would not resonate with the words.

References

American Atheists. (2017). What is atheism? https://www.atheists.org/activism/resources/about-atheism/ retrieved on November 7th 2017.
Anandarajah, G., & Hight, E. (2001). Spirituality and medical practice: Using the HOPE questions as a practical tool for spiritual assessment. *American Family Physician*, 63(1), 81–89.
Balboni, T. A., Balboni, M., Enzinger, A. C., Gallivan, K., Paulk, M. E., Wright, A., . . . Prigerson, H. G. (2013). Provision of spiritual support to patients with advanced cancer by religious communities and associations with medical care at the end of life. *JAMA Internal Medicine*, 173(12), 1109–1117.

Bekelman, D. B., Sydney, M. D. Becker, D. M., Wittstein, I., Hendricks, D. E., Yamashita, T. E., & Gottlied, S. H. (2007). Spiritual well-being and depression in patients with heart failure. *Journal of General Internal Medicine, 22*(4), 470–477.

Blanchard, J. H., Dunlap, D. A., & Fitchett, G. (2012). Screening for spiritual distress in the oncology inpatient: A quality improvement pilot project between nurses and chaplains. *Journal of Nursing Management, 20,* 1076–1084.

Borneman, T., Ferrell, B., & Puchalski, C. (2010). Evaluation of the FICA tool for spiritual assessment. *Journal of Pain and Symptom Management, 40*(2), 163–173.

Bornet, M. A., Rochat, E., & Durst, A. V., Fustinoni, S., Bula, C., vonGunten, A., & Monod, S. (2016). Instruments to assess depressive symptoms and spiritual distress investigate different dimensions. *Clinical Gerontologist, 39*(2), 104–116.

Boston, P., Bruce, A., & Schreiber, R. (2011). Existential suffering in the palliative care setting: An integrative literature review. *Journal of Pain and Symptom Management, 41*(3), 604–618.

Bussing, A., Wirth, A. G., Reiser, F., Zahn, A., Humbroich, K., Gerbershagen, K., . . . Baumann, K. (2014). Experience of gratitude, awe, and beauty in life among patients with multiple sclerosis and psychiatric disorders. *Health and Quality of Life Outcomes,12*(63). doi: 10.1186/1477-7525-12-63.

Delgado-Guay, M. O. (2014). Spirituality and religiosity in supportive and palliative care. *Current Opinions in Supportive and Palliative Care, 8*(3), 308–313.

Delgado-Guay, M. O., Hui, D., Parsons, H. A., Govan, K., De la Cruz, M., Thorney, S., & Bruera, E. (2011). Spirituality, religiosity, and spiritual pain in advanced cancer patients. *Journal of Pain and Symptom Management, 41*(6), 986–994.

Delgado-Guay, M. O., Rodriguez-Nunez, A., De la Cruz, V., Frisbee-Hume, S., Williams, J., Wu, J., . . . Bruera, E. (2016). Advanced cancer patients' reported wishes at the end of life: A randomized controlled trial. *Supportive Care in Cancer, 24*(10), 4273–4281.

Dobratz, M. C. (2013). All my saints are with me: Expressions of end of life spirituality. *Palliative and Supportive Care, 11,* 191–198.

El Nawawi, N. M., Balboni, M. J., & Balboni, T. A. (2012). Palliative care and spiritual care: The crucial role of spiritual care in the care of patients with advanced illness. *Current Opinions in Supportive Palliative Care, 6*(2), 269–274.

Elliott, B. A., Gessert, C. E., Larson, P., & Russ, T. E. (2012). Religious beliefs and practices in end-stage renal disease: Implications for clinicians. *Journal of Pain and Symptom Management, 44*(3), 400–409.

Ettema, E. J., Derksen, L. D., & van Leeuwen, E. (2010). Existential loneliness and end of life care: A systematic review. *Theoretical Medical Bioethics, 31*(2), 141–169.

Fitchett, G., & Risk, J. L. (2009). Screening for spiritual struggle. *Journal of Pastoral Care Counsel, 63*(1–2), 4–12.

Francis, L., Croft, J., & Pike, A. (2012). Religious diversity, empathy, and god image in the UK. *Journal of Beliefs and Values, 33*(3), 293–307.

Frankl, V. E. (1959). *Man's search for meaning.* Boston: Beacon Press.

Freud, S. (1927). *The future of an illusion.* Amazon Kindle Edition.

Hillman, J. (1983). *Archetypal Psychology: A brief account.* Thompson, CT: Spring Publications.

Hollins, S. (2009). *Religions, culture, and healthcare.* New York: Radcliffe Publishing.

Johnson-Bogaerts, H. (2015). Spiritual care is integral to compassionate care. *Nursing New Zealand, 21*(10), 29.

Kissane, D. W. (2012). The relief of existential suffering. *Archives of Internal Medicine, 172*(19), 1501–1505.

LaRocca-Pitts, M. (2012). FACT, a chaplain's tool for assessing spiritual needs in an acute care setting. *Chaplaincy Today, 28*(1), 25–32.

Lawrence, R. T. (1997). Measuring the image of God: The God image inventory and the God image scales. *Journal of Psychology and Theology, 25*(2), 214–226.

Loetz, C., Muller, J., Frick, E., Petersen, Y., Hvidt, N. C., Mauer, C. (2013). Attachment theory and spirituality: Two threads converging in palliative care? *Evidence-based Complementary and Alternative Medicine*. doi: 10.1155/2013/740291

Mais, L. (2010). Perspectives on death and dying from an atheist nurse. *Newsletter of the Atheist Community of Austin*, 3(1), 1–5.

Markman, K. D., Proulx, T., & Lindberg, M. J. (2013). *The psychology of meaning*. Washington, DC: American Psychological Association.

McCord, G., Gilchrist, V. J., Grossman, S. D., King, B. D., McCormick, K. E., Oprandi, A. M., . . . Srivastava, M. (2004). Discussing spirituality with patients: A rational and ethical approach. *Annals of Family Medicine*, 2(4), 356–361.

Meier, E. A., Gallegos, J. V., Thomas, L. P., Depp, C. A., Irwin, S. A., Jeste, D. V. (2016). Defnining a good death (Successful dying): Literature review and a call for research and public dialogue. *American Journal of Geriatric Psychiatry*, 24(4), 261–271.

Milstein, J. M. (2008). Introducing spirituality in medical care: Transition from hopelessness to wholeness. *JAMA*, 299(20), 2440–2441.

Neymeyer, R. A. (2006). Bereavement and the quest for meaning: rewriting stories of loss and grief. *Hellenic Journal of Psychology*, 3, 181–188.

Park, C. L. (2013). The meaning-making model: A framework for understanding meaning, spirituality, and stress-related growth in health psychology. *The European Health Psychologist*, 15(2), 40–47.

Patton, J. F. (2006). Jungian spirituality: A developmental context for late-life growth. *American Journal of Hospice and Palliative Medicine*, 23(4), 304–308.

Pearce, M. J., Koenig, H. G., Robins, C. J., Nelson, B., Shaw, S. F., Cohen, H., J., & King, M. B. (2015). Religiously integrated cognitive behavioral therapy: A new method of treatment for major depression in patients with chronic medical illness. *Psychotherapy*, 52(1), 56–66.

Peteet, J. R., & Balboni, M. J. (2013). Spirituality and religion in oncology. *CA: a Cancer Journal for Clinicians*, 63, 280–289.

Pew Foundation (2015). America's changing religious landscape. http://www.pewforum.org/2015/05/12/americas-changing-religious-landscape/ Retrieved on November 3, 2017.

Puchalski, C. M. (2010). Formal and informal spiritual assessment. *Asian Pacific Journal of Cancer Prevention*, 11(MECC Suppl), 51–58.

Puchalski, C. M., & Ferrell, B. (2010). *Making health care whole: Integrating spirituality into patient care*. West Conshohocken, PA: Templeton Press.

Puchalski, C., Ferrell, B., Virani, R., Otis-Green, S., Baird, P., Bull, J., . . . Sulmasy, D. (2009). Improving the quality of spiritual care as a dimension of palliative care: The report of the consensus conference. *Journal of Palliative Medicine*, 12(10), 885–904.

Puchalski, C., & Romer, A. L. (2000). Taking a spiritual history allows clinicians to understand patients more fully. *Journal of Palliative Medicine*, 3(1), 129–137.

Puchalski, C. M., Vitillo, R., Hull, S. K., & Reller, N. (2014). Improving the spiritual dimension of whole person care: Reaching national and international consensus. *Journal of Palliative Medicine*, 17(6), 642–656.

Richardson, P. (2014). Spirituality, religion and palliative care. *Annals of Palliative Medicine*, 3(3), 150–159.

Rizzuto, A. M. (1979). *The birth of the living God*. The University of Chicago Press.

Robinson, S., Kissane, D. W., Brooker, J., & Burney, S. (2016). A review of the construct of demoralization: History, definition, and future directions for palliative care. *American Journal of Hospice and Palliative Medicine*, 33(1), 93–101.

Saguil, A., & Phelps, K. (2012). The spiritual assessment. *American Family Physician*, 86(6), 546–550.

Schneider, K. (2008). *Existential-Integrative psychotherapy Guideposts to the core of practice*. Boston: Routledge.

Sinclair, S., & Chochinov, H. M. (2012). The role of chaplains within oncology interdisciplinary teams. *Current Opinions in Supportive Palliative Care, 6*(2), 259–268.

Sinclair, S., McClement, S., Raffin-Bouchal, S., Hack, T. F., Hagen, N. A., McConnell, S., & Chochinov, H. M. (2016). Compassion in health care: An empirical model. *Journal of Pain and Symtpom Manage, 51*, 191–203.

Smith-Stoner, M. (2007). End of life preferences for atheists. *Journal of Palliative Medicine, 10*(4), 923–928.

Smith-Stoner, M. (2007). Spiritual needs of wiccan, pagan, and nature spiritualists at end of life. *Journal of Hospice and Palliative Nursing, 9*(5), 279–286.

Speck, P. (2016). Culture and spirituality: Essential components of palliative care. *Postgraduate Medical Journal, 92*(1088), 341–345.

Sperry, L. (2012). *Spirituality in clinical practice*. New York: Routledge.

Sperry, L., & Shafranske, E. P. (2005). *Spiritually oriented psychotherapy*. Washington, DC: American Psychological Association.

Steger, M. F., Kashdan, T. B., Sullivan, B., Lorentz, D. (2008). Understanding the search for meaning in life: Personality, cognitive style, and the dynamic between seeking and experiencing meaning. *Journal of Personality, 76*(2), 199–228.

Strada, E. A., Homel, P., Tennestedt, S., Billings, J. A., & Portenoy, R. K. (2013). Spiritual well-being in patients with advanced heart and lung disease. *Palliative and Supportive Care, 11*(3), 205–213.

Strada, E. A., & Sourkes, B. M. (2015). Principles of psychotherapy. In J. C. Holland, W. S. Breitbart, P. N. Butow, P. B. Jacobsen, M. J. Loscalzo, & R. McCorkle (Eds.), *Psycho-oncology* (3rd ed., pp. 431–436). Oxford: Oxford University Press.

Sulmasy, D. P. (2006). Spiritual issues in the care of dying patients. *JAMA, 296*(11), 1385–1392.

Sulmasy, D. P. (2009). Spirituality, religion, and clinical care. *Chest, 135*(6), 1634–1642.

Sun, V., Kim, J. Y., Irish, T. L., Boerneman, T., Sidhu, R. K., Klein, L., Ferrell, B. (2016). Palliative care and spiritual well-being in lung cancer patients and family caregivers. *Psychooncology, 25*(12), 1448–1455.

Suri, R. (2009). Working with the elderly: An existential-humanistic approach. *Journal of Humanistic Psychology, 50*(2), 175–186.

Thiel, M. M., & Robinson, M. (2015). Spiritual care of the nonreligious. *PlainViews: Health Care Chaplaincy Network, 12*(7), 1–12.

Vallurupalli, M., Lauderdale, K., Balboni, M. J., Phelps, A. C., Block, S. D., Ng, A. K., . . . Balboni, T. A. (2012). The role of spirituality and religious coping in the quality of life of patients with advanced cancer receiving palliative radiation therapy. *Journal of Supportive Oncology, 10*(2), 81–87.

Waller, R., Trepka, C., Collerton, D., & Hawkins, J. (2010). Addressing spirituality in CBT. *The Cognitive Behavioural Therapist, 3*, 95–106.

Warmenhoven, F., Lucassen, P., Vermandere, M., Aertgeerts, B., van Weel, C., Vissers, K., & Prins, J. (2016). 'Life is still worth living': A pilot exploration of self-reported resources of palliative care patients. *BioMed Family Practice, 17*, 52. doi: 10.1186/s12875-016-0450-y.

Williams, J. A., Meltzer, D., & Arora, V., Chung, G., & Curlin, F. A. (2011). Attention to inpatient's religious and spiritual concerns: Predictors and association with patient satisfaction. *Journal of General Internal Medicine, 26*(11), 1265–1271.

Yalom, I. D. (1998). *Existential psychotherapy*. New York: Basic Books.

6

The Sixth Domain of Palliative Care

Cultural Aspects of Care

Focus Points

- Culture is a multidimensional construct encompassing the patient and the family background, system of beliefs, values, and practices. Culture makes individuals unique in the way they experience and interact with each other and the world.
- The patient and family culture deeply affects cognitive and psychological response to illness, communication-style preferences, and decision making.
- Care that is patient-centered and culturally competent conveys respect for values and practices and integrates what is important to the patient and the family into the interdisciplinary palliative care plan.
- All palliative care clinicians should develop awareness of their own culture, including possible biases that may affect the care they provide.
- Palliative psychologists should also reflect on how the culture of the medical system may be supportive or hindering of the patient and family experience.

Introduction

The role of culture in shaping belief systems, sense of identity, attitudes, and behaviors is well recognized. Shared and valued cultural practices can represent an important source of strength and support for the patient and the family. It is essential that palliative care be provided in a fashion that respects and validates patients' needs and values as related to all aspects of culture. Culturally competent palliative care is an expression of patient-centered care, and it can promote more effective treatment of pain and physical symptoms, as well as psychological and spiritual well-being. Cultural factors can facilitate or prevent access to palliative care and end-of-life care. Approaching the care of the patient and the family with cultural sensitivity and cultural competence can allow clinicians to address these barriers more effectively (Coolen, 2012; Gire, 2014).

Communication is a complex process of sending and receiving messages. In culturally competent and patient-centered care, it is important that patients and families feel that members of the care team are correctly receiving their messages. This will allow them to feel that not only their words but also their worldview is being understood. Similarly, clinicians must be able not only to communicate medical information, but also to convey consideration and respect for cultural values. This is especially important when it is necessary to deliver bad news related to the illness (Bousquet et al., 2015). Additionally, it is important that communication with the patient takes place in a language the patient can not only understand but also emotionally relate to. Language allows not only communication of information but also, and foremost, emotional nuances, humor, and other subtleties. Thus, the ability to express oneself to the full extent and depth needed is empowering and dignity affirming. For this reason, the use of trained medical interpreters is critical to effective verbal communication in palliative care and for facilitating the patient's active involvement in directing their care.

It is important to define some of the relevant terminology (Table 6.1).

Table 6.1 **Culture-Related Terminology**

Culture	Set of belief systems, values, practices, including spiritual and religious beliefs that are characteristic of a particular cultural group
Multiculturalism	Reality of several cultures coexisting in a society while each maintaining individuality
Multicultural focus	Necessary approach in psychology that always considers assessment and intervention as grounded in a particular cultural context
Diversity	Recognition of individual and group differences based on ethnicity, gender, sexuality, spiritual, and religious orientation
Cultural sensitivity	Respect for cultural expressions different from one's own; recognition that several approaches to assessment and intervention in psychology may not be relevant to many cultural groups
Cultural competence	Ability to provide interventions that recognize and validate different cultural experiences; ability to engage therapeutically with patients and families from cultures different from own and ability to negotiate a respectful relationship
Cultural humility	Recognition that one is not the expert on another's culture; willingness to ask questions and learn what is considered appropriate behavior in the culture; it includes not making assumptions about other cultures to explain behavior

Culture is a complex construct, and it is also fluid and dynamic. Its comprehensive focus is well described in the following words: "The word culture implies the integrated pattern of human behavior that includes thoughts, communications, actions, customs, beliefs, values, and institutions of a racial, ethnic, religious, or social group" (Cross, Bazron, Dennis & Isaacs, 1989, p. iv). A person's culture deeply influences belief systems, values, practices and social institutions, and psychological processes. Additionally, it encompasses historical, political, and economical forces that affect the way people live (Fiske, 2004).

Thus, mere knowledge of a patient and family ethnic and linguistic background is not sufficient to develop a true understanding of their worldview. It is also important to understand how patients identify themselves in all the different aspects of culture by exploring their cultural identification. According to the National Association of Social Workers and as reported in the *Clinical Practice Guidelines*, "Cultural identification may include, but is not limited to, race, ethnicity, and national origin; migration background, degree of acculturation, and documentation status; socioeconomic class; age; gender, gender identity, and gender expression; sexual orientation; family status; spiritual, religious, and political beliefs or affiliation; physical, psychiatric, and cognitive ability; and literacy, including health and financial literacy" (*Clinical Practice Guidelines for Quality Palliative Care*, 2013, p. 28).

In this view, culture and culture identification can be understood to apply to all domains of human functioning as important contributors to the way people understand their place in their community, society, and the world. It is also important to the way they understand themselves and others, and the values and implicit and explicit rules that guide their behavior.

Multiculturalism refers to the reality of the current US context, where interactions between people of different racial/ethnic/cultural backgrounds occur daily and deeply affect communication and negotiations.

Diversity is also a broad construct that refers to the importance of recognizing differences related to culture, age, sexual orientation, physical disability, role in the workplace, religious and spiritual orientation and affiliation, and family structure.

Cultural sensitivity refers to an attitude of respect for the patient and the family background, story, and cultural practices. It includes awareness that culture deeply affects the patient and the family's belief systems about health, illness, and health care, as well as their interactions with the medical system and medical providers. Respect is not dependent on whether the clinician shares the patient's cultural practices or views; rather, it is a necessary characteristic of a clinician's therapeutic stance. Cultural sensitivity does not trivialize differences; it acknowledges cultural differences and recognizes their profound impact on people's lives. In a sense, every encounter with a patient and a family could be conceptualized as a cross-cultural encounter.

Cultural competence is the result of specific knowledge and skills; these can be generic or specific, but they are necessary for a positive clinical encounter (Kemp, 2005; Chettih, 2012). Providing care that is both culturally sensitive and culturally competent can help prevent cross-cultural conflict, or it can help manage conflict effectively when it arises. Additionally, it can help increase trust and effective communication between the patient and the clinical team and improve treatment adherence.

Cultural humility involves willingness to recognize that the patient and the family are the expert about their culture and cultural practices. It also involves not making patronizing assumptions about what the patient and the family need, how they can be best supported, and what the challenges they face entail. Cultural humility is an attitude that allows the clinician to maintain a sense of curiosity and interest toward the patient and the family's culture (Foronda, Baptiste, Reinholdt & Ousman, 2016).

Competencies for Palliative Psychologists

Since the late 1980s, psychologists have recognized the importance of developing multicultural competencies to enable them to provide culturally relevant and appropriate care to minority patient populations. This impetus has prompted the development of position papers highlighting the nature of multicultural competencies and their impact in clinical practice. Practice competencies have been proposed for working with African Americans, American Indians, Latino, and people of Asian descent (Sue, Arredondo & McDavis, 1992; Arredondo et al., 1996). Palliative psychologists are also encouraged to acquire practice competencies for working with specific populations, including Jewish and Muslim patients, LGBTQQI patients (lesbian, gay, bisexual, transgender, queer, questioning, and intersex), Holocaust survivors and their families, and veterans.

Psychology graduate training programs address cultural awareness and sensitivity and cultural competence as part of the curriculum. Additionally, programs that are accredited by the American Psychological Association are required to provide doctoral students with training in cultural competence. While such training is a requirement for licensure in many states, many are now advocating for a systematic use of multicultural competencies and for making multicultural training a vital component of psychology graduate training programs and licensing requirements (Arredondo & Tovar-Blank, 2014).

The Code of Ethics of the American Psychological Association highlights the importance of developing sensitivity to patients' expression of cultural diversity. Additionally, the American Psychological Association also published *Guidelines on Multicultural Education, Training, Research, Practice, and Organizational Change for Psychologists* (APA, 2003). The guidelines emphasize that every person is a cultural being, embedded in a sociopolitical and cultural environment. Human beings do not exist and function in a vacuum—thus, the importance of applying multicultural constructs in psychological settings, including education, research, and practice. Table 6.2 summarizes the guidelines and illustrates their application to palliative psychology.

Following the development of the multicultural guidelines, APA sponsored a task force on the implementation of the multicultural guidelines (APA 2008), and the creation of psychology education and training from culture specific and multiracial perspectives. Regardless of their practice or research setting psychologists are being urged to recognize, honor, validate, and facilitate expression of cultural identity in every clinical encounter. This includes recognizing the manifestation of "white privilege" (McIntosh, 1989) and its impact on their interactions with other cultural groups, especially in the clinical setting.

Table 6.2 **APA Multicultural Guidelines**

Guidelines	Application to Palliative Care
1. Psychologists are encouraged to recognize that, as cultural beings, they must hold attitudes and beliefs that can detrimentally influence their perception of and interactions with individuals who are ethnically and racially different from themselves.	It is important that palliative psychologists maintain awareness of how their cultural background and identity impact on their ability to work with different populations. This involves awareness of any belief and biases regarding sensitive areas of palliative care, including physician-assisted death, use of life-prolonging treatments, decision-making, disclosure of diagnosis and prognosis.
2. Psychologists are encouraged to recognize the importance of multicultural sensitivity/responsiveness, knowledge, and understanding about ethnically and racially different individuals.	It is important to be informed about how different cultural groups relate to issues concerning serious and advanced illness. While general descriptions (e.g., NHPCO guidelines and brochures) can be helpful, one must recognize that profound intracultural variations exist, and it is always best to allow the family to educate the team about what practices and beliefs are important to them.
3. As educators, psychologists are encouraged to employ the construct of multiculturalism and diversity in psychological education.	Palliative psychologists invited to present or teach on palliative care topics should always address multicultural aspects of the issue. This applies to assessment and diagnosis, as well as psychological treatment.
4. Culturally sensitive psychology researchers are encouraged to recognize the importance of conducting culture centered and ethical psychological research among persons from ethnic, linguistic, and racial minority backgrounds.	Minority populations are still underrepresented in palliative and end-of-life care research. Psychologists involved in palliative care research are aware of the need to produce research that is culturally meaningful. Participatory research methods can be especially relevant when studying people of color.
5. Psychologists strive to apply culturally appropriate skills in clinical and other applied psychological practices.	Palliative psychologists ensure that their approach to assessment and treatment reflects a multicultural focus. When necessary, existing psychological models and interventions are adapted and modified accordingly.
6. Psychologists are encouraged to use organizational change processes to support culturally informed organizational (policy) development and practice.	Every palliative psychologist has the responsibility to identify gaps in the system, including policies and procedures that need revising to better meet the needs of multicultural patients and staff.

Adapted and modified from *Guidelines on Multicultural Education, Training, Research, Practice, and Organizational Change for Psychologists* (APA, 2002).

During the education leadership conference in 2005, psychologists presented the Universal Declaration of Ethical Principles, which includes among its goals that of establishing cultural competence in psychology training, research, and practice. Updated in 2007 and 2008, the declaration emphasizes the importance of recognizing and respecting diversity in all its manifestations and highlights the importance of psychologists' commitment to local communities, indigenous communities, and cultural differences (Gauthier, Pettifor & Ferrero, 2010).

Considering the focus of their training and practice, palliative psychologists are well equipped to provide patient-centered care to patients and families through a culture-focused approach to their work. Palliative psychology competencies in the cultural domain include the ability to assess and understand how culture affects the meaning attributed to illness, and communication with health-care providers. Additionally, it is necessary to explore the patient's preferences about medical treatments in advanced disease and end-of-life care, management of pain and symptoms, and utilization of life-sustaining practices. Cultural factors also impact how patients and families experience and express psychological distress, including grief reactions (Box 6.1).

In the context of assessment, rather than wondering whether there are any cultural factors that need to be considered, it is best to assume that relevant cultural factors always exist and need to be identified by the skillful clinician. Identification of sociopolitical factors that affect behavior is facilitated by broadening the focus of assessment to include this larger context. This approach can allow recognition of both overt and subtle cultural factors impacting patients' thoughts, practices, and behaviors in the health-care system. Social justice issues are especially relevant. All built-in environmental stressors, such as poverty, racism, and other forms of discrimination deeply affect perception about quality of care, response to communication from the health-care team, and the decision-making process. These factors should be recognized and not trivialized by being attributed to psychological explanations that may perpetuate blaming the victim. Clinicians guided by multicultural principles will also be more likely to recognize culture-bound elements in Western psychological theories and interventions. Thus, they will avoid pathologizing behavior or making diagnoses based on culture bound psychological theories that may be inadequate for a specific patient population.

The ability to recognize the general framework valued in a patient and family culture can provide an important context for understanding behavior. To illustrate, the focus of a collectivistic culture is mostly directed at performing and encouraging behavior that can bring honor to the entire family. Here, ensuring that the family and the community are not negatively affected by individuals' actions becomes more important than asserting one's personal decision making. However, many individuals born in the United States but raised in families with collectivistic values, may have developed a different set of values and practices from their family. It is critical that clinicians do not assume but rather use their intuition, assessment skills, and competence to identify the core values for each patient and family. Psychological care that is culturally relevant requires not only recognizing the ways in which the patient and the family share values and beliefs with members of their culture and others outside the culture but also the ways in which

Box 6.1 **Palliative Psychology Competencies in the Cultural Domain of Care**

KNOWLEDGE

- understanding of the breadth and depth of different cultural constructs and their impact on the patient and the family
- knowledge of principles of cultural sensitivity and cultural competence
- understanding of culture-bounds aspects of medical and psychological care
- understanding of bias and microaggressions in the palliative care setting
- knowledge of APA Multicultural Guidelines and Multicultural Competencies and their application to the palliative psychology

SKILLS

- ability to implement APA multicultural guidelines and competencies to the palliative care setting
- ability to conduct a cultural assessment with the patient and the family
- ability to recognize impact of cultural factors in experience and manifestation of distress, including depression, anxiety, and grief reactions
- ability to identify core cultural issues, including spiritual, that may impact on decision-making
- ability to modify psychological interventions to accommodate a multicultural focus

ATTITUDES

- maintain awareness of personal cultural beliefs, attitudes, and biases that may impact care of patients from different cultural backgrounds.
- cultivate a professional stance that reflects cultural humility and cultural sensitivity
- regard the patient and the family as the "experts" on their culture and their personal circumstances, and demonstrate willingness to be educated and informed by them about they consider valuable.
- maintain awareness of personal biases and preconceived notions that may affect the relationship with team members and other clincians

they are profoundly unique. While it is important to recognize what is important to all human beings equally, it is also critical to develop an appreciation for the unique needs of each patient.

To illllustrate, most people faced with approaching death value being free of pain and suffering; they share the desire of being in the company of loved ones and not being abandoned. In this way, every patient is "like all others" (Payne, 2015, p. 272). It is also important to recognize that shared cultural practices and backgrounds make patients "like some others." Thus, clinicians should develop an understanding of the worldview, lifestyle, and traditions of the community, geographical and otherwise, embraced by the patient and the family. And finally, palliative care clinicians must also develop the skills to recognize the uniqueness of each patient and each family, honoring the ways in which they are "like no other" (p. 273).

The importance of adapting communication style to meet the patient and the family's needs cannot be overestimated. Communication in palliative psychology is directed toward supporting, facilitating, and expanding. For this reason, both verbal and nonverbal communication should inform the psychological assessment. Active listening, observing, pausing, and sometimes sitting quietly at the bedside can provide the clinician with important information about the values important to the patient and the family. This can also facilitate the development of a culturally relevant psychological plan.

Patients with serious and advanced illness face ambiguity and uncertainty about the course of the disease and the future. The strategies they use to cope with the practical and psychological challenges are determined by their culture (Heppner, Wei, Neville & Kanagui-Munoz, 2014).

Self-awareness about a psychologist's own cultural background, history, and current cultural schemas is necessary for developing cultural sensitivity and competence. This is also recommended for every clinician. Palliative psychologists can conduct a personal self-exploration considering their answer to the questions in Table 6.3. The questions presented can also be approached as a framework for a group discussion to raise cultural awareness in the context of the interdisciplinary team. Self-awareness extends to recognizing countertransference reactions or personal biases that may negatively impact the ability to provide care. Additionally, it is also important to become aware of and uncover the cultural biases inherent in every psychotherapy framework and provide interventions that are relevant to the patient and family's life experiences and values.

Promoting the delivery of culturally competent palliative care includes addressing barriers to care. This is especially relevant for patients from minority groups that have

Table 6.3 **Exploring Personal Cultural Identity and Professional Psychological Culture**

Cultural heritage and cultural identity	• What words would you use to describe your cultural heritage?
	• How would you describe your cultural identity?
	• Can you name three aspects of your culture that you find particularly meaningful and supportive?
	• Can you describe one aspect of your culture that you do not resonate with and you have been struggling with?
	• Describe your main cultural assumptions related to family structure, interpersonal relationships, decorum and appropriate expression of emotions, role of food, meaning of life and death.
	• What are considered desirable or undesirable personal qualities in your culture?

Table 6.3 **Continued**

Professional identity	• How has your professional identity as a psychologist been integrated into your cultural identity? • Are there any aspects of your cultural identity that are not easy to reconcile with psychological culture?
Relationship with the health-care system	• Have there been times where you have been treated differently (better or worse) in the health-care system because of your cultural identity? • Have you found that medical professionals have made assumptions about you (or your family, or other people close to you) because of your cultural identity? If so, how have you responded?
Practice implications	• Have you ever experienced a cultural clash with a patient or a family? • How have you addressed cultural challenges?

been historically underrepresented and underserved. General frameworks about cultural practices and barriers in different cultural groups can provide a roadmap for exploration. However, it is critical to avoid assumptions based on broad generalizations, as profound differences exist not only among cultures but also within each culture.

Assessing Cultural Dimensions of Serious illness

From its early development, palliative care has focused on culturally determined aspects of care, including culturally appropriate ways of communicating "bad news," understanding the locus of decision making, and recognizing attitudes toward advance directives and end of life. Factors deeply influenced by cultural background and values include the role of family caregivers and manifestation of grief reactions (Table 6.4). The attention to these areas has also highlighted the complexity of approaching these issues in the clinical setting (Quill & Townsend, 1991; Searight & Gafford, 2005). The following section describes cultural factors relevant to the palliative care setting, also highlighting instances where the normative values generally accepted in Western culture may clash with the patient and the family, in overt or subtle ways.

Sociopolitical Context

The sociopolitical context of the patient and the family experience can provide important information that can help better understand their needs (Table 6.5). However, they may feel deeply uncomfortable and even unsafe sharing their experience with oppression, discrimination, and racism, or challenges related to immigration status. This may be especially true when the patient or a family member does not have citizenship or

Table 6.4 **Aspects of Care Deeply Affected by Culture**

Locus of decision making	Individual vs. collaborative and family-based decisions. Does the patient make decisions based on personal wishes even when they may conflict with the family?
Communicating "bad news"	What is the appropriate modality based on cultural values? Should bad news be communicated to family caregivers first so they can determine how to spare the patient emotional distress?
Attitudes toward advance directives	Is there a concern that by making decisions about end of life the patient will not receive the best care available? Are there cultural beliefs that consider discussions about end of life "bad luck?"
Caregiving	What is the meaning of caregiving according to the culture?
Expression of emotions	Is it appropriate to express positive or negative emotions in public and in the presence of strangers?
Spectrum of death awareness	How does the family regard good care at end of life? Are family members and friends supposed to "pretend" the patient is getting better even if everyone knows that death is close?
A good death	Is there such a concept in the culture? If not, what practices and aspects of care are considered important? (e.g., dying at home vs. dying at the hospital; symptoms management, etc.).
Relationship with medical providers	Is there a belief that authority (i.e. the doctor) should not be questioned or challenged? Are family caregivers concerned that asking questions may be perceived as a lack of trust in the medical team?

even legal status, where the profound sense of vulnerability and fear about the worsening of the patient's medical condition can become compounded by the fear and sense of vulnerability about being reported to authorities or not being able to obtain adequate medical care. If any of these factors are known, the team should reflect on their impact and not quickly dismiss them as a simple component of the psychosocial history. The goal of the team is to ensure a full appreciation of the patient's and the family's needs also based on relevant historical and social factors that impact their behaviors (Table 6.6).

Table 6.5 **Sociopolitical Aspects of the Patient and the Family Culture**

Sociopolitical stressors and trauma	Has the patient or anyone in the family experienced trauma (e.g., refugees who escaped torture, rape; political prisoners), discrimination, poverty, problems with the legal system, or any other stressors reated to sociopolitical factors?
Work situation	Being self-employed versus working for others may significantly affect the ability to take time off to attend medical appointments during caregiving, or take time to grieve in bereavement.
Levels of acculturation	Do the patient and family caregivers think of themselves as bicultural and move smoothly between different cultural realities?
English language fluency and preferred language and dialects	If fluency in English is limited, what is the impact on communication with medical providers? Are medical interpreters able to render nuances, subtleties, or humor in addition to content?
Family structure and support	Can the family support the patient? How do family caregivers find support for themselves?
Community resources	Is it appropriate to invite spiritual care providers, AA sponsors, community healers, or community advocates to participate in the plan of care?

Cultural Factors in Caregiving

Caregiving for a patient with advanced illness can be associated with significant challenges and distress (see chapter 4), but it can also represent an important expression of cultural values, such as familism and filial piety, which involve strong attachment and dedication to family members as well as a deep sense of responsibility toward them. This does not necessarily mean that distress is not present. While familism is a protective factor in caregiver burden, the presence of social support and coping style are perhaps more relevant in modulating responses to caregiving (Knight & Sayegh, 2009). Yet, if fulfilling caregiving responsibilities is identified as a core value, there may be inability or unwillingness to admit to the presence of stress or challenges by the family caregiver.

The palliative psychologist must then be able to balance validating the caregiving role with assessing for the presence of distress. Family caregivers should not receive the

Table 6.6 **Patient and Family Relationship with Medical Culture**

Construct	Examples of Cultural Variations
Relationship with the health care system	Symmetrical or asymmetrical
Experience and expression of grief	Determined by customs and community support
Direct versus indirect communication	High context vs low context culture
Physical and eye contact	Based on proxemics
Culturally appropriate defense mechanisms	Denial, avoidance, prayer, ritual, community
Meaning of hope	Acceptance of prognosis
Meaning of dignity	Physical, emotional, spiritual
Value attributed to the need of prolonging the patient's life	Impact on decisions regarding end of life care
Value attributed to disclosure of medical facts	Protective truthfulness
Value attributed to personal autonomy	Individual versus community
Style in decision making	Community and family vs. individual wishes
Expectations in the family about caring for a loved one who is ill	Responsibility and sacrifice as essential values
Appropriate ways of handling conflict with family members and with strangers	Forgiveness and tolerance may be considered more valuable than standing up for one's rights

impression they are being blamed or pathologized. A well-intentioned clinician concerned about their physical and psychological well-being may encourage the caregiver to pay more attention to their own physical and emotional needs. However, caregivers from collectivistic cultures may feel offended by such invitation, because it may be perceived as designed to create an emotional separation from the patient or detracting from the focus on the patient. Therefore, any focus on the personal well-being of the family caregiver may be resented and rejected. If indirect communication is a core value, the family caregiver in distress may want to avoid conflict and may simply withdraw, which can increase a sense of isolation. Thus, any suggestions from the clinician should be framed as intended to support the family caregiver in their role, so they can continue being effective in a manner that is consistent with their values and standards. Although this aspect may seem only a nuance, it can be important to promote effective communication and a sense of trust.

Family caregivers' expression of affect is also affected by cultural values. In some Asian cultures the ability to control not only negative feelings but also positive feelings is regarded as a sign of wisdom and maturity (Sue & Sue, 2013). Many cultural groups believe that overt expression of anger and "standing up for one's rights" is not appropriate culturally or socially. Additionally, in some cultures the family caregiver may primarily express collectivistic emotions such as shame and disgrace, rather than individual emotions, such as guilt. Thus, assessing mood based on expressed affect may be challenging and limited, with the risk of pathologizing the caregiver by inappropriately labeling someone as "passive; depressed; with blunt affect; or disengaged."

Decision-making Style

Autonomy, individualism, and ability to make one's decisions are valued in Western culture and regarded as an indication of individuation and psychological maturity. While consulting with family is considered valuable, the general belief is that the rights and wishes of the individual should not be affected by family or community decisions. In fact, the ability to make personal decisions, even when they are in contrast with those of the family, is generally considered a sign of individuation and growth.

Patients who define themselves within a collectivistic framework, however, may consider it unacceptable and inconceivable to make decisions without consulting with the family and receiving their input. Additionally, not only is consulting family considered important, but it may also be necessary to reach a decision that everyone is comfortable with, even if it is regarding personal health care. This has important implications for all palliative care clinicians in supporting decision making. Encouraging independence or individual decision making may be inappropriate and exhibits a lack of understanding and respect for important cultural norms. Supporting the patient in achieving a family-based decision making process about treatment initiation or discontinuation may require a lengthy process. It may also raise strong countertransference reactions in the clinician and questions of whether the patient is being manipulated or abused by the family. To illustrate, a patient's wish to stop chemotherapy may be strongly opposed by the family, who may perceive it as giving up, or not placing enough trust in God (see also Chapter 4). A palliative psychologist can offer much support to the team by providing assessment and clarifying issues but also by creating a therapeutic space where these aspects can be explored and decisions are reached respecting cultural values.

Awareness of Limited Prognosis

Cultural factors affect not only patients' preferences but also how they hear and understand medical information, which may directly impact on their prognostic awareness. The literature reflects the complexity of evaluating the impact of prognostic disclosure and discussions of life expectancy. The majority of participants in most studies are white, however, which obviously limits generalizability to populations of color and the ability to translate results into clinical practice.

In the advanced cancer setting, studies have indicated that patients generally have a poor or inaccurate understanding of their prognosis (Epstein et al., 2016). Patients often believe that palliative chemotherapy is designed to cure, rather than reduce symptom burden (Weeks et al., 2012). Research has also indicated that open disclosure may be associated with increased anxiety and decreased quality of life, even when physicians receive specific training in leading these discussions (Curtis et al., 2013; El-Jawahri et al., 2014).

However, identifying preferences about how much information they would like to receive about their condition and how explicit they would like it to be, and delivering information accordingly with a strong reassurance of non-abandonment, may facilitate these conversations and minimize risk of distress (van Vliet et al., 2013). In a group of predominantly (78.3%) white patients with advanced cancer, receiving prognostic disclosure by the oncologist was associated with patients' more realistic expectations about life expectancy, without compromising their relationship with the physician or their psychological well-being (Enzinger et al., 2015). Additionally, although parents of children with cancer find receiving prognostic information upsetting, they still wish to receive as much information as possible and remain hopeful even when the prognosis is poor (Mack et al., 2006; Mack et al., 2007).

Prognostic awareness is undoubtedly one of the most complex and nuanced constructs, with implications for every aspect of palliative care and virtually every clinical scenario. A palliative psychologist should welcome the opportunity to continue learning about the many influences, cultural, psychological, and otherwise, that affect it. The way a patient and a family approach and negotiate awareness of an uncertain or limited prognosis is as personal and unique as the expression of grief. For some patients, awareness of limited prognosis enhances the poignancy of the time that is left and can empower them to make important decisions about *their* life. Others may use avoidance strategies or "healthy denial" as an adaptive modality to help cope with stressful situations. In palliative psychology, it is important to differentiate between healthy denial and disruptive avoidance. It is also essential that the cultural roots of the theoretical frameworks guiding psychological assessments and interventions be examined for bias.

To illustrate, a patient diagnosed with a serious illness may choose to avoid connecting, either cognitively or emotionally, with the potential threat of the diagnosis. This may be in the service of mobilizing important physical and emotional energy in order to cope with treatment, or remain focused on a positive outcome. Patients can also display fluctuation of awareness at different times during the disease trajectory. Thus, there may appear to be a discrepancy between their stated personal awareness and their willingness to engage in discussions about a limited prognosis.

One critical assessment element is determining whether the patient's lack of knowledge of a limited prognosis or unwillingness to discuss it is preventing important treatment decisions. When this is the case, psychologists' expertise navigating complex clinical situations, realities and conflicts can be of great value as they collaborate with other psychosocial professionals to ensure the patient and family needs are adequately met.

Cultural Barriers to Palliative and End-of-Life Care

A growing body of literature indicates health disparities are prominent in the United States (Enguidanos et al., 2013; Ruiz & Brondolo, 2016). These also affect delivery and quality of palliative and hospice care for people of color. For example, among bereaved family members of veterans who received palliative and hospice care, family members of color reported receiving less quality care than their white counterparts (Kutney-Lee et al., 2016). Overall, patients from minority groups continue to be underrepresented in palliative and hospice care despite outreach efforts (LoPresti, Dement, & Gold, 2016; Park, Jang & Chiriboga, 2016). Though several factors have been described as contributing to this underutilization, each group faces unique challenges.

Studies indicate that only about 8% of patients who use hospice palliative care are from African American communities (Noah, 2012). A study explored awareness of hospice and palliative care among African American and non-Hispanic white patients (Matsuyama et al., 2011). Among all participants, only 49% were able to define hospice services. Study participants who had some awareness of palliative care were more likely to have a high school education, higher income, and be white.

Conflict with the hospice philosophy, lack of awareness of services, mistrust of the health-care system, and financial challenges have been consistently described as factors contributing to African Americans' limited use of hospice and palliative care (Taxis, 2006; Washington, Bickel-Swenson, & Stephens, 2008). Similarly, medical providers' perception of existing barriers to palliative care in this patient population include lack of knowledge about services, desire for aggressive care, insurance problems, and family members' unwillingness to accept hospice care (Rhodes et al., 2015). Advanced care planning practices and perceptions were explored in groups of African Americans with varying degrees of familiarity with palliative care and hospice (Rhodes et al., 2016). Themes that emerged from qualitative interviews indicated that while African Americans recognize the potential benefits of palliative care and advanced care planning, they also described barriers mentioned in other studies, including lack of knowledge about palliative care, concern that choosing palliative care would result in inadequate and less quality care, and perceived conflicts with religious beliefs and practices. The relatively low number of African American with knowledge of advance directives and willingness to complete them has also been attributed to mistrust of the medical system based on experiences of racism, a concept that has been further developed into the construct of healthy paranoia (Grier & Cobbs, 1968). Lack of knowledge of the existence of palliative care services, about the meaning and structure of these services, and about how to access the services are among the main barriers to utilization and are also present in Asian and Hispanic communities (Pan et al., 2015). Insufficient knowledge of palliative care services decreases the opportunity for minority patients to receive additional layers of specialized support that may benefit them and their families.

Patients of color are also less likely than white patients to discuss end-of-life care preferences and complete advanced directives (Huang, Neuhaus, & Chiong, 2016). Knowledge of patients' preferences for end-of-life care is considered an important factor for facilitating a "good death" or "successful dying." (Meier et al., 2016). Approaching this topic from a multicultural perspective reveals its complexity, because the construct of a good death has profound intracultural and intercultural variations (Gatrad et al., 2003). Western culture is increasingly valuing direct communication about prognosis and care preferences to ensure that patients' and family's wishes will be respected throughout the care, and especially at the end of life. Many non-Western cultures, however, do not value engaging in conversations about end- of-life care with family members who are ill because of the emotional distress that such conversations are likely to create. Therefore, where a Western model would encourage open communication about dying and decision making as a way to make sure individual interests are protected, non-Western cultures value protecting family members who are ill from news that they are dying, especially if they are old and frail. This approach, common in Chinese culture, has also been described as "protective truthfulness" (Pang, 1999). Additionally, it is important to note that patients and caregivers raised in Western culture may also value protecting a loved one from the distress caused by being told of a poor prognosis (Hallenbeck & Arnold, 2007). The concept of advance directives is grounded in the belief that individuals not only have the right to express health-care preferences should they become incapacitated, but that there is value for the individual, the family, and perhaps society at large in having these conversations.

The expression "goals of care" is often used to describe conversations about care preferences. When working with patients and families of color, a rushed and culturally incompetent approach to a goals of care conversation may convey the impression that the goal of the medical team is to encourage refusal or discontinuation of life-prolonging treatments. This can result in fear that the patient will not be provided the best care or that the medical team wants to "give up" too soon. Additionally, the act of signing an advanced directive document can also perceived as incompatible with a focus on living (Ko & Berkman, 2012). To illustrate, people of color are more likely to use their spirituality to cope with illness (Strada et al., 2012), believe that only God has the right to decide life and death, and believe in miracles or divine interventions. Thus, the decision to discontinue life-prolonging treatments may be seen an inconsistent with religious values. Advanced care directives as currently conceived may not represent the needs of minority groups, which contributes not only to lower rates of completion but also perpetuates discrepancies in care (Fischer, Sauaia, Min & Kutner, 2012).

When the topic of preferences and goals of care is approached in a culturally sensitive and competent manner, however, there is an indication that many patients and families from minority groups also value care consistent with the palliative care and hospice philosophy, including family support, adequate pain management and ensuring they do not receive unwanted medical treatment (Piamjariyakul et al., 2016). For many indigenous people in America and Alaska, for instance, discussing death may evoke evil spirits and promote fear and distress. However, their value placed on remaining in a familiar environment at the end of life, and on connectedness with family and community, can be consistent with the hospice care philosophy. Participatory research has been used to facilitate a culturally appropriate transition to hospice for the patient and the family in American Indian tribes (Colclough & Brown, 2014).

Clearly, promoting culturally competent palliative and end-of-life care in minority populations involves the ability to communicate in sensitive ways with each individual patient and family. It also requires maintain the focus on identifying and meeting needs, without imposing an agenda, even when the patient's wishes do not conform to the recommendations of the health care team.

CASE VIGNETTE 6.1

Brenda is a 74-year-old African American woman with end-stage congestive heart failure, admitted to the hospital for shortness of breath. She has been able to manage her disease at home for a few years; however, in the last six months she has experienced five hospitalizations for acute decompensated heart failure, and managing life at home has become increasingly difficult. Her symptoms include dyspnea and weakness, but she is alert and aware and deemed competent to make decisions. The patient has two adult daughters who are committed to her. They both work full-time, however, and can only visit a couple of times a week. The medical team makes a referral to palliative care for goals of care discussion and recommends hospice care for the patient. Brenda has a home health aide who cares for her four hours a day and prepares all the meals. The patient does not have advanced directives and has not designated an agent for health care. However, the daughters have spoken about this issue and have agreed that the oldest daughter will make decisions if their mother becomes incapacitated. They inform the medical team that their mother does not wish to discuss her illness or any issues related to death and dying. While they personally would prefer discussing these issues with her, mostly to be sure they are aware of her wishes, they have decided that the best way to honor their mother is to respect her decision to avoid the subject.

The palliative care team meets with the patient's daughters and asks them to describe their mother and the values that are important to her. They speak about her love for gardening and her attachment to her house, which has become even more important after her husband's death seven years prior. They describe her love for her church and her strong religious beliefs, which still represent her main source of strength and hope. They also describe their mother as a fighter and someone that firmly believes it is up to God to decide when her life should end. Until then, she believes she needs to do all she can medically to stay alive. She also does not believe people should discuss death and dying preferences, since it is not up to them but up to God. The daughters feel that hospice care may be a good option for their mother, but they are concerned that discussing hospice services will create emotional and spiritual distress for her.

The palliative care team agrees not to openly discuss end-of-life options with the patient, and they meet with her in the presence of the daughters to explore her needs. The team begins the meeting by asking the patient if they can have a conversation with her about her care to ensure that her wishes are respected. The patient replies that her only wish is to get better, and she cannot tell the doctors what to do, since they are the experts. The team assures the patient that everyone is committed to her care. They then proceed by asking her to describe her understanding of her medical situation and what she was told by the doctors. The patient looked puzzled and asks the team, "What do you mean my understanding? Don't you know what my disease is? Don't you people talk to each other?" The palliative care clinicians looks toward the daughters, who intervene, reassuring their mother that the doctors only want to discuss how they can best care for her. The patient does not appear convinced and remains silent. The team tries to explore further by asking the patient whether she would prefer to be cared for at home without having to go to the hospital every time there is a medical crisis. The patient replies, "Of course I want to stay home, but if I start feeling sick I will have to come to the hospital." The team attempts to ask a more direct question related to how the patient would like to be cared for if she is unable to speak for herself. The patient is now visibly irritated and tells the team, "I don't want to talk about this. My daughters are here to make sure the doctors do everything they need to do." She then turns her head and closes her eyes.

The team thanks the patient, who does not reply, and leaves the room with the daughters. After the meeting, one of the clinicians suggests that hospice services can still be contacted and explains that during admission the words "hospice" does not need to be used. They explain that the services can be described as "additional help" in the home. The daughters listen quietly and then explain that this strategy will not work. They are concerned that their mother will find out that it is hospice and feel betrayed. Although they believe hospice would be positive for their mother, they must honor her wishes to be cared for in the way she wants; they cannot force her to have a conversation about her decline. They also comment that their mother, as an African American woman, has often felt that the doctors were not as aggressive as they should have been in treating her. They comment that by making decisions for her about end of life (when she is still competent), they would betray her trust.

The team reassures the patient's daughters that they will continue to do all they can to help with symptoms management and that they will follow their mother in the outpatient palliative care clinic after her discharge. In the following three months, the team meets with the patient regularly. Both the team and the patient's daughters attempt to discuss end-of-life care wishes, especially as the patient continues to decline and become more short of breath. Nonetheless, the patient continues to refuse to discuss the topic, saying, "When God decides it is my time I will go. No need to worry about it." Only once after hearing about an acquaintance who died at the hospital she mentioned that she would be fine with that scenario; she believes the hospital is the best place for a patient to make sure they receive good medical care.

The patient remains full code and during a subsequent hospitalization is transferred to the ICU, where she received cardiopulmonary resuscitation after cardiac arrest. In spite of these efforts, the patient died in the ICU. The palliative clinicians met with the daughters and the extended family after the patient's death. While they were grieving intensely, they commented that they felt they had respected their mother's wishes, even if those wishes were not to talk about death and dying. They added that dying in the ICU was not something they would like for themselves, but they did not have the right to create distress for their mother by forcing her to engage in a conversation that was not consistent with her principles.

Recognizing Culture-Bound Values in Medicine and Psychology

An effective way of ensuring the appropriate multicultural focus in clinical practice is to approach every encounter with a patient and a family as a cross-cultural encounter. This requires awareness of the implicit and explicit contextual layers that are present. These different layers interact and are generally expressed through the verbal and nonverbal communication taking place in the encounter. In a palliative psychology clinical encounter, five main cultural contexts can be identified:

- the patient and the family's cultural context
- the psychologist's own cultural context
- the culture of Western psychology
- the culture of Western medicine

- the culture of the larger health-care system.

The culture of Western psychology is taught during training and determined by specific assumptions, beliefs, and values about the meaning of psychological health and well-being, psychopathology, and appropriate therapeutic behaviors and interventions. A palliative psychologist working in the medical system is also influenced by the culture of Western medicine, represented by another set of assumptions, values, beliefs, and desirable behaviors. Additionally, both the psychologist and the patient/family unit exist within the larger context of the health-care system. These cultural layers do not represent a problem to solve but rather a reality to be constantly aware of. When clinicians do not recognize that their communication reflects cultural values that are typical of medical and/or psychological culture that may not only lack relevance but also be in contrast with the patient and family values, conflict may occur.

Western medical culture in the United States holds overt or implicit assumptions about communication:

- Direct communication of medical facts to patients is appropriate and desirable.
- Direct communication of medical information, including prognostic disclosure, can empower the patient and the family to make the most appropriate decisions.
- The patient is in charge of decision making when it comes to health-care decisions, unless incapable of doing so.
- It is assumed that what is communicated by the health-care professional is what is heard.
- Maintaining eye contact during a conversation is a sign that the patient is fully engaged.
- Asking the patient and the family if they have any questions is sufficient to prompt asking questions.
- If patients and family members appear in agreement with the treatment plan discussed (especially if they nod), this automatically means that they have fully understood and that they are in agreement. Lack of overt disagreement is interpreted as agreement.
- When difficult information is being communicated, such as a diagnosis of serious illness, or lack of efficacy of treatment, it is generally expected that patients and families will be able to process information that is subsequently delivered to them.

It is important to note that, although it is part of the Western medical model, palliative medicine has its own, perhaps unique, culture. It focuses on understanding and managing the complexities of communication with a multicultural patient population.

Similarly, *Western psychology* also holds values and assumptions (Table 6.7). Psychological models and frameworks and interventions are not developed in a sociocultural vacuum but are the result of the philosophical, sociopolitical, and larger cultural environment. The description below is based on Sue (2010) and Sue and Sue (2013) and applied to palliative psychology.

Because Western culture generally values verbal communication above all other modalities, not surprisingly, most Western psychological approaches have focused on

Table 6.7 **Cultural Assumptions in Western Psychology and Psychotherapy**

Western Psychology Value	Implication for Palliative Psychology
Primacy of verbal modality of communication	Fluency in English and communication styles that value nonverbal communication, ritual, and shared experience will affect patients' response to psychological assessment and treatment.
At any given time, the focus of psychological treatment is either on the individual, or the couple, or the family. The same therapist does not treat both the individual and the family.	Palliative psychologists will often need to seamlessly and comfortably move from individual treatment to family treatment, or couple. The patient and family needs may warrant inviting church leaders, community healers, or family members. The framework is determined by the needs of the patient and the family, and not vice versa
Value of psychological insight in modifying behavior	In some non-Western cultures, psychological insight may not as valuable as the determination of what is appropriate or inappropriate behavior on the part of the community.
Psychological distress can be clearly described and conceptualized in words	In many non-Western cultures, psychological distress is experienced and expressed through somatic symptoms. This is especially important in palliative care when assessing patients for anxiety and depression that may not manifest through the conventional symptoms.
People benefit from talking about their feelings, emotions, and problems	This is an assumption of Western psychology that is not even valid across the board for mainstream culture. Different people have different styles in expressing distress and processing emotions, especially grief. People process kinesthetically, and through the body. In many cultures, difficult emotions need the support of the community for adequately processing.
Self-disclosure on the part of the therapist is generally discouraged.	If the therapist is accepted as part of the community, patients who belong to non-Western cultures will look at him or her suspiciously if they are not willing to disclose, for example, why they think they are the experts. In palliative care, the patient and the family may openly ask the psychologists about their experiences with death and dying and grief. Or, they may ask them for advice.
Behavior change is often the goal of therapy	Resolving conflict, especially within the community or the family is often an important goal for multicultural patients. Additionally, there is little emphasis on accomplishing personal goals. Valuable goals are those that can benefit the community.

Table 6.7 **Continued**

Western Psychology Value	Implication for Palliative Psychology
A direct style of communication is effective and appropriate	Patients and caregivers may consider direct communication as rude and a violation of their dignity
Role of caregiving	The necessity to sacrifice one's well-being and comfort for the benefit of a family member who is ill is an important value in many cultures. The caregiver often does not question the task, as it is simply what one is supposed to do. Encouraging the caregiver to exhibit good self-care can be therapeutic and necessary, but the clinicians should be particularly mindful not to communicate, implicitly or implicitly, any kind of negative bias or perception to the role of caregiving.

verbal communication as a means to facilitate psychological development and change (e.g., psychoanalysis as the "talking cure").

The majority of Western psychology models focus on the individual. Theories of psychological development value individuation as a critical tool in developing maturity and autonomy. Although several couples and family therapy models exist, the main theories of counseling and psychotherapy focus on the individual. In many cultures, however, the psychosocial unit of operation is not represented by the individual, but by the family, the group, or the community.

Because of the increasing focus on behavioral health outcomes, many psychologists have been trained to identify a specific presenting problem and develop a treatment plan of behavioral goals that will indicate that the treatment is effective. The underlying cultural assumption here is that there is a problem to define (e.g., anxiety, or depression, severe grief reaction, fear of dying, existential distress) in terms that are as precise as possible so that a plan can be developed. However, in many non-Western cultures appropriateness of communication is equally if not more important, as are subtleties and nuances. An open and direct discussion of challenges or difficulties in one's life may be perceived as rushed and rude, in spite of the therapist's intentions.

Self-disclosure on the part of the patient and the family can also be interpreted differently based on cultural values. The ability to openly and freely articulate feelings and emotions is a prerequisite for engaging in Western psychotherapy. The patient's ability to explain behavior as motivated by psychological factors has been described as psychological mindedness (Beitel, 2010) and is generally considered a desirable aspect of personality (Rai, Punia, Choudhury, & Mathew, 2015).

However, in many cultural groups it is only appropriate to disclose personal feelings and emotions with a trusted person such as a family member or a friend. In many Asian cultures, it is not appropriate to disclose personal and intimate details because they may reflect negatively on the family. Thus, the patient may be reticent to discuss any challenges and fears. As another example, a bereaved family caregiver of Asian culture may frame normal grief as the ability to return to usual routines, including eating regularly, getting adequate rest, and returning to work. They may resist discussing any emotions associated with grief. Thus, many grief counseling models that are based on expressing and exploring emotions may be culturally irrelevant for these groups.

Self-disclosure of thoughts and feelings by the psychologist is often interpreted as a sign of poor boundaries and generally not recommended. However, in certain cultural groups it is interpreted as an indication of sincerity, authenticity, and openness. Thus, instead of valuing boundaries as an expression of professionalism, patient and family may regard them with suspicion and take it as a sign that the psychologist cannot be fully trusted.

Culturally Appropriate and Relevant Palliative Psychotherapy

According to Sue and Sue (2013), the main therapeutic frameworks developed in Western culture, including psychodynamic theory, cognitive behavioral theory, or humanistic existential therapy have three main characteristics that can become problematic when serving culturally diverse groups:

All psychotherapy frameworks are culture bound. Because they were developed within a specific sociocultural framework, they may not be applicable to cultural frameworks that emphasize different life experiences and values.

The main theories of counseling and psychotherapy are class bound. They are based on a framework where a patient has the time and the means to see a therapist for a personal therapy session as a means to reflect, introspect, develop insight into their problems and subsequently solve the problems. If, however, the patient is facing discrimination or poverty, they will be primarily focused on meeting survival needs. Sitting down with a therapist to discuss problems may not be considered relevant.

The main theories of counseling and psychotherapy are linguistically bound. This means that they rely on specific use of a language, and in the United States, English is the main vehicle for the delivery of psychotherapy and for communication with the client. Psychological constructs that can be expressed in English may not be translatable into a non-Western language, because the construct may not exist in that culture.

In an effort to address these cultural limitations, attempts have been made to improve the contextual basis of the models. This has resulted in cultural adaptation of mainstream models, including cognitive-behavioral therapy, which have expanded their applicability to multicultural populations. Psychosocial interventions developed specifically to address the needs of palliative care patients are also being studied and adapted for different cultural groups. For instance, the framework of Dignity Therapy was explored in a group of older Chinese patients (Ho et al., 2013). While the main themes of the original model were supported, the study identified one subtheme that was not supported (death anxiety) and two subthemes that manifested differently in Chinese patients (generativity/legacy; resilience/fighting spirit). Additionally, new and relevant themes emerged. This information is important for the development of a culturally relevant application of Dignity Therapy for Chinese patients.

As psychological interventions are modified to reflect different cultural needs, outcome measures to evaluate the impact of the intervention should also be modified accordingly. To illustrate, the Chinese Cancer Coherence Scale (Chan, Ho, & Chan, 2007) was developed to evaluate the outcome of meaning-making interventions based on a framework culturally relevant for Chinese patients with cancer.

A professional stance reflecting cultural humility will convey to the patient and the family authenticity and true interest on the part of the clinician. Cultural humility implies that clinicians be aware that they are not the experts on the patient's culture but are focused on deepening their understanding of each interaction with the patient and the family (Comas-Diaz, 2014).

Comas-Diaz (2014) identified the core concepts in multicultural psychotherapy as reflexivity, empowerment, and pluralism (Table 6.8).

Reflexivity involves ongoing cultivation of awareness on the part of the clinician to identify not only their own cultural biases but also those psychotherapy approaches that are not meeting the needs of a multicultural population. It is essential that palliative psychologists question the psychological interventions they are using with patients and not assume these are valid. The principle of reflexivity allows clinicians to become aware of their own cultural schema and their own privilege and also the cultural schemas shared by the patient and the family.

Empowerment should always be at the core of multicultural psychotherapy, regardless of the specific models being utilized. Enhancing a sense of empowerment in the patient and the family within the boundaries of their cultural values is particularly important in the health-care setting.

Pluralism involves including several approaches and interventions in psychotherapy. It is a concept that can allow for the necessary modifications to mainstream

Table 6.8 **Core Concepts of Cultural Psychotherapy and Application to Palliative Care**

Core Principle	Meaning of the Principle	Practice Implications in Palliative Psychology
Reflexivity	Maintain self-awareness of own cultural schemas and unconscious behavior in a cross-cultural encounter	Identify triggers for countertransference and bias
Empowerment	Adopt a strength-based approach validating and affirming cultural sources of strength and support that expand options for the patient	Question cultural validity of assessment and diagnosis
Pluralism	Use a plurality of psychological approaches that have ecological and cultural validity	Develop an integrative approach

Adapted and modified from Comas-Diaz (2014).

psychotherapy models to be culturally relevant. While the ability to integrate different modalities and approaches to best meet the needs of the patient is valuable with all patient populations, it is essential with patients of color. This is especially important in the palliative care setting, where the ongoing and often sudden changes in the patient's medical condition introduce new and urgent psychosocial needs that are best-addressed by a plurality of approaches.

Avoiding Cultural Aggressions in Palliative and End-of-Life Care

All people are believed to be exposed to biases communicated by ancestors, institutions, and society at large (Sue et al., 2013; Comas-Diaz, 2014). Accordingly, a multicultural perspective recognizes that people have been socialized with individual, institutional, and societal biases associated with race, gender, sexual orientation, age, physical ability and appearance, and others. Palliative psychologists who value and pursue cultural competence are not considered to be without bias. Rather, they recognize the presence of their own cultural bias and cultivate self-awareness to adequately define, recognize, and reduce its negative impact on patient care.

Microaggressions have been described as "the everyday verbal, non-verbal, and environmental slights, snubs, or insults, whether intentional or unintentional, that communicate hostile, derogatory, or negative messages to target persons based solely upon their group membership (Sue, 2010, p. 3). The expression "racial microaggressions" was used to refer to demeaning behavior toward African Americans and it has been expanded to indicate behaviors that are culturally insensitive, invalidating, and demeaning of people not only on the basis of race, but also sexual orientation, gender, physical ability, age, sexual orientation, and sexual identity. Microaggressions have also been described as "the brief and commonplace daily verbal, behavioral, and environmental indignities, whether intentional or unintentional, that communicate hostile, derogatory, or negative racial, gender, sexual orientation, and religious slights and insults to the target person or group" (Sue, 2010, p. 5).

Microaggressions can be conscious or unconscious and are often perpetrated by well-meaning people who may not be aware of their bias and how their bias is affecting their thoughts, emotions, and behaviors toward a particular group. They represent a damaging form of discrimination, often resulting in lower quality medical care and also creating a hostile climate in the workplace (Holder, Jackson, & Ponterotto, 2015; Walls et al., 2015). While often subtle, different forms of microaggressions can have a cumulative effect resulting in depression, frustration, anger, rage, loss of self-esteem, and anxiety (Sue & Sue, 2013). Three main categories of microaggressions have been described: microassaults, microinsults, and microinvalidations.

- *Microassaults* have been described as overt verbal or nonverbal attacks aimed to damage the victim. For example, perpetrators may use derogatory expressions and engage in actions that are meant to be discriminatory. Microassaults are considered to be often conscious.

- *Microinsults* are often unconscious and refer to insensitive and rude comments about a particular groups that are demeaning and offensive.
- *Microinvalidations* are also often unconscious and refer to comments and actions that are invalidating of a person or a group's psychological reality and experience.

Although microaggressions have not been specifically described in the context of palliative care, they may occur. Personal bias can manifest in forms of microaggression that can seriously undermine communication and trust in the relationship with the patient and the family. Although overt discriminatory behaviors in hospitals and clinics are less common and can be more easily identified and addressed, microaggressions (and especially microinsults and microinvalidations) can be subtle, still creating tension and discomfort not only for the patient but also for other clinicians. Lack of awareness and work-related stress can create fertile ground for bias, especially in the context of complex case scenarios that challenge the team's resources. Consider the following examples:

The team is discussing the case of a 79-year-old Chinese patient newly diagnosed with advanced gastric cancer and referred to palliative care for pain management. The patient does not speak English and the older son has power of attorney for health care. The family is adamant that the team should not communicate the diagnosis to the patient. Their request is creating difficulties because the oncologist has recommended chemotherapy and feels the patient cannot give consent to treatment unless he is aware of all the facts. The palliative care team has been asked to help "fix" this problem. During the team discussion, the patient's oncologist rolls his eyes and comments, "It is never easy with family and especially with Chinese people; they have so many cultural issues and they want to dictate how we should do our job."

Although the clinician did not express his thoughts in the presence of the patient and the family, his comments are not only culturally insensitive, but also represent a form of microaggression. He applies his assumptions to all Chinese patients and highlights the family's request as something negative and aggravating for the team. The family's cultural preferences and values are pathologized and dismissed as inconveniences. His focus is on the clinical challenges imposed on the team by a complex case.

In presenting the palliative care referral of an 68-year-old African American woman found unconscious by her daughter and now in ICU after intubation, the nurse comments, "This patient is African American and, of course, she is full code and has no advance directives." A family meeting is requested to discuss goals of care with the patient's daughter, who is her health-care proxy agent. The daughter is distressed and animated during the family meeting, but collaborative with the team. At the subsequent team meeting, when the case is again discussed, one of the clinicians comments, "The daughter was not angry, but she was so loud; she should just calm down. I guess it's the culture."

The initial comment represents a microaggression because it dismisses and trivializes the patient's situation, implying that it should be expected that African American patients do not have advanced directives. The clinician's comment has the effect of presenting the patient in a slightly negative light based on choices attributed to her racial/ethnic background. Additionally, the daughters' affect and communication style is pathologized based on some notion of what represents appropriate communication.

The nurse manager of an inpatient palliative care unit is complaining about the behavior of the family of a patient, a 59-year-old Latino with multiple myeloma and a prognosis of days.

The patient is sedated and unresponsive. He was born and raised in Puerto Rico, although he lived in the United States most of his adult life. The nurse reports that the patient's room is always full of family members who bring food from outside and eat together at the bedside. Sometimes they play music. They have been described as "loud" by other patients, who also have complained about food smell coming from the room. The nurse explains that this behavior is disruptive and is creating challenges for the nursing staff. However, no one has approached this topic with the family yet, as the team does not want to hurt their feelings. One of the team members, who is not Latino, comments, "Well, you know, they are Latino, it's the culture."

Again, a racist and demeaning statement pathologizes behavior based on cultural background and ethnicity. Such overt demonstrations of contempt on the part of clinicians create polarization and divisiveness, instead of helping to find a way to effectively communicate with the family. Lack of training is preventing the team from approaching this issue in an effective and yet therapeutic manner. The team has labeled the family as difficult and uncooperative based on overly broad descriptions of Hispanic culture.

The team finally decided it was appropriate to discuss this issue with the spokesperson for the family. The oldest son shared the role with his older sister. A family meeting was requested and the team met with the two siblings. During the conversation they shared that watching their father slowly die was hard for them, especially because they could not take care of him at home. For this reason, they had tried to re-create the home environment with familiar sounds, smells, and presence of family. The team validated their commitment to their father and then sensitively raised concerns about the fact that the strong smells and loud noise was creating discomfort for other patients who were also trying to connect with their families in a comfortable and supportive environment. The siblings were responsive and stated they felt ashamed that they offended anyone. They asked why no one had spoken to them sooner. The team reassured them and together discussed needed adjustments that could ensure comfort for all the patients.

During a lecture on cultural aspects of palliative care presented to the oncology team and the interdisciplinary palliative care team, the presenter states that planning for one's death and completing advance directive "is the best way" to ensure a "good death." The presenter also comments that challenges in completing advance directives are caused by death anxiety and denial and encourages all clinicians to have open and direct conversations with their patients about these issues.

Respecting patients' wishes, promoting comfort, and relieving suffering at end of life are important goals of palliative care. And yet this presenter minimized the complexity of cultural aspects of palliative care. Absolute statements identifying "the best way" for promoting a good death are clearly problematic and blatantly oblivious of cultural implications. Patients and families who have not discussed advance directives are regarded negatively. The direct mode of communication is presented as optimal However, it may be perceived as harsh and disrespectful by the patient and the family increasing likelihood of conflict.

During a psychosocial assessment with a patient and her two adult daughters, the palliative care clinician discovers that the family immigrated to the United States from the Dominican Republic 15 years prior. The patient states that her older sister lives in the Dominican Republic, but most of her family lives in the United States. The patient comments that if her medical condition allows it, she would like to visit her sister, who just had a baby. The palliative care clinician nods and comments, "Of course, I completely understand you want to go home and be with your culture." The daughters look puzzled and comment, "Well, this is our home. The US is our home." The palliative care clinician explains emphatically, "Of course, of course, but you were all born and raised there, so of course that would also be home. And you speak English so well; I am really impressed." The daughters remain quiet. At the next visit, they request to see a different clinician.

One of the forms of microaggression has been referred to as "Alien in own country" (Sue, 2010). The clinician is well intentioned and is attempting to bond with the family. However, she makes inappropriate assumptions about the patient's and family's experience, which unsurprisingly are perceived negatively by the family.

During morning rounds the medical team visits a 50-year-old Korean patient diagnosed with renal cell carcinoma. The patient is rapidly declining, and her prognosis is in the order of weeks. However, she is alert and oriented and participating in the meeting. Her sister is at the bedside. An interpreter is used because both the patient and her sister speak only a few words of English and stated they would feel more comfortable with an interpreter. Two medical students on an elective rotation have also joined the team. One of the two students is Chinese American, and the other is visiting from India. The patient's main complaint is pain. The attending physician assures her that her pain will be better managed from this point on. The physician also attempts to discuss goals of care and code status, but he is quickly interrupted by the patient and her sister, who state they only want to discuss pain.

The physician tries to ask some general questions about preferences, but again, the sisters say they do not want to discuss the topic. At this point the physician smiles at the patient and turns to the interpreter saying, "You don't need to translate this." He then turns to the medical students and explains that this "resistance" discussing goals of care is common in Chinese patients and that these cases are always challenging because "they also have a lot of superstitions." The Chinese American medical student points out that the patient is Korean. The physician replies that even if that is the case, the teaching point remains valid and applies to the majority of Asian patients.

The preceding examples illustrate how assumptions, biases, and stereotyping result in microaggressions, whether the comments are expressed in the presence of the patient and the family or not. Dismissing cultural preferences about goals of care discussions is insensitive and patronizing at best, if not racist. It is certainly an aggression toward the patient's worldview. The clinician described in the preceding example was probably unaware of the bias reflecting his assumptions and communications, and even appeared unwilling or unable to reflect on his behavior after the medical student corrected his perception. This highlights the importance of constantly engaging in self-awareness related to culturally appropriate behavior.

CASE VIGNETTE 6.2

The palliative care team receives a consultation request for a 53-year-old Chinese woman diagnosed with advanced ovarian cancer. The oncologist requesting the consultation noted the patient was depressed and anxious and would benefit from psychological support. The patient is visited in her hospital room by members of the palliative care team, namely the attending physician, the social worker, and psychologist. The interpreter is present. It becomes clear that the patient is indeed anxious about future steps related to treatment options. It is not clear to her what her oncologist believes about her condition and what her options are. The patient and her family have decided that it is important to continue receiving chemotherapy, if she can tolerate it, to control the spread of the cancer and possibly prolong her life. According to the patient, the oncologist is not encouraging her to receive more chemotherapy, and she does not understand why. With the help of the interpreter, the patient explains that if the doctor is not trying to convince her to accept more treatment, the reason must be that "something is wrong" and "perhaps it means there is no hope." While the palliative care team and the patient, along with the help of the interpreter, continue exploring the patient's understanding of her options and the source of her anxiety, the interpreter is paged for an urgent need. She states she has to leave but that she will return shortly. The palliative care team members remain in the room, and using nonverbal communication primarily based on reassuring touch and smiles, they attempt to relax the patient waiting for the interpreter's return. At that point the oncologist who requested the consultation enters the hospital room. The patient appears happy to see him and the oncologist behaves warmly toward her. He stands behind her with both of his hands on her shoulder and talks to the team, even though the patient cannot understand what he is saying. He tells the team that the patient is "a very sweet woman of not great intelligence" but also kind and that he cares dearly about her. As he describes the patient as a woman with limited intelligence, he keeps his hands on her shoulders in a reassuring fashion. The patient continues smiling, unaware of what the physician is saying. The palliative care team members are feeling quite uncomfortable, and comments are made that it would be best to wait for the interpreter to come back, so that the patient can be part of the conversation. The oncologist dismisses this request, stating that he cannot wait for the interpreter; however, it is important for him to offer some context to the palliative care team about the patient's circumstances and difficulty with decisions. According to the oncologist's understanding, the patient is anxious because she wants to stop chemotherapy, while her family is pushing for her to receive more treatment. He comments that "this is typical in Chinese culture." When asked if he has information directly from the patient about her desire to stop chemotherapy, he once again dismisses the question, stating, "She didn't tell me in so many words but I understood from her affect and from the way she smiles at me and nods when I talk and I raise the issue of stopping chemotherapy."

Clearly there are several elements in this clinical interaction that are concerning from a cultural standpoint. The palliative care team should have considered leaving the room after the interpreter was called away for the emergency. The interpreter could have explained to the patient that the meeting will be resumed later in the day, and the patient would have probably felt comfortable with that arrangement. From the description of the case, it appears that the palliative care team created some positive nonverbal, implicit bonding through smiling, but it is really not possible to determine if the patient felt comfortable. When the oncologist came into the room and saw that the interpreter was not there he also should have avoided engaging in a medical conversation about treatment decisions without the patient understanding the communication.

Although well intentioned—he expressed caring deeply about this patient—he adopted a paternalistic approach that included openly insulting her by making disparaging and patronizing comments about her intelligence. There is a disconcerting discrepancy between his affectionate and warm nonverbal communication and his comments about her intelligence.

The oncologist was clearly in charge and represented the medical hierarchy in the room. The members of the palliative care team felt uncomfortable with his approach and timidly suggested that it would be best to wait for the interpreter to return before continuing the discussion. They were quickly dismissed by the oncologist and were not able to successfully negotiate a comfortable exit from that awkward situation. Perhaps most important, it appears that the oncologist's erroneous assumptions about Chinese culture and his reliance on an incorrect interpretation of some elements of the patient's body language (e.g., smiling and nodding) prevented him from fully and meaningfully exploring the patient's understanding and wishes. It appears he based his understanding of the wishes of the patient on nonverbal communications, which he interpreted with cultural bias. He assumed the patient's smile meant that she is in accordance with the plan.

Subsequent interviews with the patient in the presence of the interpreter and the family revealed that the patient and the family smile at the doctor and nod as a way of demonstrating respect. Because of her cultural values, she will consider it disrespectful to just listen quietly. Furthermore, it appears that the patient and the family are in perfect agreement when it comes to making decisions. The patient stated clearly, with the help of the interpreter, that she wishes to receive more chemotherapy to control the spread of her cancer. What the oncologist interpreted as a family conflict causing anxiety for the patient, is anxiety about the discrepancy between the oncologist's understanding on the one hand and the patient's and family's understanding on the other. Further exploration reveals that the patient and the family are actually becoming anxious because plans are not being made for her to receive further chemotherapy, even after it has been suggested that could be helpful.

Professional humility on the part of clinicians is important in recognizing that they and are not experts on the patient's cultural background. This can prevent making quick assumptions about the meaning of communication. Cultural sensitivity and basic respect would have prevented disparaging comments the patient could not understand. Cultural competence would have prevented the conversation about the patient's medical needs from occurring in the absence of an interpreter.

References

American Psychological Association. (2003). Guidelines on multicultural education, training, research, practice, and organizational change for psychologists. *American Psychologist, 58*(5), 377–402.

American Psychological Association. (2008). Report of the task force on the implementation of the multicultural guidelines. Washington, DC: APA. Retrieved from http://www.apa.org/pi.

Arredondo, P., Toporek, R., Pack Brown, S., Jones, J., Locke, D. C., & Stadler, H. (1996). Operationalization of the multicultural counseling competencies. *Journal of Multicultural Couseling and Development, 24*, 42–78.

Arredondo, P., & Tovar-Blank, Z. G. (2014). Multicultural competencies: A dynamic paradigm for the 21st century. In F. T. L Leong (Ed.), APA handbook of multicultural psychology: Applications and training (Vol. 2, pp. 19–34). Washington, DC: American Psychological Association.

Beitel, M. (2010). *Psychological mindedness: The Corsini encyclopedia of psychology*. New York: John Wiley & Sons.
Bousquet, G., Orri, M., Winterman, S., Brugiere, C., Verneuil, L., & Revah-Levy, A. (2015). Breaking bad new in oncology: A metasynthesis. *Journal of Clinicial Oncology*, 33(22), 2437–2443.
Chan, T. H. Y., Ho, R. T. H., & Chan, C. L. W. (2007). Developing an outcome measurement for meaning-making intervention with Chinese cancer patients. *Psycho-Oncology*, 16(9), 843–850.
Chettih, M. (2012). Turning the lens inward: Cultural competence and providers' values in health care decision making. *The Gerontologist*, 52(6), 739–747.
Colclough, Y. Y., & Brown, G. M. (2014). American Indians' experiences of life-threatening illness and end of life. *Journal of Hospice and Palliative Nursing*, 16(7), 404–413.
Comas-Diaz, L. (2014). Multicultural psychotherapy. In F. T. L Leong (Ed.), *APA handbook of multicultural psychology: Applications and training* (Vol. 2, pp. 419–441). Washington, DC: American Psychological Association.
Coolen, P. R. (2012). Cultural relevance in end of life care. *EthnoMed*. http://ethnomed.org/clinical/end-of-life/cultural-relevance-in-end-of-life-care.
Council of National Psychological Associations for the Advancement of Ethnic Minorities Interests. (2009). *Psychology education and training from culture-specific and multiracial perspectives: Critical issues and recommendations*. Washington, DC: American Psychological Association. Retrieved from http://www.apa.org/pi/oema.
Cross, T. L., Bazron, B. J., Dennis, K. W., & Isaacs, M. R. (1989). *Towards a culturally competent system of care*. Washington, DC: CASSP Technical Assistance Center, Georgetown University Child Development Center.
Curtis, J. R., Back, A. L., Ford, D. F., Downey, L., Shannon, S. E., Doorenbos, A. Z., . . . Engelberg, R. A. (2013). Effect of communication skill training for residents and nurse practitioners on quality of life communication with patients with serious illness: A randomized trial. *JAMA*, 310(21), 2271–2281.
El-Jawahri, A., Traeger, L., Park, E. R., Greer, J. A., Pirl, W. F., Lennes, I. T., . . . Temel, J. S. (2014). Association among prognostic understanding, quality of life, and mood in patients with advanced cancer. *Cancer*, 120(2), 278–285.
Enguidanos, S., Vesper, E., & Goldstein, R. (2013). Ethnic differences in hospice enrollment following inpatient palliative care consultation. *Journal of Hospital Medicine*, 8(10), 598–600.
Enzinger, A., Zhang, B., Schrag, D., & Progerson, H. (2015). Outsomes of prognostic discplosure: Association with prognostic understanding, distress, and relationship with physician among patients with advanced cancer. *Journal of Clinical Oncology*, 33(32), 3809–3816.
Epstein, A. S., Prigerson, H. G., O'Reilly, E., & Maciejewski, P. K. (2016). Discussions of life expectancy and changes in illness understanding in patients with advanced cancer. *Journal of Clinical Oncology*, 34(20), 2398–2403.
Fischer, S. M., Sauaia, A., Min, S. J., & Kutner, J. (2012). Advanced directive discussions: Lost in translations or lost opportunities? *Journal of Palliative Medicine*, 15(1), 86–92.
Fiske, S. T. (2004). *Social beings: A core motive approach to social psychology*. New York: John Wiley & Sons.
Foronda, C. L., Baptiste, D., Reinholdt, M., & Ousman, K. (2016). Cultural humility: A concept analysis. *Journal of Transcultual Nursing*, 27(3), 210–217.
Gatrad, A. R., Brown, E., Notta, H., & Sheikh, A. (2003). Palliative care needs of minorities: Understanding their way is the key. *British Medical Journal*, 327:176–177.
Gauthier, J., Pettifor, J., & Ferrero, A. (2010). The universal declaration of ethical principles for psychologists: A culture-sensitive-model for creating a reviewing and code of ethics. *Ethics and Behavior*, 20(3–4), 179–196.
Gire, J. (2014). How death imitates life: Cultural influences on conceptions of death and dying. *Online Readings in Psychology and Culture*, 6(2), 1–22.
Grier, W. H., & Cobb, P. M. (1968). *Black rage*. New York: Basic Books.
Hallenbeck, J., & Arnold, R. (2007). A request for nondisclosure: Don't tell my mother. *Journal of Clinical Oncology*, 25(31), 5030–5034.

Helms, J. E., & Talleyrand, R. M. (1997). Race is not ethnicity. *American Psychologist*, 52(11), 1246–1247.

Heppner, P. P., Wei, M., Neville, H. A., & Kanagui-Munoz, M. A. (2014). Cultural and contextual model of coping. In FTL Leong (Ed.), *APA handbook of multicultural psychology: Applications and training* (Vol. 2, pp. 83–106). Washington, DC: American Psychological Association

Ho, A. H., Chan, C. L., Leung, P. P., Chochinov, H. M., Neimeyer, R. A., Pang, S. M., & Tse, D. M. (2013). Living and dying with dignity in Chinese society: Perspectives of older palliative care patients in Hong Kong. *Age and Ageing*, 42(4), 455–461.

Holder, A. M. B., Jackson, M. A., & Ponterotto, J. (2015). Racial microaggression experiences and coping strategies of black women in corporate leadership. *Qualitative Psychology*, 2(2), 164–180.

Hook, J. N., Davis, D. E., Owen, J., Worthington E. L., Jr., & Utsey, S. O. (2013). Cultural humility: Measuring openness to culturally diverse clients. *Journal of Counselling Psychology*, 60(3), 353–366.

Huang, I. A., Neuhaus, J. M., & Chiong, W. (2016). Racial and ethnic differences in advance directive possession: Role of demographic factors, religious affiliation, and personal health values in a national survey of older adults. *Journal of Palliative Medicine*, 19(2), 149–156.

Johnson, K. D. (2013). Racial and ethnic disparities in palliative care. *Journal of Palliative Medicine*, 16(11), 1329–1334.

Johnstone, M. J. (2012). Bioethics, cultural differences and the problem of moral disagreement in end of life care: A terror management theory. *Journal of Medicine and Philosophy*, 37, 181–200.

Kemp, C. E. (2005). Cultural issues in palliative care. *Seminars in Oncology Nursing*, 21, 44–52.

Knight, B. G., & Sayeg, P. (2009). Cultural values and caregiving: The updated sociocultural stress and coping model. *The Journal of Gerontology*, 65B(1), 5–13.

Ko, E., & Berkman, C. S. (2012). Advance directives among Korean American older adults: Knowledge, attitudes, and behavior. *Journal of Gerontology and Social Work*, 55(6), 484–502.

Kutney-Lee, A., Smith, D., Thorpe, J., Del Rosario, C., Ibrahim, S., & Ersek, M. (2016). Race/ethnicity and end-of-life among veterans. *Medical Care*. doi: 10.1097/MLR.0000000000000637.

Lalonde, R. N., Cila, J., Lou, E., & Cribbie, R. (2015). Are we really that different from each other? The difficulties of focusing on similarities in cross-cultural research. *Peace and Conflict: Journal of Peace Psychology*, 21(4), 525–534.

Lijtmaer, R. M. (2001). Countertransference and ethnicity. *Journal of Academy of Psychoanalysis*, 29(1), 73–84.

LoPresti, M. A., Dement, F., & Gold, H. T. (2016). End-of-life for people with cancer from ethnic minority groups: A systematic review. *American Journal of Hospice and Palliative Care*, 33(3), 291–305.

Mack, J. W, Wolfe, J., Cook, E. F., Grier, H. E., Cleary, P. D., & Weeks, J. C. (2007). Hope and prognostic disclosure. *Journal of Clinical Oncology*, 25(35), 5636–5642.

Mack, J. W., Wolfe, J., Grier, H. E., Cleary, P. D., & Weeks, J. C. (2006). Communication about prognosis between parents and physicians of children with cancer: Parent preferences and the impact of prognostic information. *Journal of Clinical Oncology*, 24(33), 5265–5270.

Marchioli, J. (2008). African American outreach guide. National Hospice and Palliative Care Organization, Alexandria, VA: NHPCO.

Matsuyama, R. K., Balliet, W., & Ingram, K., Lyckholm, K., Wilson-Genderson, M., & Smith, T. J. (2011). Will patients want hospice or palliative care of they don't know what it is? *Journal of Hospice and Palliative Nursing*, 13(1), 41–46.

McIntosh, P. (1989). White privilege: Unpacking the invisible backpack. http://code.ucsd.edu/pcosman/Backpack.pdf. Retrieved on January 1, 2017.

Meyer, O. L., Nguyen, K. H., Dao, T. N., Vu, P., Arean, P., & Hinton, L. (2015). The sociocultural context of caregiving experiences for Vietnamese dementia family caregivers. *Asian American Journal of Psychology*, 6(3), 263–272.

Meier, E. A., Gallegos, J. V., Montross-Thomas, L. P., Depp, C. A., Irwin, S. A., & Jeste, D. V. (2016). Defining a good death (successful dying): Literature review and a call for research and public dialogue. *American Journal of Geriatric Psychiatry*, 24(4), 261–271.

Migrant Information Center Eastern Melbourne Community Partners Program.(2009). Palliative care for culturally and linguistically diverse communities. Retrieved from http://www.miceastmelb.com.au

Nadal, K. L., Mazzula, S. L., Rivera, D. P., & Fujii-Doe W. (2014). Microaggression and latin/o americans: An analysis of nativity, gender, and ethnicity. *Journal of Latina/o Psychology, 2*(2), 67–68.

Nadal, K. L., Griffin, K. E., Wong, Y., & Hamit, S. (2014). The impact of racial microaggressions on mental health: Counseling implications for clients of color. *Journal of Counseling and Development, 92*, 57–66.

Noah, B. A. (2012). The role of race in end of life care. *Journal of Health Care Law & Policy, 15*(2), 349–378.

Pan, C. X., Abraham, O., Giron, F., LeMarie, P., & Pollack, S. (2015). Just ask: Hospice familiarity in Asian and Hispanic adults. *Journal of Pain and Symptom Management, 49*(5), 928–933.

Pang, M. C. (1999). Protective truthfulness: The Chinese way of safeguarding patients in informed treatment decisions. *Journal of Medical Ethics, 25*(3), 247–253.

Park, N. S., Jang, Y., & Chiriboga, D. A. (2016). Factors affecting willingness to use hospice in racially/ethnically diverse older men and women. *American Journal of Hospice and Palliative Care, 33*(8), 770–776.

Payne, R. (2015). Culturally relevant palliative care. *Clinics in Geriatric Medicine, 31*, 271–279.

Periyakoil, V. S., Stevens, M., & Kraemer, H. (2013). Multicultural long-term nurses' perceptions of factors influencing patient dignity at the end of life. *Journal of the American Geriatric Society, 61*(3), 440–446.

Periyakoil, V. S., Neri, E., & Kraemer, H. (2015). No easy talk: A mixed method study of doctor reported barriers to conducting effective end of life conversations with diverse patients. *PLoS ONE, 10*(4), e0122321.

Periyakoil, V. S., Neri, E., & Kraemer, H. (2016). Patient-reported barriers to high quality end of life care: A multiethnic, multilingual, mixed-method study. *Journal of Palliative Medicine, 19*(4), 373–379.

Piamjariyakul, U., Smith, C., Werkowitch, M., Thompson, N., Fox, M., Williamson, K. P., & Olson, L. (2016). Designing and testing an end of life discussion intervention for African American patients. *Journal of Hospice and Palliative Nursing, 18*(6), 528–535.

Quill, T. E., & Townsend, P. (1991). Bad news: Delivery, dialogue, and dilemmas. *Archives of Internal Medicine, 151*, 463–468.

Rai, S., Punia, V., Choudhury, S., & Mathew, K. J. (2015). Psychological mindedness: An overview. *Indian Journal of Positive Psychology, 6*, 1.

Rhodes, R. L., Batchelor, K., Lee, S. C., & Halm, E. A. (2015). Barriers to end of life care for African Americans from the providers' perspective: Opportunities for intervention development. *American Journal of Hospice and Palliative Care, 32*(2), 137–143.

Rhodes, R. L., Elwood, B., Lee, S. C., & Tiro, J. A. (2016). The desires of their hearts: The multidisciplinary perspectives of African Americans on end of life care in the Africal American Community. *American Journal of Hospice and Palliative Medicine, 34*(6), 510–517.

Ruiz, J. M., & Brondolo, E. (2016). Introduction to the special issue disparities in cardiovascular health: Examining the contributions of social and behavioral factors. *Health Psychology, 35*(4), 309–312.

Searight, H. R., & Gafford, J. (2005). Cultural diversity at the end of life: Issues and guidelines for family physicians. *American Family Physician, 71*(3), 515–522.

Smith, C., & Brawley, O. (2014, July 30). Disparities in access to palliative care. *Health Affairs Blog.*

Strada, E. A., Homel, P., Tennestedt, S., Billings, J. A., & Portenoy, R. K. (2012). Spiritual well-being in patients with advanced heart and lung disease. *Palliative and Supportive Care, 11*(3), 205–213.

Sue, D. W., Arredondo, P., & McDavis, R. J. (1992). Multicultural counseling competencies and standards: A call to the profession. *Journal of Counseling and Development, 70*, 477–486.

Sue, D. W., Nadal, K. L., Capodilupo, C. M., Lin, A. I., Torino, G. C., & Rivera, D. P. (2008). Racial microaggressions against Black Americans: Implications for counseling. *Journal of Counseling and Development, 86*(3), 330–338.

Sue, D. W. (2010). Microaggression, marginality, and oppression. In D. W. Sue (Ed.) *Microaggressions and marginality* (Chapter 1 p. 3–22). Hoboken, NJ: John Wiley & Sons. Kindle Edition.

Sue, D. W. & Sue, D. (2013). *Counseling the culturally diverse* (6th ed.). Hoboken, NJ: John Wiley & Sons.

Taxis, J. C. (2006). Attitudes, values, and questions of African Americans regarding participation in hospice programs. *Journal of Hospice and Palliative Care Nursing, 8*(2), 77–85.

Van Vliet, L. M., van der Wall, E., Plum, N. M., & Bensing, J. M. (2013). Explicit prognostic information and reassurance about non abandonment when entering palliative breast cancer care: Findings from a scripted video vignette study. *Journal of Clinical Oncology, 31*(26), 3242–3249.

Walls, M., Gonzalez, J., Gladney, T., & Onello, E. (2015). Unconscious bias: Racial microaggressions in American Indian care. *Journal of the American Board of Family Medicine, 28*(2), 231–239.

Washington, K. T., Bickel-Swenson, D., & Stephens, N. (2008). Barriers to hospice use among African Americans: A systematic review. *Health & Social Work, 33*(4), 267–274.

Weeks, J. C., Catalano, P. J., Cronin, A., Finkelman, M. D., Mack, J. W., Keating, N. L., & Schrag, D. (2012). Patients' expectations about effects of chemotherapy for advanced cancer. *New England Journal of Medicine, 367*, 1616–1625.

White, D. B., Ernecoff, N., Buddadhumaruk, P., Hong, S., Weissfeld, L., Curtis, J. R., . . . & Lo, B. (2016). Prevalence of and factors related to discordance about prognosis between physicians and surrogate decisions makers of critically ill patients. *JAMA, 315*(19), 2086–2094.

Williams, D. R., & Priest, N. (2016). Understanding association among race, socioeconomic status, and health: patterns and prospects. *Health Psychology, 35*(4), 407–411.

7

The Seventh Domain of Palliative Care

Care of the Patient at the End of Life

> ## Focus Points
>
> - Palliative psychologists participate in the interdisciplinary care of the patient at the end of life, which requires adequate management of physical and psychological symtpoms, including pain, anxiety, and agitated delirium.
> - Palliative psychologists need to be familiar with the medical processes involved in disease progression and dying, including methods for evaluating prognosis and recognizing signs that death is near.
> - The ability to engage in sensitive and effective communication with family caregivers as the patient enters the active dying phase is an essential component of specialist palliative care.
> - End-of-life care includes ensuring that cultural and religious preferences are honored and facilitating bereavement support for surviving family caregivers.
> - Palliative sedation is different from euthanasia and physician-assisted dying, and it is an accepted legal and ethical medical practice for relieving refractory suffering in patients at the end of life.

Introduction

This domain of palliative care was previously known as "Care of the Imminently Dying Patient" in the earlier edition of the *Clinical Practice Guidelines*. The current name, "Care of the Patient at the End of Life," reflects a desire to "expand the focus of care" and includes the period prior to final days or hours of life (*Clinical Practice Guidelines*, p. 6). End of life can refer to the months leading up to the moment of death. Accordingly, "dying" can be conceptualized as a process, with important physical, psychological, social, cultural, and spiritual implications.

Caring for the patient who is dying and the family requires a complex set of skills in the areas of medical management, communication, and psychological and spiritual support. Patients and families frequently develop questions and concerns about the dying process. Some may not feel comfortable expressing them openly. Others may have difficulty integrating the reality that death is near and may choose to avoid thinking and talking about it to protect themselves and the patient from emotional distress.

In coping with worsening illness and approaching death, family caregivers are required to constantly adjust to ongoing change and establish a sense of a "new normal" in their relationship with the patient and their own life as caregivers. Every patient and family story is unique, with each individual approaching death and the awareness of death differently. Therefore, communication with family caregivers must reflect great sensitivity and awareness of their psychological pain after receiving news that their loved one is "really" dying. Poor communication between the patient, the family, and the medical team can be particularly disruptive in end of life. Not only does it undermine their ability to process grief during bereavement, but it also has the potential to negatively affect the collective experience of care received during the entire illness.

The palliative care team has a responsibility to recognize signs that a patient is approaching death: this recognition is vital not only to adequately manage symptoms, but also to provide expanded psycho-education and support to the family during the dying process. Specialist palliative care continues after death by honoring patients and families' cultural and religious practices related to caring for the patient's body. This may include supporting the family by providing practical help in making arrangements for funerals and other aspects of post-death care. Additionally, ensuring adequate bereavement follow-up for family members, including management of urgent clinical situations due to severe grief reactions, is a fundamental component of care that should never be considered of a lesser importance or approached casually.

Specialist palliative care clinicians do not idealize or romanticize the dying process and avoid promoting a personal agenda about what should happen at the end of a patient's life. Rather, they are committed to ensuring that the patient and family goals are recognized and respected based on their unique circumstances.

Competencies for Palliative Psychologists

Physicians and nurses become accustomed to witnessing death early in their professional training. Hospital chaplains and hospice social workers also have experience with the dying process and are frequently present with patients and families during the last days, hours, and moments of life. Exposure to the dying process is an important component of training and competency development in providing care to the patient at the end of life.

Historically, however, psychologists have not been involved in end of life care. Graduate psychology programs do not routinely provide opportunities for supervised training with dying patients and their families. Additionally, psychology internships at sites providing palliative and end-of-life care are not yet widely available. Therefore, many licensed and practicing psychologists may have limited experience supporting patients and families during such a sensitive time. Psychologists practicing in a medical setting may also lack experience with the dying process if they perform most of their work on an outpatient basis.

Palliative psychology competencies in end-of-life care involve knowledge of the medical context of dying and signs that death is approaching, and the skills to support family caregivers during the dying process. Most important, the ability to provide a calming and reassuring presence can allow the psychologist to normalize the experience for family members, while continuing to assess their need for information and psychological support.

Palliative psychologists can also offer an important contribution by providing integrative medicine interventions that can help relieve stress for patients and family caregivers as death nears. For instance, hypnosis, imagery, and contemplative/meditative practices have been safely and effectively used around the time of death, especially when there is anxiety. There is also growing indication that energy-based practices, including Reiki and Therapeutic Touch, can relieve distress. Additionally, the palliative psychologist's ability to work collaboratively with music therapists, massage therapists, and other practitioners of mind-body modalities is an important skill.

This chapter describes some of the knowledge, skills, and attitudes that are relevant to developing competency in providing psychological support to the patient who is approaching the end of life, the patient who is actively dying, and the family who accompanies the patient during this experience (Box 7.1).

Box 7.1 **Palliative Psychology Competencies in Care of the Patient at the End of Life**

KNOWLEDGE

Understand the medical context of dying
Recognize the difference between a death in the home versus the hospital or other facility
Familiarity with aspects of prognostication and its psychological impact on the patient and family caregivers
Knowledge of the main physiological changes at the end of life
Recognize signs of imminent death
Describe diagnosis and management of delirium
Recognize the psychological and spiritual impact of dying process on family members
Understand grief reactions throughout the continuum of disease in the patient and the family

SKILLS

Provide nonpharmacological interventions in terminal delirium
Provide integrative medicine modalities to relieve distress in the patient and the family, when indicated and appropriate
Support family members during palliative extubations
Actively participate in family meetings aimed at goals of care
Provide grief support to the family and assess for urgent needs
Coordinate bereavement care

> **ATTITUDES**
>
> Calm and mindful presence that can support the patient and family members
> Respect and validation of patient and family cultural and spiritual practices
> Openness toward different manifestations of grief during and after the dying process
> Willingness to recognize when a patient's death has been particularly impactful and willingness to process emotions associated with it

Expected Psychophysical Changes in the Period Preceding the Dying Process

Advanced illness causes several changes in patients' cognitive and psychological, as well as physical, state. While some of the changes can begin a few months before death, they become more pronounced in the last weeks of life (Table 7.1). Both patient and family caregivers need information about the meaning of these changes. The knowledge that they are signs and symptoms that death is approaching can trigger intense grief reactions. However, the awareness that these changes are caused by illness can also provide important clarification for family caregivers and prevent additional distress.

To illustrate, in the last weeks of life a patient with advanced cancer may report feeling progressively more fatigued with decreased appetite. Family caregivers who are unaware that these symptoms are caused by the illness may feel a responsibility to encourage the patient to eat, or to "fight" and engage in activities despite the progressive fatigue. These family caregivers may express regret after the death of the patient

Table 7.1 **Physical, Cognitive, and Psychological Changes in Patients Approaching End of Life**

Physical Changes	Cognitive/Neurologic changes	Psychological Changes
Decrease in energy levels	Cognitive impairment	Emotional withdraw
Progressive difficulty performing daily activities	Decrease in attention and concentration	Possible increase in fear and anxiety
Decrease in overall activity level	Easily distracted, fatigues easily	Grief reactions
Decrease in food and fluid intake	May appear uninterested in surroundings	Less engaged with family members
Becoming progressively bedbound	Confusion	May begin talking about loved ones who have died

for missing the opportunity to be present and connect because they were focused on changing an irreversible course.

The expectation that the patient "will get stronger," reflects an understandable and natural hope that the progressive effects of the illness may be somehow reversed. Holding the hope that the patient's condition will improve may represent an adaptive mechanism; however, it may also become an impediment to nurturing close relationships and connections if patients and caregivers become unable to live in the moment and are postponing important conversations or opportunities for experiencing deep connection.

PHYSICAL CHANGES

Patients with advanced illness may experience a significant fluctuation in their energy level, mood, desire to engage with loved ones, and interest in normal activities. Dramatic differences can occur during the day. The patient may wake up with good amounts of energy and plan some activity for the day. Only a couple of hours later, she may feel exhausted, uninterested in pursuing the same activities, and may become irritable if family members try to encourage her. These rapid changes in physical, cognitive, and emotional energy should be normalized for the patient and the family. Furthermore, allowing for sleep and rest one day does not necessarily mean patients will have more energy and can engage more the following day, because in advanced illness, different organ systems can be thought of as progressively shutting down. Witnessing these changes can be quite distressing for family caregivers. The patient may become withdrawn and may not wish to engage, and family caregivers may worry they have upset the patient. The main communication style in the family affects how family caregivers will respond to these scenarios. Some may approach the issue directly with the patient. Others may not want to create further upset by raising the question. In all circumstances, there is potential for feelings of confusion, guilt, and disconnect at a time when close connection and support are most important. Therefore, it is necessary that palliative care clinicians normalize the changes by providing the patient and family caregivers with information and the emotional support necessary for coping with the meaning of the changes.

Some patients with advanced cancer receive palliative chemotherapy or radiation for the purpose of slowing progression of disease or reducing overall symptom burden. The doses are usually lower than those used for cure, but may still cause toxic effects. While in earlier stages of illness the patient's condition allows him or her to "bounce back" from treatment, this becomes increasingly difficult in more advanced illness. Significant difficulty recovering from treatment and coping with adverse effects may prompt the medical team to discuss the need to stop treatment.

Fluctuation in energy level progresses to increased fatigue, weakness, and somnolence, which is likely to cause the patient to become bedbound. As the illness continues its course, even sitting in a favorite chair watching television or reading a book may require more energy than can be mobilized. Simply getting out of bed and walking to the bathroom may become a major task. Interacting with others, even beloved family members can become physically and emotionally draining. Moreover, patients may feel obligated to receive visits from close friends and family, but they may become easily anxious and overwhelmed, due to their fragile cognitive and emotional state. Similarly, family caregivers may feel a responsibility to welcome friends who wish to express their support but may fear the visits will be draining and will prevent them from spending precious private time with the patient. If they do not feel comfortable addressing this issue, a skilled clinician who recognizes this situation could simply ask the family and/or the patient if they are experiencing any difficulties managing the flow of visitors. Normalizing the ambivalence that is common in these circumstances can help identify strategies that promote connections while respecting boundaries. This applies whether the patient is cared for at the hospital or at home.

Advanced illness is also generally characterized by anorexia and cachexia. *Anorexia* refers to the lack of appetite, even if food has not been eaten for an entire day. *Cachexia* refers to progressive weight loss and muscle wasting in advanced illness, even when patients can eat. While cachexia is often described in the context of advanced cancer, it can also be present in other diseases, such as AIDS, chronic obstructive lung disease (COPD), or heart failure (Vigano, Del Fabbro, Bruera & Borod, 2012; Wagner, 2008). Lack of appetite, decreased desire for food and fluids, and weight loss can be caused by either the inability to process the food, as is frequent in advanced cancer, or the inability to swallow or digest food due to obstructions, digestive problems, or decreased alertness and cognitive decline. Furthermore, in cancer the body may become catabolic, resulting in a metabolic consumption of its own muscle tissue and fat, rather than utilizing nutrients in food to become anabolic and build up the body. This becomes more common as cancer progresses. Thus, even patients who make efforts to eat, despite their lack of an appetite, can continue to lose weight. Anorexia, in particular, generally raises great alarm in family caregivers, as it may appear to them that the patient is giving up or "starving to death." They may hold the belief that if the patient could eat more, he could become stronger and ultimately fight the disease or prolong his life. And they may request that medically assisted nutrition be administered.

If the patient is experiencing problems related to swallowing or digestion that can be bypassed, and it is believed the patient may benefit from nutrients, feeding tubes or parenteral nutrition can be considered. This can occur in patients with cancer who are unable to eat due to the disease or treatment-related complications but are not in the terminal phase of the disease. However, when anorexia and cachexia are considered an expected development of advanced disease and approaching death, physicians usually recommend against artificial nutrition. This is because of the risks of adding burden to the patient, without any significant benefits. To distressed family caregivers, however, a physician's recommendation against medically assisted nutrition may appear as lack of compassion or care.

In many cultures, the value of food is not only important for nourishment and physical strength but also for its symbolic meaning as an expression of love and care. Accordingly, palliative care and hospice clinicians address these issues frequently. Helping family members understand when anorexia and cachexia are part of the illness progression, and not an independent medical complication, may require several conversations. Furthermore, using the expression "natural part of the illness" may not necessarily resonate with family caregivers or reassure them.

The topic of hydration in patients who are close to death is similarly complex. Family caregivers may ask that the patient receive IV fluids, for fear the patient will "die of thirst." Furthermore, patients and family caregivers may also consider medically assisted hydration as associated with comfort, pain control, and increased quality of life, even when they understand it will not change the course of the disease (Cohen, Torres-Vigil, Burbach, de la Rosa & Bruera, 2012).

Two systematic reviews concluded that the available studies do not allow for any practice recommendations regarding medically assisted nutrition and hydration for adult palliative care patients (Good et al., 2014a; Good et al., 2014b). Thus, decisions about interventions should be the result of a collaborative approach between the patient, family caregivers, and medical providers. In some cases, medically assisted hydration is approached on a trial basis, to determine whether the patient is experiencing benefits.

Family caregivers who have difficulty accepting, cognitively and emotionally, that death as inevitable may, however, reject the team's explanations about the expected course of the illness. Therefore, it is necessary that these issues about changes in food and fluid intake be approached with great sensitivity and with enough time to allow family caregivers to make sense of the information and emotionally adjust to its meaning. Some family caregivers may appear singularly focused on nutrition and hydration as ways to express their devotion to the patient. Psychological support may include redirecting family caregivers toward expressing care for the patient in alternative, yet tangible, ways. Gently rubbing lotion on the patient's hands and feet, singing to the patient, and ensuring that her lips are kept moist can be calming and can help promote physical comfort. Most important, psychological support can help family caregivers identify practical care strategies that are not only soothing and unharmful to the patient, but also consistent with their cultural and spiritual values.

PSYCHOLOGICAL AND COGNITIVE CHANGES

Psychological changes can occur concurrently with physical changes or precede them in some patients. Family caregivers may report that while the patient's energy level has not significantly changed, he appears less engaged or less present emotionally. A psychologist who is providing therapy to a patient who is seriously ill may notice similar subtle changes, even before major physical changes become evident. For instance, addressing issues that had been considered important, such as family dynamics and old conflicts, may be now dismissed by the patient as no longer worthy of discussion. Or the patient may engage in a sort of psychological life review with a sense of urgency, by simply describing several relationships and events in rapid succession, with little input from the therapist. The patient may express relief and a sense of completion afterward and may not want to revisit the topic again. The patient may also appear preoccupied or distractible and may have difficulty engaging.

These cognitive and emotional changes can occur progressively over weeks, but they can also become evident within days. In the presence of mood changes and fluctuation of consciousness and confusion, it is necessary to evaluate the patient for depression and delirium. For some patients, a progressive emotional detachment and withdrawal can be an expected part of the decline and dying process, even if it occurs weeks prior to death.

To illustrate, a lack of strong emotions, sometimes a sense of numbness that is not distressing, may occur. A patient with advanced cancer described these emotional shifts about two months before his death. He started feeling like a spectator or an observer and enjoyed spending time in quiet contemplation. While he felt sad about dying, he was not depressed or distressed. His approach was in stark contrast with his spouse and his three daughters, who felt the need to talk and openly grieve with him. The patient commented that while he was very sad about dying and leaving his family, he did not find comfort in expressing this sadness openly and asked them to allow him space. His spouse and daughters felt emotionally abandoned and began fluctuating between resenting him and subsequently feeling guilty.

Family therapy helped the patient and his family caregivers understand the changes associated with advanced illness and the dying process. It helped them reframe the meaning of these changes in ways that preserved love and connection in the family. While most of the sessions also included the patient, some were focused on providing his wife and daughters with a safe space to express and process their grief. Additionally, the entire family participated in identifying ways of expressing grief and receiving support that would not create distress for the patient. For instance, the patient suggested that his wife and daughters could express their emotions in writing in the form of emails. This way, the patient could pace himself reading about their experience and would not be overwhelmed. After reading each email, he would then reconnect with his family and express his love by hugging and holding his wife and daughters, a healing experience for all. Most important, this and other helpful strategies emerged organically from the therapy session and were the result of the family's effort to find creative ways to express love while also respecting boundaries.

The Medical Context of the Dying Process

A comprehensive discussion of the medical aspects of advanced illness and dying is beyond the scope of this book or the scope of practice of a palliative psychologist. This section highlights aspects that are especially relevant to the psychological care plan for the patient at the end of life and the family. The recognition of the constant interplay of medical and psychological factors in end of life allows for more effective and compassionate care (Table 7.2).

Chronic progressive diseases are associated with patterns of functional decline that ultimately lead to the patient's death. Four patterns, also known as illness trajectories, have been described, each with different physical, social, and psychological implications (Lunney et al., 2003; Murray et al., 2005). The first trajectory is sudden death, which can occur as a result from complications in any disease. The second trajectory, common in cancer, is characterized by a steady progression and preservation of function, followed by a rapid decline in the advanced and terminal stages. To illustrate, a patient with advanced cancer may experience functional decline that starts months before his or her death, with increased severity in the last weeks and days of life.

The third trajectory, common in respiratory disease and heart failure, is marked by a gradual decline with several episodes of acute exacerbations leading to hospitalization. After each episode, the patient may not recover to the previous level of function. In these

Table 7.2 **Interplay of Medical and Psychological Factors in the Dying Process**

Patient experiences a progressive decline into active dying	Patient experiences an acute complication, expected or unexpected, which significantly alters prognosis
Decline over weeks or months	The patient may die suddenly
Risk of it not being appreciated by treating team	Potential trauma for the family even if death was expected
Tendency to overestimate prognosis	Psychological timeline followed by family does not always match that of the medical team
Consideration of performance status	Consideration of performance status
Can offer the opportunity to optimize medical treatment plan	Can trigger guilt in family members if they were not present
Psychological support to the patient and/or the family can be provided over a longer period of time.	Difficult process of meaning-making of abrupt change
Offers the opportunity for a longer relationship with the team	May trigger sense of anger at medical team for decisions made (e.g., agreeing to increase pain medication for the patient is followed by an unrelated sudden event, and the family makes the connection between the two events)
Can offer the patient and the family the opportunity to accomplish goals and take full advantage of services offered by palliative care health care systems, such as hospice	Visually traumatic (e.g., in the case of hemorrhage)
Can translate into a prolonged death and additional caregiver distress	Family may need support with many practical tasks
When patient suffers from a disease that interferes with emotional connection, such as dementia, there may be additional distress for family caregivers	Disappointment if patient was about to enroll in hospice after extensive discussion and then dies before enrollment
Bereavement	Bereavement

patients, death generally occurs during one of the exacerbations. Therefore, while death may have been expected at some later time in the future, it may be perceived by family caregivers as sudden. The fourth trajectory is typical of patients with Alzheimer's and is characterized by a slow and progressive decline from an already low level of functioning.

An understanding of illness trajectory can provide the patient and family caregivers with broad answers to sensitive questions (e.g., How much time do I have left? What will dying look like? What can I expect?). It is also important to remember that acute complications that are not part of the illness (e.g., hemorrhage, stroke, embolism, or sepsis) can occur, altering the expected trajectory and causing a rapid decline into the active dying phase.

Acute complications that significantly change prognosis have the potential of causing severe emotional distress when the patient and the family expected to have more time. Family caregivers may subsequently also feel that death was sudden, even if the patient had been ill for some time and death was somewhat expected. Palliative psychologists can provide important feedback to other clinicians about the family's expectations about prognosis. Additionally, when there is an acute complication or rapid decline, they can represent an important resource for the patient and the family experiencing a psychological emergency.

THE PSYCHOLOGICAL IMPACT OF PROGNOSTICATION

Prognostication is an area of medicine often discussed using technical medical language, but it has tremendous psychological impact on the patient and the family. While it involves a certain degree of inaccuracy, it provides a time framework that allows the patient and the family to make decisions about end-of-life-care and to plan accordingly. The formulation of a prognosis can also allow medical providers to determine the appropriateness of medical treatment and to coordinate care. This can include stopping medications that may be no longer indicated in the context of the patient's life expectancy (Kutner et al., 2015).

It is well recognized that prognostication is challenging for the medical professional and that clinicians tend to overestimate survival (Lamont, 2003). Clinicians may want to remain optimistic and hopeful when they communicate with family members and only focus on the best-case scenario of the patient's survival. This is particularly likely when family caregivers appear distressed and unable to tolerate accurate prognostic information. Paradoxically, there is indication that physicians who are less emotionally involved with the patient and have less patient contact may provide more accurate prognoses (Christakis & Lamont, 2000).

Medical professionals use several approaches to formulate prognosis, including performance status scales, prognostic scores and models, the patient's symptoms, and quality of life. Nonetheless, it has been estimated that about 5% of hospice patients and 10% of patients in the palliative care setting have unexpected deaths, meaning that they die sooner than anticipated by the medical team (Hui, 2015). Family caregivers planning their presence based on the prognostic information received from the medical team may feel deprived of the opportunity to be with the patient during the final moments of life. Even family caregivers who had prepared emotionally and practically for the death may perceive it as a surprise and a shock when it occurs sooner than anticipated. Several strategies have been suggested for medical providers to minimize these occurrences and their negative impact (Hui, 2015):

- maximizing prognostication accuracy by using validated models and performance scales

- optimizing communication with patients and the family by not being overly optimistic about prognosis and describing both the best and the worst case scenario, encouraging the family to prepare for both
- minimizing iatrogenic causes of unexpected death by limiting medical interventions at the end of life that can cause significant burden with questionable benefits
- providing psychosocial care for family caregivers by ensuring adequate bereavement care, especially after an unexpected death

Studies of patients with cancer have suggested the presence of signs that can provide an indication that death is imminent (generally within three days). These include a decreased response to visual and verbal stimuli, an inability to close eyelids, drooping of the nasolabial fold, Cheyne-Stokes breathing, decreased urine output, and noisy breathing due to secretions (Hui et al., 2014; Hui et al., 2015).

Appropriate communication about prognostic disclosure is the result of an understanding of cultural, emotional, and religious factors related to patients and family preference (see also Chapter 6). However, identification of signs of decline may allow the family to complete important planning. Family members who feel they were not aware of how rapidly the decline of their loved one could continue and how soon death could occur often report this as a source of distress during bereavement, with distressing feelings of guilt, regret, and missed opportunities.

Exploring how patients and families understand signs of decline can help assess prognostic awareness and their meaning-making process regarding these changes. Providing gentle but ongoing psychoeducation about the physical and psychological changes common in advanced illness should be an important goal for palliative care clinicians. Additionally, a discrepancy between the family and the medical team's perceptions about prognosis should be promptly addressed because it is a likely cause of confusion and distress.

Because prognostication is based on the medical evaluation of the patient, this information should be discussed by medical providers with the patient and the family. Palliative psychologists can play an essential role assisting the family in adjusting to the information they have received. If the patient and family ask the psychologist for information about estimated survival, it is important to act promptly to arrange for this topic to be discussed with a member of the medical team, either in the hospital, or at home if the patient is receiving hospice care. In the hospital setting it could mean telling the family that their questions will be shared immediately with the doctor who will meet with them to answer questions and address concerns. Psychologists who are making a home visit as hospice clinicians can promptly leave a phone message for the patient's nurse relating the family's questions. Making this phone call during the visit will convey to the family that the clinician appreciates the importance of having questions addressed as soon as possible.

If a patient or a family is distressed after receiving news that death is close, it is important to quickly put in place a psychological plan for support. This may include psychoeducation, cognitive and relaxation strategies and clinical hypnosis interventions to decrease the sense of being overwhelmed and to relieve severe anxiety. Subsequent interventions, including psychotherapy, can help the patient and the family develop and consolidate self-management strategies and process grief in a safe, therapeutic space.

The psychological plan should be broad and flexible enough to allow for the rapid evolution of the clinical scenario. The plan should include bereavement care and consideration of risk factors for complications of bereavement, including complicated grief and depression (Burton, Haley & Small, 2006; Lobb et al., 2010; Keyes et al., 2014).

While dying often involves a process of variable length, the final moments of the patient's life will often have a profound impact on family caregivers' quality of life and bereavement. Witnessing physical, psychological, or spiritual distress in a loved one has a direct impact on caregivers' well-being. Caregivers who perceive that their loved one died in pain often report traumatic memories. They may report having felt fearful and helpless witnessing uncontrolled symptoms. Additionally, family caregivers of patients with delirum report high levels of distress. In essence, optimal management of physical and psychological symptoms will not only comfort the patient during the dying process, it can also represent an important protective factor in bereavement for surviving family caregivers (Monin & Schulz, 2009; Pace et al., 2009; Zelenikova et al., 2016).

Facilitating Transitions and Optimizing Communication

Ideally, ongoing and supportive communication between the patient, the family, and the medical team can facilitate decision making, minimize distress, and convey an overall sense of safety. However, challenging end-of-life care scenarios can occur, often caused by unexpected changes in the prognosis that allow the patient and the family little time to adjust. For instance, a patient who is hospitalized for management of acute needs (e.g., symptom exacerbation in advanced COPD) may expect to return home. The family may have mobilized energy and resources to allow for a safe home discharge. However, sudden complications may cause a rapid transition to end of life with the patient remaining in the hospital during the dying process. This and similar scenarios can cause great distress to the patient and family caregivers. A palliative care consultation may be requested at this time by the primary medical team caring for the patient to assist with symptom management and psychological support. Palliative psychologists can play an important role by helping the patient and family caregivers adjust to unexpected changes and focus on identifying new needs, hopes, and wishes that can be realistically met. If the palliative care consultation indicates that the patient is hospice eligible, and if this is acceptable to the patient and to the family, the main function of the palliative care team may be facilitating a smooth transition to hospice care, ensuring that relevant psychological, cultural, and spiritual factors are adequately communicated to the hospice team. However, if the patient and family have not interacted with the palliative care team previously, they may not feel comfortable accepting recommendations from them about transitions of care. For this reason, involving the primary team in these discussions is always recommended, as it can create a more comfortable decision-making process for the family.

Conflict and tension may also occur if the family feels pressured to make end-of-life decisions about their loved one without the opportunity to process the information provided to them (Radwany et al., 2009). Family members often struggle with decisions they have made for the patient and want to feel confident they made the right one. Many find it challenging to balance advocacy for the loved one with trust in the medical professionals' plan.

A good understanding of the family's preferred communication style, coping and grieving style, and emotional processing, including defense mechanisms against distress, can help clinicians develop a bond with the family. To illustrate, one family may be private in their ways of expressing grief and other emotions and may wish to receive only clear and open medical information from the team, refusing any kind of emotional support. Another family may feel deeply hurt by medical providers who convey medical information in a direct manner without balancing every medical fact with hopeful reassurance and support. Additionally, while one family member may appear more outspoken and in charge of communicating with medical providers, it should not be assumed they speak for the rest of the family. This is especially important in extended families, with siblings, in-laws, stepchildren, and others. Although it is always important to remember that there may be a clearly determined decision-maker in the family, the team provides support to every family member, and consensus building should be supported to avoid conflict. Psychological and social factors that may further hinder communication should also be addressed. These include each individual's history of traumatic and unprocessed loss or presence of mental illness in the patient or in a family member.

As the patient approaches end of life, communication with family caregivers should clarify their expectations including specific aspects of care. For example, if a family caregiver requests to be kept informed about any changes in the patient's condition, the team should clarify what type of changes they would like to be notified about. The team should ask openly and clearly, to avoid or minimize misunderstandings or conflict. This applies to patients cared for in a hospital setting and also hospice.

CASE VIGNETTE 7.1

Belinda was a 79-year-old African American woman with end-stage COPD and moderate cognitive decline, admitted to an inpatient palliative care and hospice unit. Her 50-year-old daughter was the primary caregiver. At the time of admission, she communicated to the attending physician that she should be notified of any changes in her mother's condition. The team agreed, and the daughter, who lived about 30 minutes from the hospital, was also to receive regular updates about changes in medication to address pain and dyspnea. Her mother had been able to use the restroom with assistance, and possible changes in that ability were never discussed. About two weeks after admission the patient developed a fever and increased shortness of breath and became unable to get out of bed to use the restroom. The nurse started using diapers for the patient. She did not believe the daughter should be notified of this change in the mother's condition and did not call to notify her. When the daughter arrived at the hospital and saw the mother in diapers she became angry with the staff. She stated she should have been notified about the decision to start using diapers for a woman who had been fairly independent up to that point. She angrily explained that as a caregiver she was also in charge of protecting her mother's dignity and that being in diapers, while perhaps necessary, was a significant transition. As the primary caregiver, the daughter felt she should have been notified ahead of time so she could adjust to the change or discuss options. The daughter was still trying to process her anger about the diapers when the mother had a sudden decline and died the following day. At the time of death the daughter was participating in a meeting with her mother's doctor to discuss her dissatisfaction with the team's handling of the situation. This situation and series of events greatly impacted on the daughter's grieving process, as it became focused on anger and regret. The anger was directed at the team for what she felt was a failure to respect her request. However, she also regretted that she not been able to be present during her mother's last hours because she had been focused on letting the team know how upset she was. The team, on the other hand, became defensive and attributed the daughter's behavior to maladaptive personality and labeled her as "entitled" and "borderline." In an attempt to avoid being the recipient of the daughter's anger, many clinicians on the team kept their distance after the patient's death. They thought the daughter needed privacy and that interacting with the team would only worsen the situation. The daughter, on the other hand, perceived this behavior as further evidence of abandonment and lack of caring, and complained that the team had not been there for her after her mother's death.

This case highlights the importance of communication and ongoing assessment of the patient and caregiver preferences without making assumptions about the impact of changes in the patient's condition. As patents approach the end of life, family caregivers may feel more distressed and their grieving may become more intense. Some may be reluctant to express their emotions due to cultural factors or personality style, fearing that expressions of their own distress will be interpreted as complaining about caregiving. It is important to continue assessing needs because as the patient's condition may rapidly change, so may the psychological state of the caregiver. Each change represents an additional loss, carrying the symbolic meaning of approaching death. Preferences about communication should be fully explored—what should be communicated to the family caregiver, when it should be communicated, and how it should be done. Expectations should be clarified, and the team should determine whether the requests are feasible. If they do not appear feasible given the staff time constraints (e.g., "I would like to receive a phone call after every meal and review what my mother ate, and how much"), the team should discuss alternative options that can still reassure the caregiver. The agreed-upon plan should be documented for reference by all staff.

It is important to be aware of the psychological and symbolic impact of changes in the patient's medical condition and level of functioning, however small they may appear to nursing or medical staff. In the case above, the patient's nurse thought that maintaining comfort by controlling pain and symptoms was the most important aspect of care and would promptly inform the daughter after every increase in pain medication. When using the commode became too burdensome for the patient, she thought that using diapers was a natural and noninvasive way of allowing the patient to be comfortable while preserving her dignity. However, she did not consider the symbolic impact of the change on the patient's primary caregiver. To the daughter, the change from complete independence to being in diapers represented an abrupt and shocking indication that her mother was indeed deteriorating. It also presented an image of her mother as completely vulnerable and dependent (like a child) for which she felt unprepared.

Most important, it must be considered that every aspect of care can directly impact on the caregiver's bereavement. Traumatic images or experiences may significantly affect the grieving process by increasing the risk for complications of bereavement. Despite all best efforts, however, negative interactions with families and complaints may occur, raising clinicians' risk for distress, guilt, and burnout. In these circumstances, the role of leadership and team support are critically important to help frame challenges as opportunities for improving care and to avoid placing blame or becoming defensive.

CASE VIGNETTE 7.2

Emily was a 53-year-old Chinese woman with breast cancer that was metastatic to her bones and her brain, admitted to the hospital for pain and delirium. Over the past two weeks her gait had become unsteady and her vision blurred; she had become bedbound with recurring episodes of agitation.

The patient was transferred from a different hospital by her younger sister, who was also her primary caregiver and health-care proxy agent. The reason for the transfer was the sister's belief that Emily was being overmedicated, and the hospital staff was trying to hasten her death. Given the history with the previous hospital, a meeting with the attending oncologist and the palliative care service was arranged. The patient was drowsy after receiving medication for pain and a neuroleptic for agitation, so she did not participate, leaving instructions that her sister could make all necessary decisions. The patient's sister spoke English, but some team members had the impression that there were gaps in her ability to understand. They suggested the presence of an interpreter, but the sister adamantly refused, saying she felt insulted that they did not think her English was good enough. During the family meeting the team discussed that the patient's prognosis was short and that the delirium and agitation were a result of the worsening of disease and the presence of brain metastases. They explained that using enough medication to control the pain and agitation was not intended to hasten her life but to control symptoms and prevent her from suffering. The impact the medication may have on the patient's ability to interact and be alert was not described in detail, as the emphasis was placed on the importance of preventing her from suffering. The patient's sister asked few questions during the meeting. At the end, the team summarized the meeting and emphasized that they would continue to actively manage the patient's symptoms. The sister agreed. After the meeting, some team members commented they were pleased that the meeting had such a positive outcome. The following evening the sister asked to speak urgently with the physician in charge of the treatment plan. She explained that the patient had been sleeping for over 10 hours, and she had not been able to have a conversation with her. She expressed concern that she was being overmedicated. The physician attempted to reassure her, explaining that they were only using enough medication to keep the patient comfortable as was discussed at the meeting and as the sister had agreed. The sister became angry and stated she never agreed to keep Emily sedated for hours without being able to speak with her. The physician continued to explain that since the prognosis was so poor it could be expected that the patient would continue to be increasingly sleepy, and that was probably more a result of the disease than the medication. The sister repeated that she had never agreed to a plan to keep her sister sedated, and she expected to be able to interact with her. She frantically explained that she had been put in charge of caring for her sister here in the United States and that her family trusted her with this task. She now felt she had been set up to fail by the physician who had tricked her into agreeing to a plan that was different from what she expected. She felt she had brought shame to the family and failed her sister.

In debriefing this challenging case after the patient's death, the team reflected on the importance of clarifying family caregivers' understanding and expectations about prognosis and about the goals and expected outcomes of medical care at the end of life. Additionally, it is important to clarify the meaning of commonly used but somehow vague expressions (e.g., keeping the patient comfortable). Discrepancies between the team and family caregivers' understanding can result in confusion and distress.

When Death Is Imminent

The presence of multiple irreversible physical changes occurring at the same time generally indicates that the death can occur in hours or in a few days. Educating the family about the approaching dying process is often a process that requires clinicians to carefully balance the necessity to deliver medical information clearly, while understanding the family culture and recognition of their unique emotional needs. Even though the patient may have been steadily deteriorating and even been bedbound for days, it should be considered that the family may have significant difficulties hearing and fully integrating information about the patient's approaching death.

Studies have indicated that in the hospital setting, family caregivers value consistency of nursing presence, a calm and relaxing hospital room that allows for connection and shared experience, and receiving adequate information and guidance during the dying process (Cronin, Arnstein & Flanagan, 2015). Similarly, when family caregivers do not feel prepared for the death (e.g., they are not aware of the meaning of changes in the patient's condition) they report less satisfaction and may be at increased risk for a complicated bereavement process. The last place where the patient received care impacts on how caregivers' needs are met, with hospice care being associated with fewer unmet needs.(Gallagher & Krawczyk, 2013).

Family members' responses to imminent death will depend on many factors, including how much time they had to prepare emotionally, their history of prior losses and how they handled those losses, and the type of relationship they have with the patient (i.e., loving and supportive versus conflictual with a high level of ambivalence). During the dying process, the focus of the clinical team is to provide information, reassurance, and comfort to the family while controlling physical and cognitive symptoms in the dying patient (Smith-Stoner, 2011).

CASE VIGNETTE 7.3

Nancy was a 35-year-old woman with non-small-cell lung cancer metastatic to the brain. Nancy lived with her partner of two years, Anna. Her mother had not been supportive when Nancy came out as a lesbian, and this had been a source of conflict between them.

Despite this conflict, Nancy and her mother remained close, but they would often begin arguing after about 30 minutes together. At the hospital, Nancy became progressively weaker and periodically agitated. At every visit, her mother would express her love to her daughter, but she would also express negative comments about her relationship. Nancy found these comments distressing and was unsuccessful in asking her mother to stop. She did not feel she could be more assertive because her mother was in her late seventies and suffered from severe anxiety. Upon Nancy's request, members of the palliative care team met with her mother and discussed the importance of keeping the visits short and focused on positive communication. They explained that the spread of the cancer to the brain made Nancy's emotional condition particularly vulnerable and susceptible to stress. It was also suggested to Nancy that she could tell her mother she needed to rest if her mother made uncomfortable comments, and she could close her eyes to indicate her need for rest. In this way, Nancy's need to avoid a confrontation with her mother was honored, but her need to be protected from distress was also met.

Clarifying the goals of psychological support is especially important when death is close. Unless specifically stated as a wish by the caregivers or the patient, the dying process may not be the time for an in-depth resolution of an old family conflict. And even when the patient desires such a resolution, it may not be attainable. The role of the psychologist then becomes assisting the patient in identifying strategies that can represent an acceptable compromise, in the moment, in the service of emotional comfort (Strada, 2008). In these situations, the patient leads the way, while careful assessment and coordination are provided.

CASE VIGNETTE 7.4

Ramon was a 47-year-old Latino hospitalized with end-stage cirrhosis of the liver. He was completely bedbound, and his main complaints were pain and nausea. The primary team requested a palliative care consultation for help with management. Ramon lived with his partner and had been involved in his community until his health began to deteriorate. He was known for his cheerful personality, which he maintained at the hospital. He enjoyed reviewing his life and his travels, and he spontaneously initiated conversations about these memories and spoke about them at length with every clinician who would spend time with him. Ramon also valued open and direct communication about his condition. After a conversation with his doctor he became aware of his poor prognosis, in the order of a few weeks. He was told that death would not be painful, which reassured him. Hospice care at home was suggested as an option, but his partner did not feel he could provide the patient with the level of care he needed. Most important, the partner had read that patients with cirrhosis can hemorrhage when they die, and he was concerned this could happen at home and thus felt it would be too traumatic for him. The patient's mother and brother were also involved in his care and visited daily but stated repeatedly that the patient would not die and were convinced he would improve because he was always in such good spirits. The relationship between the partner and the family was strained, though they did not exhibit overt conflict. The brother was upset that he was not chosen as the health-care proxy agent and felt the patient's partner was unreliable and unwilling to make real sacrifices for the patient. The patient appeared somewhat oblivious to this underlying conflict and stated clearly that negative feelings and negative words were not allowed in his room. He explained to the psychologist that he had chosen to focus his attention on the positive memories of his life and felt that by describing them over and over he was keeping them alive and real. He admitted that concerns and worries sometimes "crept up" but he was able to "push them down." The psychologist and the patient discussed whether acknowledging those concerns could be beneficial and the pros and cons were carefully considered. The patient was concerned that discussing those concerns could cause some emotional distress. The psychologist validated his concerns and commented that acknowledging that concerns did exist may generate both discomfort and relief, and it was agreed this would be approached slowly. The clinician also taught the patient two hypnosis exercises involving interactive guided imagery for decreasing the negative impact of the concerns. In one exercise, the patient developed an image that represented his concerns. He imagined a red ball, hot to the touch. He decided he needed to wear special heat-resistant gloves for handling it. In the exercise, he placed the ball into a thick wood box, locked it, and buried it deep into the cool earth. In the second exercise, he imagined having a cannon and shooting the ball far into space, so that it could be retrieved only with a spaceship. For the next two days, the patient resumed his positive life review and did not mention his concerns. He also continued to decline, feeling weaker and progressively sleepier. On the third day, he told the psychologist he needed her help to plan what he called "an important event." He mentioned he thought it was time to express his concerns before he died and wanted to gather all his relatives and a few close friends at the hospital. He also asked the psychologist to help him ensure that people would listen to him and not become distressed. During a preparatory meeting with the friends and family the psychologist expressed the patient's wishes. She framed the event as witnessing and honoring the patient. During the meeting with the family the patient told them he knew he was dying and he needed them to know, too. He stated that he did not want to die pretending he was getting better because that would make him feel alone. He asked his family to welcome his partner after his death if they could, and reassured them that despite some troubles in the relationship, he had been very happy with him.

This case indicates the importance of following the patient's lead and tailoring psychological interventions to their needs. This may involve embracing a perspective of unlimited time available for therapy. In the case, above, it was clear that it might not have been possible for the patient and the psychologist to explore his concerns before his death. However, both patient and therapist had a shared understanding that comfort and positivity were the main values the patient held, and should be preserved above all.

SUPPORTING THE PATIENT AND THE FAMILY DURING THE DYING PROCESS

Health-care professionals experienced in working with patients at the end of life may have become accustomed to the changes in appearance during the dying process and may describe these changes as a natural component of dying. However, family members who have not witnessed death previously may consider these changes frightening and distressing, and this may prevent them from maintaining an emotional connection with the patient. They may think the patient is experiencing pain or distress. While explaining the nature of the changes and normalizing them for family members is important, it does not necessarily relieve grief and emotional distress. Though becoming overly detailed in the explanation or too didactic (or pointing out every change in the patient) would not be therapeutic, sensitivity to any signs of discomfort in family members related to the patient's physical appearance should prompt gentle exploration of emotions, clarification, and reassurance.

It is also possible that some family caregivers may refuse to consider that the patient is dying and become upset, anxious, and even agitated at any attempt to discuss prognosis. If the patient is receiving hospice services at home, it is important to assess family caregivers' ability to safely care for themselves and the patient—or whether the inability to psychologically integrate impending death is compromising their ability to make decisions, communicate with the medical team, and to support the patient. In the latter case, it may be necessary to provide more support at home or facilitate the patient's admission to an inpatient facility for safety.

Several physical and cognitive changes occur during the dying process (Crow, 2014). As blood circulation changes and slows, the patient's lower extremities become cold and may develop a purple color. The patient's food and fluid intake decreases and finally completely stops. Thus, patients at the end of life do not have bowel movements. While managing constipation is an important element of symptom management in advanced illness, it is not believed to be as important in the last days of life. Urine production also decreases until it completely stops. Changes in rate and patterns of breathing are also normal, and they often are an important indicator that death is close. Patients who are close to dying usually become progressively drowsy, to the point of being unresponsive. When patients are unresponsive or comatose, it is still important to ensure that they are not experiencing distress, in the form of pain or other symptoms. Clinicians usually rely on nonverbal signs to determine if the patient is in distress. In absence of grimacing, frowning, or agitated behavior, changes in breathing patterns or oxygen levels are not necessarily considered measures of distress. It should be explained that if the patient's face appears peaceful and relaxed, then he or she is not likely to be in pain or distress.

If the patient is experiencing shortness of breath, the medical team may administer corticosteroids, bronchodilators, or opioids in low doses. Neuroleptics are also used. Benzodiazepines may be used to relieve the anxiety associated with dyspnea. However, it is not uncommon for weak patients to have rapid or shallow breathing or to use shoulders and neck muscles to help their breathing. A medical evaluation can determine if the patient is in distress. Also, periodic cessation of breathing for short periods of several seconds, called "periodic" breathing or Cheyne-Stokes breathing, can be distressing for those at the bedside. Breathing can also become very noisy due to the accumulation of secretions in the throat or lungs and the patient's inability to cough, or swallow, due to general weakness. Sometimes referred to as a "death rattle," it can occur in many patients. While this symptom is believed not to cause distress to the patient who is unconscious, it can be addressed by non-pharmacological and pharmacological means. Non-pharmacological means include repositioning the patient and/or suctioning. However, if the secretions are not easy to reach because they are beneath the pharynx, deep suctioning is usually avoided because it can cause discomfort and pain to the patient. Medications with anticholinergic effects, such as scopolamine, atropine, and glycopyrolate are often utilized to reduce production of secretions. Respiratory symptoms are particularly stressful for family. After medical evaluation, the palliative psychologist may be helpful to family caregivers by providing reassurance and support.

Some family caregivers may find it beneficial to use simple breath-based meditation practices at the bedside. For instance, the caregiver may imagine that during the inbreath, she is receiving healing and soothing energy from a power source meaningful to her (e.g., the earth, the universe, or God, or a deceased family member). During the outbreath, she may be invited to imagine that this healing and soothing energy through the breath is sent to the patient, promoting comfort and ease during his transition. This practice and the evocative language used to describe it can be modified to incorporate images and beliefs meaningful to the family. It can help family caregivers channel their own anxiety about the dying process, which is sometimes augmented by holding vigil and waiting at the bedsite.

Patients very close to dying can lose control of sphincter muscles and may become incontinent. Patients who are still conscious may experience a sense of loss of dignity and control that can be distressing. Similarly, family members who are not aware that this is also part of the normal dying process may feel uncomfortable and embarrassed for the patient. Nursing interventions are critical to manage these symtpoms and promote comfort. Insertion of soft, flexible catheters are used in the most challenging cases to manage fecal incontinence (Kyle, 2011). It is also important to attend to patient's and family members emotional distress. While minimizing the emotional impact of the symptom may result in the patient feeling not understood and consequently more distressed, providing gentle reassurance and listening deeply to the patient and caregivers' concerns will help them feel heard and supported.

Appropriate psychological interventions at this stage should focus on promoting a peaceful and tranquil environment for the patient and the family. Psychological approaches based on verbal communication may become less relevant and feasible for the patient, while continuing to represent an important source of support for family members. Integrative medicine approaches, such as music therapy, guided imagery, and energy-based interventions such as Reiki and Healing Touch may become the primary modality for psychological support of the patient and may promote connectedness between the patient and the family.

During the days before death it is also be helpful to clarify the expectation of the family and other caregivers about who will be present at the moment of death. It should be noted to the family that a rapid change in the patient's condition may occur and not allow this type of planning to be implemented. However, some family members may fear that planning for the patient's death is an indication they are giving up on the possibility of a miracle, especially if there are spiritual or religious beliefs involved.

A discrepancy may develop between the clinicians' perception that the family is reasonably prepared for the patient's death and the family's actual psychological state. Psychologists working with the family can help recognize and identify these discrepancies and alert the team. Spiritual, sociocultural, and psychological factors affect the way family caregivers approach the period surrounding the dying process. For some, the process of holding vigil continues until the actual death of the patient. For this reason, they may take few breaks from the bedside, concerned that they may not be physically present at the moment of death. Not infrequently, however, family caregivers leave the bedside briefly, finding the patient has died during their short absence. When family members have attached a special meaning to being present at the time of death, it is important to explore this meaning and how they think not being physically present would affect them and the patient. It can valuable to explain that the exact moment of death cannot be predicted, and it is not uncommon for patients to die when there is no one present.

However, by exploring the importance of this process for the family, it is possible to develop a plan for minimizing distress. For example, the family caregiver can ensure that someone remains in the room with the patient during their absence. One spouse found it helpful to record a loving and reassuring message for her husband during his dying process. She would play the recorder when she could not be in the room and felt reassured that her husband felt her presence through her voice. Thus, while it is essential to support and validate family choices and needs, it is also valuable to provide information the can help with planning and decision-making.

Profuse bleeding or hemorrhage occasionally occurs near the time of death. It is a particularly frightening and distressing experience for the patient and the family. If the medical team determines there is a likelihood of bleeding, an interdisciplinary plan is usually put in place to minimize distress. Generally, family members are forewarned that bleeding may occur and the causes are explained. It is important to have several dark towels available to minimize the view of blood. If the patient is conscious and becomes anxious and distressed, even in the absence of pain, the medical team may decide to administer a benzodiazepine, such as midazolam, which also causes amnesia. The awareness that profuse bleeding may occur around or at the moment of death may affect family members' decisions about caring for the patient at home or in a different setting. The decision to die at home or in a facility is ideally made jointly by the patient and the family. However, family caregivers who are older, live alone, and are frail may not feel emotionally and/or physically able to handle what could be a potentially traumatic dying process.

If the patient is dying in the hospital and a family member is in distress, it may be necessary to find a quiet room or corner and provide support. It is necessary to be clinically and personally comfortable providing support to family member in any setting and circumstances. Psychologists accustomed to the private practice model may value the ability to speak in private as essential for family members. However, family caregivers often feel overwhelmed by their distress and may not even notice who is around them. Additionally, they may want to remain in the proximity of the patient's room. Finding a quiet corner on the hospital floor, even if it is just outside the room, may be more beneficial than trying to find a suitable place for a session.

Family members living in a different state or in a different country may not be able to make plans to visit the patient before the death. Or the patient's decline has been more rapid than expected and family members living far away are forced to make quick preparations for the visit only to arrive at the hospital or at the home to find out that the patient has died. This situation can be difficult for family members, especially for those who may have hoped to heal a previously difficult relationship with the patient. Depending on the circumstances, it may be desirable to facilitate an opportunity for them to spend time with the deceased and ask if they would prefer to be alone or would like the presence of a team member in their room with them.

Supporting family members during the patient's dying process always includes skillfully and unobtrusively monitoring their levels of grief and identifying any risk factors that should be addressed. At this stage, they may need even more intense help and support with processing grief while at the same time maintaining self-care and the ability to connect emotionally with the patient (Box 7.2). For example, when grief in family caregivers becomes unmanageable, they may exhibit life-threatening self-neglect, such as stopping important medication or refusing to eat or drink. This behavior is particularly concerning in older family members and in those with a prior history of psychiatric illness, including major depression, bipolar disorder, or psychotic disorder. Passive suicidal ideation in family members should never be discounted as a merely understandable expression of distress. An empathic but thorough suicidal assessment should be part of the ongoing monitoring and follow-up. This is especially important in the case of family caregivers who live alone and have comorbid medical illness—or have been the primary caregivers for the patient—and those without adequate social support.

Family caregivers' behavior and expression of grief during the dying process is based on their values, and well as cultural, spiritual, and psychological factors. For some, the environment surrounding the dying person should be as peaceful and quiet as possible, without overt manifestations of grief in the room, because it may cause distress for the patient. Accordingly, they may request that everyone around the patient, including health-care professionals, maintain a serene and peaceful attitude. Others may gather as a family, sit around the bed, and begin sharing uplifting and even humorous stories about the family, openly referring to the patient even if they are no longer conscious. There may be important moments of review of family life and even laughter.

For some, the moments following death becomes focused on quiet prayer and ritual, with little overt manifestation of grief. For others, grieving is openly manifested, including crying, calling out the name of the patient, and letting themselves fall on the floor or

---

Box 7.2 **Supporting Family Caregivers during the Dying Process**

- understand impact of physical place of death
- work with staff to ensure maximal comfort
- explore what is important to the patient and the family
- follow the caregiver's lead in providing support
- provide therapeutic and supportive presence
- contain anxiety, reassure, and promote connectedness
- empower family caregiver to express grief as feels appropriate to them
- educate team members about cultural differences in expression of grief
- reassure, normalize, explain
- support family members when distressing EOL symptoms occur (i.e. agitated terminal delirium)
- maintain awareness of countertransference to avoid burdening the family

on the bed. If the family caregivers are safe, it is important to respect grieving practices and behaviors. Emotional preparation for a loved one's death can be protective for the development of bereavement complications, but it should not be assumed that manifestations of grief will be attenuated.

Psychologists by training are focused on identifying ways of improving, modifying, problem solving, and addressing maladaptive thoughts and behaviors. While it may be tempting to use these approaches to address family members' distress during the patient's dying process, clinicians may quickly find that patients and families do not respond positively, as they may feel that the clinician is out of touch with the reality of the situation. The importance of providing psychological evidence-based interventions needs to be balanced by a focus on developing a strong therapeutic presence. When patients are very close to death, a psychologist's role is to identify what concrete actions can be taken to increase everyone's comfort but especially, to provide a respectful, reassuring, and comforting therapeutic presence in the hospital room or in the home.

Developing a compassionate presence that is focused on "being" rather than "doing" is an important combination of knowledge, skills, and attitudes. A therapeutic and compassionate presence at the bedside to assist patients and families during the dying process is an important element of the attitude and skills that clinicians should develop. The dying process is not something that can be fixed; family members' grief and distress cannot be avoided or prevented. The ability to bear witness and be human, without preconceived notions or judgments, can allow psychologists to provide a healing presence, truly honoring the patient's and the family's unique and irreplaceable story.

Delirium at End of Life

CASE VIGNETTE 7.5

Ellie was a 73-year-old African American woman with ovarian cancer metastatic to the kidneys. After a course of palliative radiation, she was discharged from the hospital and sent home. Palliative care and hospice service were not available in the rural area where she lived. The patient's daughter and granddaughter were the primary caregivers and were convinced the course of radiation had stopped the disease. Open conversations about prognosis, goals of care, and what the patient and the family could expect did not take place before discharge. After three weeks at home, Ellie began to complain of increasing pain and nausea. She was bedbound except for using the restroom. Her primary care physician prescribed large doses of NSAIDs but with minimal improvement. Ellie had no appetite, and would only sip a few tablespoons of hot milk. Her family caregivers focused on trying to convince her to eat, because they thought she needed to eat to become stronger; however, they felt increasingly unable to manage her care at home. The patient's daughter worked three jobs to support the family, and the granddaughter was in school most of the day. Ellie became increasingly confused one day, with restlessness and agitation. She called out in pain, crying that her back and abdomen were "on fire." She became unable to recognize her daughter and granddaughter and reacted to their verbal attempts to calm her by accusing them of wanting to kill her. Distressed, her daughter asked the primary care physician to make a home visit. He evaluated the patient and described the situation as "normal, under the circumstances, as she is dying." The family received the news as a shock and commented that no one had even mentioned that Ellie would not improve. The primary care physician recommended a transfer to the hospital, as management at home seemed no longer possible. Ellie was admitted to the hospital, with agitated delirium and complaining of pain. The medical team told the family that Ellie's kidneys had stopped working and that her agitation was a sign that she was dying. They also suggested that she should be sedated to be kept comfortable. Ellie's daughter, who was also the health-care proxy agent, asked if the patient could be started on dialysis and was adamant her mother was not dying, because no one had told her so during the prior hospitalization. The medical team requested a palliative care consultation to help with discussion of goals of care and assistance with what was described as "family's denial." When the palliative care physician, social worker, and psychologist met with the patient's family caregivers, it became clear that they had experienced significant distress, they lacked information about the patient's illness trajectory and life expectancy, and felt upset and frightened by Ellie's suffering with pain and delirium. The palliative physician told the team that the large dose of NSAIDs used to manage her advanced cancer pain had been not only ineffective but may also have contributed to the patient's delirium. The palliative care psychologist and social worker had several meetings with Ellie's family to help them process grief and distress. They deeply regretted focusing on encouraging Ellie to eat more, rather than creating positive memories together. They felt severe guilt for not being able to better advocate for adequate pain management, and also felt anger at the primary care physician for prescribing medication that was ineffective. They had felt helpless in attempting to manage Ellie's agitation and were relieved she was now sedated and not in distress. However, the realization that they would not be able to interact with her before she died caused great sadness.

Delirium is a neuropsychiatric disorder that requires immediate assessment and management.

Diagnosis. Based on the DSM-5 criteria, delirium is a disturbance of consciousness (i.e., a disturbance of awareness of the environment and level of arousal) with reduced ability to focus, sustain, or shift attention. It involves changes in cognition (such as memory deficit, disorientation, language disturbance, perceptual disturbance) that are not accounted for by a preexistent dementia. The onset of delirium is typically acute, evolves over a short period of time (usually hours to days), and tends to fluctuate during the course of the day. Additionally, evidence from the history, physical examination, or laboratory findings indicates the presence of a general medical condition that can trigger the condition. Subtypes of delirium can be described as *hyperactive/agitated, hypoactive/lethargic, or mixed* (American Psychiatric Association, 2013).

Hyperactive delirium is commonly characterized by restlessness, agitation, hallucinations, and delusions. As illustrated in the case vignette, hyperactive delirium is traumatic for the patient and the family, and it prevents nurturing and peaceful connection (Breitbart, Gibson, & Tremblay, 2002; DiMartini, Dew, Kormos, McCurry & Fontes, 2007). This is especially important when there is an expectation that the patient will have a peaceful death at home, without distress. Instead, family caregivers may subsequently experience intrusive thoughts and memories about the delirium episode. They may also feel resentment toward medical providers, blaming them for their loved one's distress. These traumatic symtpoms and negative emotions can severely impact the grieving process during bereavement.

Hypoactive delirium is characterized by psychomotor retardation, lethargy, and reduced awareness of surroundings. It is common in the palliative care and hospice setting, but it can be misdiagnosed as depression or severe fatigue. In distinguishing delirium from depression, clinicians must evaluate the onset and the temporal sequencing of depressive and cognitive symptoms. To illustrate, while disturbance in level of arousal and consciousness is present in delirium, it is not usually present in depression. Additionally, while patients with hypoactive delirium are often perceived to be in less distress, they are likely to experience perceptual disturbances that can become distressing (Breitbart & Alici, 2008, 2012).

While delirium is a common complication occurring in up to 85% of patients with advanced illness in the last weeks or days of life, it is often under-recognized or misdiagnosed (Close & Long, 2012). Because a diagnosis of delirium is frequently missed by the primary team referring a patient for a palliative care consultation, universal screening has been recommended (de la Cruz et al., 2015; Senel et al., 2017).

It is important to appreciate that delirium is associated with increased morbidity, distress, and mortality in patients, and distress in family caregivers and staff. Patients who are able to recall a delirium episode often describe it as distressing. Family caregivers report even higher levels of distress (Bruera et al., 2009). Family caregivers who witnessed delirium in a loved one report negative emotions (e.g., sadness, guilt, fear), anxiety, and hopelessness (Finucane, Lugton, Kennedy & Spiller, 2017).

Palliative psychologists can have an important role in the diagnosis and nonpharmacological management of delirium. They can identify prodromal symptoms, help differentiate between delirium, depression, and anxiety, and facilitate timely pharmacological and nonpharmacological treatment by communicating their diagnostic impressions to the medical team. Additionally, they can promote communication and collaboration between the family and medical providers. Supporting family caregivers is essential. Receiving psychoeducation about delirium and learning strategies for nonpharmacological management can help family caregivers experience a sense of control and less distress. As in the preceding case vignette, family caregivers also need help processing grief and guilt resulting from the abrupt change in the relationship caused by delirium. This is especially important when the patient dies without regaining the ability to connect meaningfully with family caregivers.

Etiology. There are several causes of delirium in advanced disease. In cancer, there are direct causes such as primary brain tumors and presence of metastases. There are also indirect causes of delirium, such as hypoxia and metabolic encephalopathy due to organ failure, or electrolyte imbalance. Among indirect causes of delirium are also side effects from chemotherapy agents, steroids, radiation, opioids, anticholinergic drugs, and antiemetics. Other indirect causes are infections, immunologic abnormalities, nutritional deficiencies, and paraneoplastic syndromes. The diagnostic workup in patients with a short life expectancy must be minimally invasive and minimally burdensome or distressing. In palliative care, the presence of delirium is often described as pre-terminal delirium, or terminal delirium. In pre-terminal delirium, the management is focused on preventing or reversing the etiology. Terminal delirium, on the other hand, is irreversible, and management is focused on controlling symptomatology and relieving suffering for the patient and family caregivers (Alici & Breitbart, 2009).

It is important to note that patients who are very close to death often report seeing and interacting with deceased family members and other loved ones, and even beloved pets. These experiences are generally described as deathbed visions, and are not uncommon in the palliative care and hospice setting in the last days or hours of life. Patients generally report that these experiences are meaningful, comforting, and relieve anxiety and fear of dying (Kerr et al., 2014). Deathbed visions can also inform provision of spiritual care at the end of life. Framing these experiences to the patient and family caregivers as perceptual disturbances in the context of hypoactive delirium would be not only insensitive, but also clinically contraindicated. Different clinicians can offer different explanations for these experiences (Chang et al., 2017), but they point to an element of mystery and sacredness in the dying process that is experienced by many and should never be trivialized. A clinician should, however, continue to gently monitor the patient's response to ensure that the images and visions continue being supportive and do not become frightening or threatening. Pharmacological treatment may be considered as an option to calm and comfort the patient.

Management of delirium. Nonpharmacological interventions to promote safety and comfort should always be considered. Whenever possible, family caregivers should become involved in the plan. Reassuring and reorienting can be achieved by maintaining visual and hearing aids, and creating an environment with familiar objects that is quiet and well lit. It is also important to avoid physical restraints and to minimize the use of immobilizing catheters and IV lines. Ensuring adequate pain control is essential.

When patients develop delirium at the end of life, as part of the dying process, management can be challenging. Presently, there are no FDA-approved medications for treatment of delirium. Low-dose haloperidol and selected atypical antipsychotics such as olanzapine have been described as effective in managing the symptoms of delirium (Breitbart & Alici, 2012). However, a placebo-controlled randomized control trial showed that distressing symtpoms of delirium, including perceptual disturbances and behavioral symptoms, were greater in patients treated with antipsychotics (Agar et al., 2016). In this study, midazolam was used to address severe distress and agitation. The authors of the study recommend an individualized approach to managing delirium, by screening patients for early detection, and providing supportive care.

The literature shows that 30% of dying patients with delirium do not have their symptoms adequately controlled by antipsychotic medications (Leonard et al., 2008). In these cases, the use of sedative agents may be necessary to minimize distress and suffering for the patient and family caregivers. Hyperactive agitated terminal delirium that requires the use of sedating agents often results in the dying patient's inability to communicate. Therefore, having missed the opportunity to re-establish their connection with the patient, family caregivers may perceive the death as abrupt and traumatic. Additionally, as the final words they have heard from their loved one may have been words of anger or agitation, careful reframing may be especially important. Psychologists can have an important role in helping caregivers adjust to what appears as an abrupt transition in their relationship with the loved one by providing immediate and long-term psychological support.

Understanding Palliative Sedation

Despite receiving quality and attentive medical care, advanced disease for some patients can be associated with suffering, which can be so severe as to be considered unbearable. Palliative sedation therapy is an approach currently widely accepted for refractory symptoms at the end of life. It consists of the administration of a sedative non-opioid drug to a patient who is at the end of life and suffering due to symptoms that are not responding to other types of medical management. The goal is to relieve the patient's suffering (Gurschick, Mayer & Hanson, 2014). Palliative sedation remains a sensitive topic, and it is important that palliative psychologists be aware of the relevant ethical principles and clinical implications (Schildman & Schildman, 2014).

Part of the controversy is related to confusion about the meaning of palliative sedation. It is also essential to carefully differentiate between palliative sedation, physician assisted dying (PAD; also called physician assisted suicide), and euthanasia, because they are substantially different from a practice, intent, and legal standpoint. Serious ethical and legal implications surround any action that can hasten death in the context of a terminal illness. A patient's wish to hasten death has been defined as a reaction to suffering, in the context of a life-threatening condition, from which the patient can see no way out other than to accelerate his or her death. This wish may be expressed spontaneously or after being asked about it, but it must be distinguished from the acceptance of impending death or from a wish to die naturally, although preferably soon. The wish to hasten death may arise in response to one or more factors, including physical symptoms (either present or foreseen), psychological distress (e.g., depression, hopelessness, fear, etc.), existential suffering (e.g., loss of meaning in life), or social aspects (e.g., feeling that one is a burden) (Balaguer et al., 2016).

Euthanasia involves the "administration of a lethal agent by another person to a patient for the purpose of relieving the patient's intolerable and incurable suffering" (AMA, 2003). In euthanasia it is a third party, generally the physician, who directly administers the lethal dose of medication. The intent is to cause the patient's death, and this is reflected in the lethal dose of medication administered. Euthanasia is illegal in the United States. It is currently legal in the Netherlands, Belgium, and Luxembourg.

In PAD, the physician's intent is to facilitate the death of the terminally ill patient by providing the patient with necessary means (i.e., a prescription for a *lethal dose of medication*) so that the patient will be able to perform the life-ending act. The agent in PAD is the terminally ill patient, and the intent is to cause death. PAD in only legal in California, Oregon, Washington, Vermont Colorado, and Washington. In Montana PAD has not been legalized, but according to a Supreme Court ruling it is not considered criminal if the physician was following a competent patient's request.

On the contrary, in palliative sedation the intent is to relieve unbearable suffering, not to cause the death of the patient. This is reflected in the dose of medication, which is *titrated to effect and adjusted accordingly based on the desired outcome, of symptom relief*. Indeed, palliative sedation is administered following three important principles (McCrate Protus, Kimbrel & Grauer, 2015). These are

- *Intent.* The intent of palliative sedation is to relieve symptoms that have been refractory to any other treatment attempt.

- *Proportionality.* The dose of medication administered to the patient is based on the necessary amount to relieve symptoms.
- *Criterion for success.* The criterion for success in palliative sedation is relief from symptoms that are causing suffering. The death of the patient is not a criterion for success.

The most common refractory symptoms addressed with palliative sedation are

- terminal delirium
- pain
- bleeding
- hiccups
- myoclonus
- nausea and vomiting.

It is important to emphasize that palliative sedation is a last resort for symptoms that are refractory to available treatments, when there are no further treatments available, when available treatments would not be tolerated by the patient, or when the treatments are not likely to be effective in quickly relieving the patient's suffering (Box 7.3). The use of palliative sedation therapy for terminal patients with unbearable existential and psychological suffering is, however, considered highly controversial. A study conducted in Belgium, the Netherlands, and the United Kingdom indicated that physicians who used continuous palliative sedation for psychological and existential distress had tried several pharmacological and psychological interventions that were either inappropriate or ineffective (Anquinet et al., 2014).

Benzodiazepines and barbiturates are the classes of pharmacological agents used for palliative sedation. Midazolam is often chosen due to its short half-life, its efficacy, and its ease of administration. Drug combinations are also used, depending on the experience and practice in a particular setting. When opioids are used, it is for their analgesic effect and not for sedation purposes.

It is important to consider the impact of palliative sedation on family caregivers. An observational questionnaire study compared levels of well-being reported by caregivers of 151 patients who had received palliative sedation and 90 patients who had not been

---

Box 7.3 **Characteristics of Refractory Symptoms**

- All the known and available treatments have been used and have been ineffective in controlling the symptoms (e.g., pain).
- The medical team is convinced that there are no further treatments that could provide relief.
- Potential treatments are not tolerated or expected to be tolerated by the patient.
- Potentially beneficial treatments are not expected to bring relief within an acceptable time frame.

sedated. Also considered was caregiver assessment of the patient's quality of life in the weeks before their death and the quality of their death (Bruinsma et al., 2016). Results revealed no difference in caregiver assessment and reports about their own quality of life and well-being after the death, suggesting that experiencing palliative sedation of a loved one did not have a negative impact on caregiver bereavement.

One of the early definitions describes palliative sedation as the "action of deliberately inducing and maintaining deep sleep, but not deliberately causing death, for the relief of one or more intractable symptoms, (often called refractory symptoms) when all other possible interventions have failed, and the patient is perceived to be terminally ill" (Cherny & Portenoy, 1994). This definition identifies the goal or intent of palliative sedation as inducing and maintaining deep sleep, addressing refractory symptoms, and consideration of the medical context, which is a patient being perceived as terminally ill. Palliative sedation is legal across the United States.

More recently, palliative sedation has been referred to as palliative sedation therapy (PST) and described as the "use of specific sedative medications to relieve intolerable suffering from refractory symptoms by a reduction in patient consciousness by using appropriate drugs carefully titrated to the cessation of symptoms" (De Graeff & Dean, 2007). Here, the key element remains the presence of refractory symptoms that cause intolerable suffering to a patient *who is very close to death*. A more recent definition by the American Academy of Hospice and Palliative Medicine describes palliative sedation as "the intentional lowering of awareness towards, and including, unconsciousness for patients with severe and refractory symptoms . . . after careful interdisciplinary evaluation and treatment of the patient when palliative treatments that are not intended to affect consciousness have failed or, in the judgment of the clinician, are very likely to fail; where its use is not expected to shorten the patient's time to death and only for the actual or expected duration of symptoms" (AAHPM, 2014).

This definition introduces the need for interdisciplinary evaluation as a new critical element. Here, the decision to consider and implement palliative sedation in the context of intractable suffering no longer rests exclusively with the medical professional but is the result of interdisciplinary collaboration and discussion. In this expanded view, the input of palliative psychologists and psychosocial clinicians about their evaluation of the patient and the family can add an important dimension to the discussion.

Palliative sedation does not indicate a fixed modality but is based on the patient's clinical needs. It can be administered as a respite from intractable pain and other symptoms, in which case it can be brief (24–48 hours) or intermittent, generally followed by reversal of sedation to evaluate symptoms. Or it can be administered as continuous sedation that continues until the patient's death. Thus, the level of sedation can range from superficial to deep sedation where the patient in unconscious and unable to communicate.

In the palliative care setting, the decision to administer palliative sedation is the result of extensive considerations of alternatives and discussions within the palliative care team, with patients able to participate and express their preferences, and with family caregivers. Palliative sedation may be considered when the patient or their healthcare proxy agents or surrogate decision makers have provided informed consent. Ethics committees generally review every case prior to initiation of palliative sedation and may be consulted in the course of the case. It is essential that family members be given detailed information about the process and that clinicians take the time to ensure effective communication has occurred.

Even with careful planning and preparation, the dying process retains elements of unpredictability that cannot be controlled. Most family members who have been preparing for the patient's death hope for a peaceful process, with little or no distress. This is especially true if they have had traumatic experiences caring for other family members in the past. When the circumstances do not allow for emotional and practical preparation, there may be guilt and distress. This is also true when even careful planning does not translate into the peaceful death families may have hoped for. For all of these reasons, it is important to ensure the highest level of physical, psychological, and spiritual support for the patient and the family through collaborative efforts. To use an expression commonly used in hospice, clinicians have one chance to get it right, and need to get it right the first time (Sykes, 2015).

References

Agar, M. R., Lawlor, P. G., Quinn, S., Draper, B., Caplan, G., Rowett, D., . . . & Curroe, D. C. (2017). Efficacy of oral risperidone, haloperidol, or placebo for symtpoms of delirium among patients in pallaitive care: A randomized controlled trial. *JAMA Internal Medicine, 177*(1), 34–42.

Alici, Y., & Breitbart, W. (2009). Delirium in palliative care. *Primary Psychiatry, 16*(5), 42–48.

American Academy of Hospice and Palliative Medicine. (2014). Statement on Palliative Sedation. http://aahpm.org/positions/palliative-sedation. Retrieved on August 20, 2017.

American Medical Association. (2003). Glossary: End-of-life care: Do not harm. *AMA Journal of Medical Ethics. Vurtual Mentor, 5*(1). http://journalofethics.ama-assn.org.

American Psychiatric Association. (2013). *Diagnostic and statistical manual of mental disorders,* DSM-5, Fifth edition. Washington, DC: Author.

Anquinet, L., Rietjens, J., van der Heide, A., Bruinsma, S., Janssens, R., Deliens, L., . . . & Seymour, J. (2014). Physician's experience and perspectives regarding the use of continuous sedation until death for cancer patients in the context of psychological and existential suffering at the end of life. *Psychooncology, 23*(5), 539–546.

Balaguer, A., Monforte-Royo, C., Porta-Sales, J., Alonso-Barbarro, A., Altisent, R., Aradilla-Herrero, A., . . . & Voltz, R. (2016). An international consensus definition of the wish to hasten death and its related factors. *PLoS One, 11*(1). http://doi.org/10.1371/journal.pone.0146184

Breitbart, W., & Alici, Y. (2008). Agitation and delirium at the end of life: "We couldn't manage him." *JAMA, 300,* 2898–2910.

Breitbart, W., & Alici, Y. (2012). Evidence-based treatment of delirium in patients with cancer. *Journal of Clinical Oncology, 30*(11), 1206–1214.

Breitbart, W., Gibson, C., & Tremblay, A. (2002). The delirium experience: Delirium recall and delirium-related distress in hospitalized patients with cancer, their spouses/caregivers, and their nurses. *Psychosomatics, 43*(3), 183–194.

Bruera, E., Bush, S. H., Willey, J., Paraskevopoulos, T., Li, Z., Palmer, J. L., . . . Elsayem, A. (2009). Impact of delirium and recall on the level of distress in patients with advanced cancer and their family caregivers. *Cancer, 115*(9), 2004–2012.

Buinsma, S. M., van der Heide, A., van der Lee, M. L., Vergouwe, Y., & Rietjens, J. A. (2016). No negative impact of palliative sedation on relative's experience of the dying phase and their wellbeing after the patient's death: An observational study. *PLoS ONE, 11*(2). doi: 10.1371/journal.pone.0149250.

Burton, A. M., Haley, W. E., & Small, B. J. (2006). Bereavement after caregiving or unexpected death: Effects on elderly spouses. *Aging and Mental Health, 10*(3), 319–326.

Chang, S. O., Ahn, S. Y., Cho, M. O., Choi, K. S., Kong, E. S., Kim, C. G., . . . Kim, N. C. (2017). Identifying perceptions of health professionals regarding deathbed visions and spiritual care in end-of-life care: a Delphi consensus study. *Journal of Hospice and Palliative Nursing, 19*(2), 177–184.

Cherny, N. I., & Portenoy, R. K. (1994). Sedation in the management of refractory symptoms: Guidelines for evaluation and treatment. *Journal of Palliative Care, 10*(2), 31–38.

Christakis, N. A., & Lamont, E. B. (2000). Extent and determinants of error in doctors' prognoses in terminally ill patients: Prospective cohort study. *British Medical Journal, 320*, 469–472.

Close, J. F., & Long, C. O. (2012). Delirium: Opportunity for comfort in palliative care. *Journal of Hospice and Palliative Nursing, 14*(6), 386–394.

Cohen, M. Z., Torres-Vigil, I., Burbach, B. E., de la Rosa, A., & Bruera, E. (2012). The meaning of parenteral hydration to family caregivers and patients with advanced cnacer receiving hospice care. *Journal of Pain and Symtpom Management, 43*(5), 855–865.

Cronin, J., Arnstein, P., & Flanagan, J. (2015). Family members' perceptions of most helpful interventions during end of life care. *Journal of Hospice and Palliative Nursing, 17*(3), 223–228.

Crow, F. M. (2014). Final days at home. *Canadian Family Physician, 60*(6), 543–545.

De Graeff, A. & Dean, M. (2007). Palliative sedation therapy in the last weeks of life: A literature review and recommendations for standard. *Journal of Palliative Medicine, 10*(1), 67–85.

De la Cruz, M., Fan, J., Yennu, S., Tanco, K., Shin, S., Wu, J., . . . Bruera, E. (2015). The frequency of missed delirium in paitents referred to palliative care in a comprehensive cancer center. *Supportive Care in Cancer, 23*(8), 2427–2433.

DiMartini, A., Dew, M. A., Kormos, R., McCurry, K., & Fontes, P. (2007). Posttraumatic stress disorder caused by hallucinations and delusions experienced in delirium. *Psychosomatics, 48*(5), 436–439.

Finucane, A. M., Lugton, J., Kennedy, C., & Spiller, J. A. (2017). The experiences of caregivers of patients with delirium, and their role in its management in palliative care settings: an integrative literature review. *Psycho-Oncology, 26*, 291–300.

Fritz, L., Dirven, L., Reijneveld, J., Koekkoek, J. A., Stiggelbout, A. M., Pasman, H. R. W., & Taphoorn, M. J. B. (2016). Advanced care planning in glioblastoma patients. *Cancers, 8*(11), 102.

Gallagher, R., & Krawczyk, M. (2013). Family members' perceptions of end of life care across diverse locations of care. *BMC Palliative Care,12*, 25.

Good, P., Richard, R., Syrmis, W., Jenkins-Marsh, S., & Stephens, J. (2014a). Medically assisted nutrition for adult palliative care patients. *Cochrane Database of Systematic Reviews, 4*. Doi: 10.1002/14651858.CD006274.pub3.

Good, P., Richard, R., Syrmis, W., Jenkins-Marsh, S., & Stephens, J. (2014b). Medically assisted hydration for adult palliative care patients. *Cochrane Database of Systematic Reviews, 4*. Doi: 10.1002/14651858.CD006273.pub3.

Gurschick, L., Mayer, D. K., & Hanson, L. C. (2014). Palliative sedation: An analysis of international guidelines and position statements. *American Journal of Hospice and Palliative Medicine, 32*(6), 660–671.

Hui, D., Dos Santos, R., Chisholm, G., Bansal, S., Silva, T. B., Kilgore, K., . . . Bruera, E. (2014). Clinical signs of impending death in cancer patients. *Oncologist, 19*, 681–687.

Hui, D., Dos Santos, R., Chisholm, G., Bansal, S., Crovador, C. S., & Bruera, E. (2015). Bedside clinical signs associated with impending death in patients with advanced cancer: Preliminary findings. *Cancer, 121*(6), 960–967.

Hui, D. (2015). Unexpected death in palliative care: What to expect when you are not expecting. *Current Opinion in Supportive and Palliative Care, 9*(4), 369–374.

Kerr, C. W., Donnelly, J. P., Wright, S. T., Kiszczak, S. M., Banas, A., Grant, P. C., & Luckzkiewicz, D. L. (2014). End-of-life dreams and visions: A longitudinal study of hospice patients' experiences. *Journal of Palliative Medicine, 17*(3), 296–303.

Keyes, K. M., Pratt, C., Galea, S., McLaughlin, K. A., Koenen, K. C., & Shear, M. K. (2014). The burden of loss: Unexpected death of a loved one and psychiatric disorders across the life course in a national study. *American Journal of Psychiatry, 171*(8), 864–871.

Kutner, J. S., Blatchford, P. J., Taylor, D. H., Ritchie, C. S., Bull, J. H., Fairclough, D. L., ... Abernethy, A. P. (2015). Safety and benefit of discontinuing statin therapy in the setting of advanced, life-limiting illness. *JAMA Internal Medicine, 175*(5), 691–700.

Kyle, G. (2011). End of life: A need for bowel care guidance. *Nursing Times, 107,* 17.

Lamont, E. B. (2003). Complexities in prognosticating in advanced cancer. *JAMA, 290*(1), 98–104.

Leonard, M., Raju, B., Conroy, M., Donnelly, S., Trzepacz, P. T., Saunders, J., & Meagher, D. (2008). Reversibility of delirium in terminally ill patients and predictors of mortality. *Palliative Medicine, 22*(7), 848–854.

Lobb, E. A., Kristjanson, L. J., Aoun, S. M., Monterosso, L., Halkett, G. K., & Davies, A. (2010). Predictors of complicated grief: A systematic review of empirical studies. *Death Studies, 34*(8) 673–698.

Lunney, J. R., Lynn, J., Foley, D. J., & Guralnik, J. M. (2003). Patterns of functional decline at the end of life. *JAMA, 289*(18), 2387–2392.

McCrate Protus, B., Kimbrel, J. M., & Grauer, P. A. (Eds.). (2015). *Palliative care consultant.* Montgomery, AL: HospiceScript.

Monin, J. K., & Schulz, R. (2009). Interpersonal effects of suffering in older adult caregiving relationships. *Psychology & Aging, 24*(3), 681–695.

Murray, S. A., Kendall, M., Boyd, K., & Sheikh, A. (2005). Illness trajectories and palliative care. *British Medical Journal, 330*(7498), 1007–1011.

Pace, A., Di Lorenzo, C., Guariglia, L., Jandolo, B., Carapella, C. M., & Pompili, A. (2009). End of life issues in brain tumor patients. *Journal of Neurooncology, 91*(1), 39–43.

Radwany, S., Albanese, T., & Clough, L., Sims, L., Mason, H., & Jahangiri, S. (2009). End-of-life decisions making and emotional burden: Placing family meetings in context. *American Journal of Hospice and Palliative Medicine, 26*(5), 376–383.

Schildman, E., & Schildman, J. (2014). Palliative sedation therapy: A systematic literature review and critical appraisal of available guidance on indication and decision-making. *Journal of Palliative Medicine, 17*(5), 601–611.

Senel, G., Uysal, N., Oguz, G., Kaya, M., Kadioullari, N., Kocak, N., & Karaca, S. (2017). Delirium frequentcy and risk factors among patients with cancer in palliative care unit. *American Journal of Hospice and Palliative Medicine, 34*(3), 282–286.

Smith-Stoner, M. (2011). Teaching patient-centered care during the Silver Hour. *Online Journal of Issues in Nursing, 16*(2), 6. doi: 10.3912/OJIN.Vol16No02Man06

Strada, E. A. (2008). Preserving life at the end of life: Shifting the temporal dimension of hope. *Palliative and Supportive Care, 6*(2), 187–188.

Sykes, N. (2015). One chance to get it right: Understanding the new guidance for care of the dying person. *British Medical Bulletin, 115*(1), 143–150.

Vigano, A., Del Fabbro, E., Bruera, E., & Borod, M. (2012). The cachexia clinic: From staging to managing nutritional and functional problems in advanced cancer patients. *Critical Reviews in Oncology and Hematology, 17*(3), 293–303.

Wagner, P. D. (2008). Possible mechanisms underlying the development of cachexia in COPD. *European Respiratory Journal, 31,* 492–501.

Zelenikova, R., Ren, D., Schulz, R., Given, B., & Sherwood, P. R. (2016). Symptoms as the main predictors of caregivers' perception of the suffering of patients with primary brain tumors. *Cancer Nursing, 39*(2), 97–105.

8

The Eighth Domain of Palliative Care

Ethical and Legal Aspects of Care

Focus Points

- One of the main goals of palliative care is to ensure that each patient receives medical care during illness and at end of life that is consistent with his or her preferences, as well as cultural and spiritual values.
- Palliative care clinicians can facilitate conversations with the patient and family caregivers to explore their preferences about care throughout the illness trajectory, including end of life.
- Ethical issues that frequently arise in palliative care are related to medical decision-making, communication about prognosis, and withholding or withdrawing medical treatment.
- Conflict may develop when they is disagreement between members of the health-care team, patients, and families about what kind of care should be provided and what type of information should be communicated.
- Palliative psychologists working in teams carefully balance the patient's right to confidentiality with the need to share information essential to the care plan.
- The palliative care team carefully assesses any indications that the patient may be the victim of neglect or physical, emotional, or fiduciary abuse, and takes steps to minimize distress for the patient while following the requirements of the law.

Introduction

One of the main goals of palliative care is to preserve patient autonomy and ensure that decisions about medical treatments are reflective of the patient's and the family's preferences and values. It is a basic right for every patient to accept or refuse medical treatment. If the patient is unable to make decisions due to cognitive or physical decline, the person appointed is required to make decisions consistent with the patient's values.

Although obtaining consent is an essential component of the patient-provider relationship, it is not always a straightforward process. It can be complicated by a combination of psychosocial and cultural factors, especially when illness is advanced and the patient is approaching end of life (Ditto, 2006). For instance, the family may hold specific values about how much information should be provided to the patient about prognosis. Additionally, conflict within families may negatively affect decision-making. As a result, disagreements may develop between medical providers, who feel it is their responsibility to provide the patient with clear information, and the family, who may wish not to disclose this information in an effort to protect the patient from distress. Conflict may also arise if the health-care team believes that medical intervention requested by the family may harm the patient. In all circumstances, the delivery of care by the palliative care team is the result of careful consideration of medical, psychological, and cultural needs, as well as ethical principles.

This chapter begins by discussing some application of psychology principles and standards to the palliative care setting. This is important, because psychologists practicing in medical settings have a responsibility to follow their discipline-specific guidelines, in addition to the general principles of biomedical ethics. This chapter also reviews examples of case scenarios that required consideration of different ethical, professional, and clinical issues, with a focus on medical decision-making.

Competencies for Palliative Psychologists

Palliative psychologists, as all licensed psychologists providing clinical services, follow the ethical guidelines developed by the American Psychological Association (2003, 2010) and the laws and regulations developed by the Board of Psychology of the state where they are practicing. Additionally, palliative psychologists should be familiar with the *Guidelines for Psychological Practice in Health Care Delivery Systems* (APA, 2013). These apply to all psychologists working in health care. For example, the importance of preserving confidentiality while also providing important input to other providers is an ethical concern shared by all psychologists working in the health-care setting, and especially those working in institutional settings as consultants or as members of a health-care team.

Palliative psychologists may face additional challenges, however, because the urgency of a patient's medical condition often demands a rapid and concerted effort on the part of the team. It is important that they reflect on how their professional ethical standards can be applied specifically to the palliative care setting, in rapidly evolving and complex clinical scenarios. Seeking peer consultation or supervision may be necessary. Ethical recommendations for psychologists working with patients who are dying have been offered and should be reviewed by every palliative psychologist (Werth & Kleespies, 2006). As an increasing number of psychologists become palliative care practitioners, it is likely that continuing education programs and professional publications will focus specifically on the ethical dilemmas that may be unique to palliative psychologists.

A familiarity with legislation related to palliative care and end-of-life care is necessary to develop competence in the legal and ethical domain of care. It is especially important that psychologists update their knowledge of any development in the field of palliative and end-of-life care that have ethical and clinical implications. For example, psychologists who practice in a state where physician-assisted death is legal are more likely to become involved in these discussions with the patient, family, and the health-care team. Therefore, they should be aware of the impact of cultural and religious issues on patient's preferences in this regard (Periyakoil, Kraemer, & Neri, 2016). Palliative psychologists should be knowledgeable in the main principles of biomedical ethics regarding decision-making capacity and the broad topic of advance care planning. It is also necessary that they develop the ability to facilitate therapeutic conversations in which patients and family caregivers can explore their wishes and preferences for medical care during the entire illness trajectory, and not just at end of life (Box 8.1). Competence in the ethical and legal domain of palliative care will allow palliative psychologists to become involved in family meetings when ethical issues are discussed and also to become members of ethics committees. They may be called to provide evaluation for decisional capacity and provide psychological intervention to support a family in distress when conflict arises regarding care. A psychologist's ability to engage with the team and the patient and family in this comprehensive manner may be compromised if there is a lack of knowledge of the application and implications of legal and ethical issues. As in all domains of palliative care, a psychologist does not function independently or as a solo practitioner. When complex ethical issues are at stake, the presence of the interdisciplinary palliative care team represents an invaluable resource for all clincians. Here, the assessment and perspectives from different disciplines can allow for a full appreciation of the issues involved and the development of a care plan that balances the respect for ethical principles with the best interest of the patient and the family.

Following the Psychology Ethics Code in the Palliative Care Setting

This section briefly reviews principles and ethical standards relevant to the palliative care setting and discusses their clinical applications. Importantly, palliative psychologists should seek consultation or supervision when guidance is needed.

The ethics code developed by the American Psychological Association contains aspirational goals (the "General Principles") and enforceable rules (the "Ethical Standards"). The ethics code does not provide grounds for determining liability, as these decisions are made by the boards of psychology in each state. Additionally, while APA membership is voluntary and does not affect a psychologist's licensure status or ability to practice, actions that clearly violate the APA ethics code can be reported to licensing bodies and others, irrespective of APA membership, and can result in sanctions for psychologists. Of note, boards of psychology in certain states may place more emphasis on the ethics code. For example, the book of laws and regulations related to the practice of psychology developed by the California Board of Psychology specifically includes a copy of the ethics code (California Board of Psychology, 2015).

BENEFICENCE AND NON-MALEFICENCE

This principle requires that psychologists be committed to do no harm to the people with whom they work and to protect the welfare of all those with whom they interact. In the palliative care setting, psychologists use their training and expertise in communication

> *Box 8.1* **Palliative Psychology Competencies in the Ethical and Legal Domain of Palliative Care**
>
> **KNOWLEDGE**
>
> - principles of medical ethics
> - decision-making process about consent to medical treatment, withholding and withdrawing life-sustaining treatments
> - meaning of goals of care
> - cultural and religious factors relevant to medical decision making
> - cultural factors affecting requests regarding disclosure of prognosis
> - advance directives
> - psychology ethical principles and standards and their application to the palliative care and end-of-life care setting
>
> **SKILLS**
>
> - provide supportive education to the patient and the family regarding decision-making and facilitate discussions about medical care preferences
> - actively participate in family meetings designed to discuss goals of care and medical prognosis
> - provide evaluations for decisional capacity and assess for instances of abuse or neglect
> - work collaboratively as a member of the palliative care team to support the patient and the family during difficult transitions (e.g., palliative extubations)
>
> **ATTITUDES**
>
> - respect for patients and families' cultural values with regard to medical treatment in advanced illness and end of life
> - awareness of own values and biases with regard to end-of-life care
> - appreciation for the complexity of ethical issues during the illness trajectory, including end of life

to ensure that information is presented to the patient and the family in a manner that is always respectful and validating of personal and cultural values. Therefore, they do not participate in or condone jokes or comments designed to perpetuate stereotypes and racism about ethnic or minority groups. Awareness of personal bias and countertransference reactions are important protective factors to avoid harmful communication (see also Chapter 6).

Psychologists are particularly aware of the impact of *language* on the patient and family. Certain expressions used in the medical setting may convey an unsupportive, blaming, or disrespectful attitude toward the patient and the family. They should be avoided. For instance, it is not appropriate to say "the patient has failed the chemo" when cancer recurs, or "the patient has failed the weaning process" when an extubation is not successful. Additionally, the use of broad negative labels, including "the patient is in denial," should be avoided. These expression have minimal clinical value unless they are fully contextualized and explained and risk alienating the patient and the family. Most important, their use reveals poor appreciation of psychological and cultural factors that may affect the understanding of diagnosis and prognosis.

The use of metaphors and expressions about the illness that may not reflect the values of the patient and the family should also be avoided. For instance, describing the reaction to a diagnosis of cancer as a "fight," or a battle, or encouraging the patient to "fight" to promote coping, is not appropriate, *unless* this language is used by the patient and the family, and it is recognized by them as a source of support. Additionally, clinicians should be cautious about using expressions that may be perceived as patronizing, superficial, and dismissive about the need to "let go," or "resolving unfinished business," or achieving "life closure."

While these and other expressions may be used with benign intentions, they trivialize the complexity and uniqueness of the patient and the family experience. They also reveal a paternalistic attitude about what people should accomplish or focus on at the end of life.

The ethical principle of "beneficence" also involves the need for psychologists to maintain awareness of how their physical or emotional condition may affect their work with patients and families. Burnout and other manifestations of professional stress prevent being fully present for the patient and family caregivers. Furthermore, losses and transitions in the psychologist's personal life can certainly trigger a grieving process that must be recognized, acknowledged, and supported. This will allow the psychologist to sustain the patients and families she cares for, while she sustains herself. Accordingly, maintaining self-care should be considered a professional and ethical responsibility for psychologists. Below is a description of the principles.

FIDELITY AND RESPONSIBILITY

This principle involves developing professional and trusting relationships with all colleagues and professionals. While a psychologist may be familiar with working in a multidisciplinary team, he may be unfamiliar with the interdisciplinary approach, where boundaries are more fluid. Becoming an integral part of an interdisciplinary palliative care team requires developing a trusting relationship with other team members, validating and supporting others' work, and understanding the unique nature of interdisciplinary teamwork. This is not expressed by hierarchy and territory but rather by recognizing everyone's skill, competence, and creativity. Ultimately, the focus should be on how each member of the team can contribute to the development of a care plan that truly meets the patient's and the family's needs.

While each clinician on the interdisciplinary team provides unique contributions to the care of the patient and the family, the focus is on coordinated team action. Experienced palliative care clinicians do not emphasize their own work with the patient, or the special relationship they may have established; rather, they think in terms of teamwork. They recognize that the team is the necessary infrastructure and platform that allows each clinician to express competency and creativity and receive support to manage challenges. Adopting this framework may require adjustment by psychologists who are accustomed to working in private practice and focusing on their individual work with patients, but it is a necessary aspect of working in palliative care.

Another expression of the fidelity and responsibility principles involves taking any commitment made to a patient very seriously. For instance, a palliative psychologist working in an inpatient setting should avoid telling a patient she will visit him at a specific time (e.g., I will come back this afternoon) unless the time frame is realistic. Patients who are hospitalized, especially those with limited family support, often look forward to the visit from the psychologist and will likely feel disappointed and confused if the clinician does not show. This is especially important to avoid ruptures in the therapeutic alliance if the patient and the psychologist have been meeting regularly even for a few sessions, and there is a reasonable expectation of predictability. Psychologists who are new to palliative care work or new members of the team may wish to be identified as a valuable resource and may develop the tendency to overload their schedule. This may interfere with their ability to sustain a reasonable workload and keep appointments with patients, ultimately creating conditions that may lead to burnout.

JUSTICE

Following this principle, psychologists ensure that their countertransference, personal biases, and limits of competence do not interfere with the services that patients and families receive. To illustrate, strong spiritual and religious beliefs about end of life may turn into bias if they are used as a reason for judging the behavior of patients and families.

Ongoing reflective practice is necessary to recognize engrained bias that can negatively affect psychological interventions. Additionally, the ability to promptly identify and address countertransference will also ensure that the principle of justice is fully embodied and that patient and family care is not affected by any clinician's personal factors.

The principle of justice also requires clinicians to operate within the boundaries of their competence. Palliative psychologists should exercise caution discussing medical information without involving medical providers. This also applies if family caregivers ask specific questions about the patient's medical condition or prognosis, or the reason for a specific medical treatment. Because psychologists hold a doctoral degree, they are generally referred to as "doctor." Some patients and family caregivers may assume that the psychologist is also a medical doctor and may begin asking medical questions or believe that the psychologist can offer medical insight. Clarifying roles and responsibilities will prevent confusion and not create an additional burden for the patient.

Furthermore, new psychological modalities of interventions should not be used with patients or family caregivers unless the clinician has skillfully practiced the approach, obtained clinical supervision, and is able to ensure a safe administration or safely address any complications. This is especially important where the modalities have the potential of eliciting strong responses, as Eye Movement Desensitization and Reprocessing (EMDR) or other exposure-based modalities, and clinical hypnosis (see also discussion of competence further in this chapter).

RESPECT FOR PEOPLE'S RIGHTS AND DIGNITY

This principle is especially important in advanced illness and end of life because it emphasizes the importance of respecting the patient's dignity, privacy, confidentiality, and self-determination. Psychological assessment and intervention should be culturally relevant and should respect diversity in all its manifestations, including age, gender, sexual orientation, ethnicity, race, socioeconomic status, disability, and language.

A comprehensive psychological assessment can reveal important information about the values that are important to the patient and the family and need to be respected (see also Chapters 4 and 6). The values related to decision making, communication, goals of medical treatment and wishes for care at the end of life, and meaning of quality of life are especially relevant. The interdisciplinary palliative care team carefully considers the unique circumstances of each patient and family to ensure respect for values and dignity.

Is decision-making driven by the individual or by the family? Is there a family member other than the patient who appears to be in charge of making decisions? How should important medical information be conveyed if a family favors indirect versus direct communication? How can clinicians conduct a sensitive exploration of the patient's goals for medical care when disease is progressing and prognosis is poor?

Respecting people's rights and dignity is especially important in the case of vulnerable patients when autonomous decision-making may be impaired. This aspect can become challenging when the patient has a diagnosis of psychiatric illness or is experiencing the physical and cognitive decline of advanced illness. While the presence of psychiatric disorders is not specifically mentioned in the ethical principle, psychologists are aware of the potential stigma associated with certain diagnoses, especially when the symptoms are not adequately controlled. For example, patients with poorly controlled bipolar disorder or schizophrenia may present agitated, uncooperative, or explosive. Similarly, patients with personality traits in the borderline range may easily be labeled by staff as "demanding," "difficult," and "disruptive." Patients with an active substance use disorder may easily evoke negative emotions in staff, due to impulsive and drug-seeking behaviors.

Because of their extensive professional training and experience in diagnosing and treating patients with psychiatric diagnoses, psychologists are often better equipped to establish rapport with these patients and help develop an adequate care plan. They can educate medical and nursing staff about using adequate behavioral and communication strategies. They can also model a professional demeanor that competently blends compassion and appropriate boundaries. As patients with mental illness represent an especially vulnerable population, all efforts need to be made to improve the therapeutic alliance between the patient and the medical team.

Ethical Standards

Ethical standards represent enforceable rules of conduct that must be followed. This section reviews selected ethical standards with applications to palliative psychology.

Competence. Palliative psychologists have a responsibility to develop and maintain competence in providing services to palliative care patients and their families in inpatient and outpatient settings. Because palliative psychology is an emerging field, specific best practice guidelines may not be available. Therefore, the *Clinical Practice Guidelines for Quality Palliative Care* should be followed to identify specific competencies and skills. Each domain of palliative care can be used to provide a general framework for competency in each area. This book has proposed and described relevant competencies for psychologists in each domain, identifying specific roles. Continuing education, supervision, and consultation are important tools to maintain and further develop competency. As palliative psychology continues to develop as a specialty, it is anticipated that formal practice guidelines will become available.

Privacy and confidentiality. This is a core and critical issue for all psychologists providing clinical service. Palliative psychologists recognize patients' and families' right to privacy and confidentiality in psychological treatment. However, they are also aware of the unique nature of interdisciplinary teamwork and the importance of sharing information and input that is relevant to the care plan. The ability to determine what information should be kept confidential and what is relevant to the interdisciplinary care plan is key, because interdisciplinary palliative care work cannot be approached as a psychotherapy private practice.

Problems can be avoided if the palliative psychologist clarifies her role to the patient and the family at the onset by identifying herself as a member of the team, and working with the team to support them. In a sense, palliative psychologists working in hospital or clinic settings maintain a dual role that involves providing confidential psychological intervention to patients and families, while also serving as members of an interdisciplinary team or as consultants. It is important to note that *dual role* does not imply *dual relationship*.

Confidential information shared in the context of a therapy session that does not have direct impact on medical treatment and the rest of the care plan does not need to be disclosed during team meetings. For example, as part of the session, the patient may disclose being abused as a child by a deceased relative. If this information has no foreseeable impact on the care plan, it should be kept confidential. However, the information shared with the psychologist may directly impact the care plan by helping identify necessary changes. To illustrate, a patient may share with the psychologist that as a result of being the victim of a sexual assault, she is distressed by receiving care from a nurse of the same sex as the perpetrator. In this case, the psychologist may share with the team that due to past trauma, the patient needs to be cared for by a female (or male) nurse. The important outcome in this case is the patient's sense of safety and comfort, and these goals can often be accomplished without sharing confidential information in detail.

Obviously, any mention of suicidal ideation, even though fleeting or passive, should be shared with the team to ensure adequate follow-up and safety, even if the patient does not appear to be in imminent danger.

Approaching the patient and the family with openness and honesty will help establish good rapport and therapeutic alliance. And in many cases the patient will feel encouraged to share much of his or her emotional experience. During a clinical interview or psychotherapy session, patients may discuss several aspects of their experience that may require further action. For example, they may reveal that physical symptoms are not adequately controlled or report a worsening of depression and anxiety. Family caregivers may share that they are confused about some elements of the treatment plan that they do not fully understand, requiring follow-up by the medical team. Difficulties with the hospital system in itself or difficulties with staff can also be discussed during the psychology session.

A strategy for explaining to patients what will be shared with the team is to summarize the meeting and present a possible plan. For example, the psychologist could say, "It sounds as if we have a few issues that we need to work on to help you feel better. You described to me this new pain deep in your abdomen, and it is important that your doctors know about this so that they treat it. I would like to mention this to them, so they will come to see you sooner and ask you more questions about this new pain. You have also described very difficult experiences you had in the past while you were in the hospital. I would like for us to work together to help you deal with the anxiety that comes up when you think about those memories. Does this sound like a good plan? Am I leaving anything out?"

Record-keeping. Psychologists have the obligation to provide accurate documentation in the electronic chart of any encounter with a patient or family member. Additionally, phone conversations with other professionals contacted for the purpose of obtaining collateral information should also be documented. Many psychologists have been trained to write extensive notes that include a detailed description of the session. In the busy hospital setting, however, notes have the purpose of conveying information that the rest of the team can utilize to develop an effective treatment plan. Therefore, it is best to write notes that are succinct but contain all essential elements. A comprehensive clinical description of the patient's emotional processing as in a detailed psychotherapy note or process note may not serve the best interest of the hospitalized patient. It may unnecessarily compromise confidentiality, and it may prevent other professionals not particularly interested in detailed descriptions of emotional aspects from actually reading and benefiting from the clinical note.

At a minimum, however, psychology notes in the inpatient setting should communicate the following:

- identifying information
- patient's main medical diagnosis
- reason for consultation request and referral question
- presenting complaints and problem list
- brief previous psychiatric history
- assessment considerations, including diagnosis, if applicable, and mental status exam
- psychological intervention provided (e.g. psychotherapy, clinical hypnosis, relaxation training, grief therapy, etc.)
- treatment plan including elements of psychological treatment and collaboration with other team members.

Confidentiality is especially relevant to record-keeping. The challenge is to determine not only what information should be documented in the chart because it is relevant to the plan, but also what information should be protected because sharing it would violate the patient's confidentiality. After a therapy session, patients may wonder whether the content of the session will be recorded in a note, especially after disclosing difficult personal experiences, such as a history of abuse, trauma, family conflict, or other. In some cases, patients may also disclose criminal behavior they have perpetrated in the past.

Psychologists are not required to document in detail the content of therapy sessions or sensitive elements of the patient's history that have no direct impact on the care plan. They have an obligation to protect the patient's confidentiality, even when working in a hospital setting. The medical chart can be accessed by various clinicians, including some who may evaluate the patient only once, as can be the case for a physical therapy evaluation or a swallowing evaluation, and these clinicians do not need access to a sensitive psychological history.

Therapy. The importance of obtaining consent for treatment is a fundamental requirement for all psychologists. Psychologists working in a primary care setting who are part of a medical group may include their psychotherapy consent form with the documentation the patient signs during the first visit. In other outpatient settings, patients sign a general consent form that applies to all and any services provided and received by the patient, including psychological consultations, evaluations, and psychotherapy. This form of general consent is generally also obtained during patient hospitalizations.

This does not imply that palliative psychologists should not obtain consent from a hospitalized patient. Consent starts by asking permission before entering a patient's room. Even though patients are in a way a "captive audience" because they cannot leave their hospital room, they can choose to decline psychological support. However, due to their vulnerable physical and emotional state, they may not feel empowered to clearly state their preference. Some patients may feel uncomfortable refusing the visit because they do not want to be considered rude, or because they are concerned that a refusal will somehow negatively impact their medical treatment. Therefore, psychologists should rely also on their clinical judgment to determine if conducting a visit is appropriate.

In discussing consent, it is important to note the difference between ongoing psychotherapy and a psychological consultation for evaluation or crisis intervention. A palliative psychologist may be asked by the palliative care team or the primary medical team to conduct an evaluation to assess the patient for possible depression, anxiety, cognitive disorders, and for differential diagnoses, such as grief reactions and demoralization. The consultation can be a one-time-only event with the understanding that the medical team needs the results of the evaluation to implement a treatment plan.

In this case, the psychologist will use clinical skills and judgment to engage with patients who do not wish to talk to anyone. If at the onset of the conversation the patient says, "I don't want to talk to anybody; I don't want to talk to you," the psychologist can attempt to use strategies to diffuse the situation and form some rapport with the patient that will allow the evaluation to take place, if at all possible. For instance, the psychologist could say, "Yes, I am aware that this hospitalization is giving you a really hard time and you don't want to talk to anybody. I just have one question, though: do you think it would be possible to help you feel better while you are here? I am thinking that if we could just try to figure out what is making this experience so difficult for you, perhaps we can improve things. It seems that things are not going in a way that is helpful for you, and I would like your help understanding what the problem is, so we can do something about it." A confident but compassionate presence is helpful in establishing rapport with patients.

Ongoing psychotherapy during the hospitalization implies that the patient is consenting to each session. Consent is basically informally given every time the psychologist visits the patient, and it is appropriate to ask if he or she is ready for the session. Of course, the patient can not only refuse a session, but also end the session at any point, for any reason. Although the psychologist should follow the patient's wishes, it is appropriate to ask the patient if he or she is experiencing any physical or emotional discomfort that may require immediate attention.

Understanding Medical Decision-Making in Palliative and End-of-Life Care

Patients, family caregivers, and medical providers often feel reluctant to discuss the kind of care desired at the end of life. Yet, without this conversation, the patient's wishes may not be known and may not be honored. Introducing palliative care early in the disease course may provide an opportunity for the patient and family caregivers to begin these sensitive conversations and to discuss the concerns brought by serious illness.

For many, good quality care at the end of life is associated with less aggressive care. A study of 1,146 bereaved family members of patients who died with advanced lung or colorectal cancer explored the family members' perception of the quality of end-of-life care received. Results showed that a rating of "excellent" for end-of-life care was associated with death outside the hospital, hospice care longer than three days, and avoidance of ICU admission within 30 days of death (Wright et al., 2016). However, if a patient's wishes about end-of-life care preferences are not known, there may be more hospitalizations and ICU admissions. This can translate to perception of poor care and can have significant negative implications for bereaved family members. Another study found that while the number of patients 65 and older likely to die at home has increased, so has the rate of admissions in ICUs in the last month of life. Also, while there has been an increase in the utilization of hospice services, almost 30% of patients were on hospice for three days or less (Teno et al., 2013).

A telephone survey of 1,851 residents of Massachusetts who experienced the death of a loved one indicated that one in five felt that the end-of-life care provided was only fair or poor (Freyer, 2016). The survey revealed that poor communication between medical providers and patients was often the cause of confusion and misunderstanding. Of note, while 85% of people surveyed stated that physicians should discuss end-of-life care preferences with patients, it was reported in this survey that only 25% of those with a serious illness had this conversation with their doctors.

Choosing less aggressive care at the end of life for some patients involves the issue of withdrawing or withholding treatment. For instance, palliative or terminal extubation involves cessation of mechanical ventilation to allow the patient a natural death (O'Mahoney, McHugh, Zallman & Selwyn, 2003). While it is an ethical and legal practice, making the decision of allowing the patient to die can cause distress for family members who are making this decision for a patient who is no longer able to make decisions. Or patients who are receiving mechanical ventilation may also decide they wish to be allowed to die. This decision can become a source of disagreement among family members. The key point here is that an open conversation about prognosis and end-of-life care with medical providers is necessary to allow patients and families to make decisions that are difficult, but that reflect important values. Palliative extubations always involve extensive preparation to avoid physical distress for the patient and to provide emotional support for the family (Billings, 2011, 2012; Campbell, 2004).

Medical ethics has evolved significantly in the way it considers how physicians should give patients information about their health. According to the American Medical Association's *First Code of Medical Ethics* (1847): "The life of a sick person can be shortened not only by the acts, but also by the words or the manner of the physician. It is, therefore, a sacred duty to guard himself carefully in this respect, and to avoid all things which would have a tendency to discourage the patient and to depress his spirits" (p. 2639–2640).

This approach focused on protecting patients from "bad news" that may deprive them of the will to live. In some cultures, physicians still follow an indirect mode of communication that avoids communicating clearly and directly about diagnosis and prognosis. Similarly, family members may feel a responsibility to protect the patient from bad news (see also Chapter 6).

The increased focus on individual rights and autonomy has resulted in significant changes to this approach in the United States. The Patient Self-Determination Act of 1991 addresses a patient's right to make decisions for his or her medical care, including the right to decide what kind of treatments would be acceptable at the end of life. The ability to make an informed decision implies having the necessary information. Although this process may appear straightforward, it is actually quite complex. The medical culture mandate to provide direct and clear information to the patient about their diagnosis and prognosis may clash with the culture of the family, where the most important value is protecting the patient from distress irrespective of circumstances. These situations can generate great distress in the family and create conflict with the medical team.

All palliative care clinicians guide their actions according to the main principles of biomedical ethics (Beauchamp & Childress, 2001):

- The principle of *autonomy* recognizes the individual's right to make personal decisions based on core values that define the meaning of his or her existence.
- According to the principle of *beneficence*, the health-care provider should always consider the risks and benefits of a treatment and try to determine which course of action benefits the patient.
- The principle of *non-malevolence* implies that the health-care professional should not harm the patient. Since medical treatment may involve some degree of harm, this should not be higher than the benefits.
- Finally, the principle of *justice* involves that all patients in similar circumstances should receive similar treatment, though their choice to refuse such treatment is preserved.

Advance care planning is a general term that refers to the process of identifying patients' goals and wishes concerning end-of-life care and informing health-care providers. Ideally, this process includes conversations between physicians, patients, and their surrogates or health-care agents. End-of-life care wishes are a sensitive and emotionally stressful topic and, in order to make informed decisions, the patient and the family need to evaluate information about medical procedures that can be provided to patients at the end of life, including cardiopulmonary resuscitation and intubation, tube feeding and artificial nutrition and hydration, and use of antibiotics.

A clear understanding about how a patient would like to be treated at the end of life can be beneficial in several ways. It relieves family caregivers and others from the responsibility and burden of having to make difficult decisions for the patient if he or she becomes unable to express his or her wishes. Additionally, it may prevent conflict among family members and between medical providers and family caregivers when the patient's wishes are known and they are unequivocal. Most important, making patients' wishes about end-of-life care known ensures that their autonomy, dignity, and values are respected and followed, especially at a time when caregivers may feel overwhelmed by the reality of their loved one's impending death.

Specialist palliative care clinicians have training, experience, and expertise navigating these difficult conversations with patients and families by engaging them directly or by assisting other medical providers. The key element of this expertise is the ability to communicate in supportive and therapeutic ways during an emotionally charged and difficult time. Many patients and families have never thought about their wishes for the time when death is near. Engaging them in a gentle and competently guided conversation eliciting their values and preferences can promote a decision-making process that truly honors personal wishes.

To summarize, earlier conversations about advance care planning can offer patients and their families the opportunity to consider several important issues:

- personal values about what makes living meaningful
- understanding of their current medical condition and decisions they may foresee in the future
- specific concerns over wishes they may have regarding life support or aggressive interventions, hospice, or long-term care
- main concerns about death and dying
- wishes for how the patients would want to spend the last month, weeks, or days of life.

For some, advance care planning conversations are better tolerated when the patient is feeling relatively well physically and there is no pressure to make decisions due to physical decline or sudden complications of the disease.

Palliative psychologists can play an important role in facilitating these discussions. These can occur in several contexts: in the hospital setting during a family meeting with the palliative care team; during the course of ongoing psychotherapy in an outpatient practice; in the primary care setting where the psychologist engages in advanced care planning discussions with the patient, the primary care physician, and the family. Psychologists can also be members of ethics committees and actively participate in discussions of complex cases when ethics consultations are requested.

If these issues and concerns are raised during psychotherapy, palliative psychologists can facilitate their exploration by providing background information to the patient and the family about the decision-making process and support them as they are considering options. While psychologists would not express their personal opinions about what the patient should do, they may help the patient discern his or her values and goals of care. They can also facilitate these difficult conversations with the patient's family members and medical providers.

The final result of advance care planning can be the creation of a legal document such as an *advance directive*. Or patients can express their wishes verbally to their physician in the presence of witnesses. These wishes should be documented in the medical record. An advance directive, also called an "advance health-care directive" is a legal document that indicates what kind of medical treatments and interventions a patient would like to receive at the end of life if he or she is unable to speak for him- or herself. The essential principles at the base of advance directives are the value of patients' *autonomy* and the recognition that they have *control over medical decisions.*

The advance directives become effective when the patient lacks the capacity to make decisions about medical care. The determination that a patient lacks decisional capacity should be made by the attending physician, and it should be confirmed by another physician in writing. It is important to note that competence to make decisions is domain specific. In other words, a patient may be competent to make some decisions but not competent to make decisions for medical care.

Patients may become incapacitated before having had the opportunity to discuss their wishes. To address these concerns, in most states there are provisions in the law for *surrogate decision-making,* by which family members are empowered to make medical decisions if the patient is unable to do so.

HEALTH-CARE PROXY

A health-care proxy is a document that designates someone to be an "agent" with authority to make medical decisions for the patient. The person identified by the health-care proxy should be aware of the patient's end-of-life preferences, based either on specific conversations or long-term knowledge of the patient. The health-care proxy agent is supposed to use "substitutive judgment," by attempting to make decisions as the patient would have if he or she could have, consistent with the patient's past behavior and how he or she has reacted when others have faced end-of-life decisions. In the circumstance where the patient's preferences are not known because end-of-life care decisions have never been discussed, the health-care proxy agent is charged with making medical decision that are in the *best interest of the patient.* At the end of life, the concept of best interest generally refers to ensuring that the patient's values are respected.

The health-care proxy must contain some basic information in order to be valid. It should include a statement that the patient intends the agent to have authority to make health-care decisions on his or her behalf. The document must be signed and dated by the patient, and it must be signed and dated by two witnesses. An alternate agent can be designated if the original agent is unwilling or unable to perform. The document should contain a statement of the patient's wishes regarding artificial hydration and nutrition; alternatively, it can also simply state that the agent knows the patient's wishes as to artificial nutrition and hydration and will make the appropriate decision if such a situation should arise.

It is important that patients understand the role of health-care proxy agents in order to make an informed decision about whom they should appoint. A close relationship between the patient and the proxy prior to the illness does not necessarily guarantee better decision-making. Friends and family members may have beliefs and personal agendas that can be in conflict with the ability to make decision in the patient's best interests. For instance, family members and friends may hold religious beliefs not shared by the patient; these beliefs may emphasize the importance of continuing treatment or life-prolonging treatments even when the patient is not expected to recover or improve as a result of these treatments. Or family members may have prior conflict with the patient related to estate and other financial issues, which may cloud their ability to decide about stopping life-prolonging treatment. In essence, while a prior close relationship with the patient may be helpful, it may also create additional challenges.

As mentioned previously, in absence of advance directives, family members are usually asked to make decisions if the patient becomes unable to do so. This is a complex task with emotional and ethical implications. Some of the factors considered important by family surrogates in decision-making include the following: ensuring that their decision respects the patient's preferences; being able to use knowledge of the patient and past experience to determine what decision he or she would make currently; and considering what decision represents the patient's best interest. However, family surrogate decision-makers also use their personal preferences and religious and spiritual beliefs as guiding principles when making decisions for the patient (Fritch, Petronio, Helft & Torke, 2013), which could result in the surrogates making decisions primarily based on what they would like for themselves or what they believe is morally or religiously right, rather than what represents the best interest of the patient. Palliative psychologists can help ensure that ethical standards are followed by helping family surrogates constantly focus their attention on the patient's preferences as separate from their own.

Preferences about end-of-life care should also be periodically reviewed with the patient and the family, to ensure that they are still consistent with the content of the advance directive. This is important; some patients and family caregivers may incorrectly remember what preferences were documented and may be under the impression that the advance directive still represents their current wishes, even when this is no longer the case (Sharman, Garry, Jacobsen, Loftus & Ditto, 2008).

Addressing Complex Scenarios

When there is disagreement among the patient, the family, and medical providers, issues can rapidly escalate from conflict to crisis. Ethical consultations are an important resource for addressing complex cases that raise ethical dilemmas and the associated distress. The ability to carefully evaluate all the issues involved requires in-depth assessment skills. Once the issues involved have been uncovered, a comprehensive plan can be implemented. Palliative psychologists can contribute a level of psychological sophistication in assessment and interventions that can greatly benefit the patient and the family (Table 8.1).

UNDERSTANDING FAMILY REQUESTS TO WITHHOLD PROGNOSTIC DISCLOSURE

As mentioned previously (see also Chapters 4 and 6), the patient's and family's values about communication of diagnosis and prognosis may be in conflict with the medical team. While physicians often feel it is their duty to disclose this information to the patient, family members may strongly disagree. This can occur frequently when adult children are caring for an aging parent. In an effort to protect the patient from emotional distress, the children may feel that the physician should communicate with them and not directly with the patient.

The request for nondisclosure should be approached with an open mind, flexibility, and willingness to understand the family's viewpoint. It is generally motivated by the desire to protect the patient from distress and is considered part of the obligations

Table 8.1 **Common Ethical Reasons for Referrals to Palliative Care**

Ethical Scenario	Possible Causes of Distress to Patient, Family, Health-care Providers	Role of Palliative Psychologist
The family is considering withdrawing life-sustaining treatments.	Family caregivers' stress is caused by the awareness that the decision will result in the patient's death; concern that perhaps with more time the patient could recover; difficulty reconciling ambiguity and finality.	Assess family need for additional information that could support decision-making; participate in and help manage family meetings to provide education and support to families.
Supporting the patient and the family during and after a palliative extubation	Family caregivers may fear that the patient will suffer during the procedure; witnessing physical changes (twitching or involuntary movements) after extubation may cause distress.	Provide support to the family together with other team members, especially music therapists, Reiki therapists, spiritual care providers, and social workers; help clarify family wishes for who will attend extubation and how support should be provided to different family members; facilitate referrals to community bereavement resources if the patient was not on hospice—if the patient was on hospice, alert bereavement counselors about the case and consider requesting early bereavement outreach.
The clinical team believes family is not acting in the best interest of the patient.	Clinician countertransference and feeling the need to protect patient; possible polarization and overreaction on the part of the clincians	Assess the patient and the family for any presence of coercion; work with the team to develop a plan that minimizes distress for all and prioritizes patients' preferences and wishes.
Patient and/or family request palliative sedation (see Chapter 7)	The medical team may feel that not all treatments have been attempted; clincians may be concerned that the family is pressuring the patient to request palliative sedation.	Whenever possible, conduct clinical interview with the patient and the family to understand nature of the request and determine nature of patient's unbearable suffering.

(continued)

Table 8.1 **Continued**

Ethical Scenario	Possible Causes of Distress to Patient, Family, Health-care Providers	Role of Palliative Psychologist
Family members do not want medical providers to disclose diagnosis or prognosis to loved one.	Concern that request is motivated by ulterior motive; risk of overreaction on the part of the team and inability to empathize with the family's point of view	Assess the patient to determine preferences; work with the family to understand reason for request; discuss practical implications of request and support the family.
Patient is victim of intimate partner violence but does not wish to report abuse or change living situation.	Clinician countertransference may prompt a strong desire to save the patient; hopelessness and anger on the part of the team	Ensure safety for the patient and any children present and follow the law regarding reporting; carefully evaluate together with the team whether an adult patient is a vulnerable adult and if a report should be made; consider all options that can ensure safety and minimize suffering for the patient.
The patient is competent but is being pressured by family caregivers to make certain medical decisions or to change previously made decisions.	Challenge of evaluating the situation from all perspectives; possible anger toward family on the part of health-care team with additional distress for the patient	Evaluate the meaning of the patient's decision to comply with family's request (e.g., desire to help a spouse emotionally by agreeing to aggressive care). Conduct meetings with the patient and the family both separately and together for a more accurate assessment.

imposed by their role as family caregivers. The processes leading up to these requests should be carefully assessed to ensure they reflect the patient's wishes. Palliative psychologists can play an important role conducting patient and family assessments to determine the patient's capacity to make decisions for health care, their willingness to do so, and the extent to which they would like family caregivers to be involved. Additionally, they can provide much-needed psychological support to the patient, the family, and the team (even when there is disagreement) with a focus on ensuring that the patient's autonomy is being respected.

CASE VIGNETTE 8.1

Ben is a 71-year-old widower who presented to the emergency department for severe abdominal pain, vomiting, and altered mental status over a three-day period. He has been progressively losing weight and feeling fatigued for over three months but continued working full time. He saw his primary care physician who prescribed a course of vitamin B_{12} but did not recommend further studies. Imaging studies conducted in the emergency room show extensively metastatic colon cancer. Because the patient is severely dehydrated and debilitated, the oncologist asks to speak to a family member. Ben has no children but is very close to his nephew, with whom he also shares a business. His nephew was designated as the health-care proxy agent even before the patient's wife died, 15 years prior. The oncologist shares the diagnosis with the patient's nephew and only recommends supportive care. He is confident that the patient's altered mental status was caused by severe dehydration and can be reversed. However, he thinks the patient will continue to deteriorate rapidly with a prognosis of weeks. The nephew asks the oncologist not to share the news with his uncle, stating it would only upset him further. For the past nine years Ben has been in a stable relationship with a woman who is 20 years younger. They have been living together, but her presence has not been well accepted by the rest of the family, and she has not been welcome in the nephew's home. Upon hearing about the diagnosis, she states that Ben would like to know the truth about his condition and about his diagnosis. She states he has always been independent and values being in control. The patient's nephew adamantly disagrees and accuses her of wanting his uncle's financial assets. The conflict rapidly escalates, and an ethics consult is requested. In the meantime, the patient's mental status has significantly improved and, while he is still weak, he is not complaining of pain, and his cognition is assessed within normal limits. As part of the ethics consult, the palliative psychologist is asked to evaluate the patient's capacity and preferences. During the evaluation, the psychologist focuses on understanding what core values are meaningful to Ben and his preferences regarding medical decision-making. The patient states that his nephew should be the one making decisions if he is incapacitated but also stated that until that day comes, he (the patient) is in charge, and that doctors should speak directly with him. He also clearly states that he wants to know exactly what his health condition is, because he has a large business, and he needs to make decisions regarding assets allocation. During the conversation the patient presents alert and oriented to person, place, time, and situation. He speaks with a stutter and states he has stuttered since he was a child. He describes his mood as "anxious to know what is going on and get out of the hospital." His affect is somewhat anxious, but he is otherwise engaged with the psychologist and able to sustain attention. His answers are appropriate, and when asked the same question twice, he comments that the question has already been asked. His thought process is linear and congruent; his thought content is focused on his health situation and anger at the primary care physician who apparently did not understand the seriousness of his complaints. He denies visual and auditory hallucinations and other perceptual disturbances. His insight and judgment are within normal limits. He is aware that his health has not been good for some time and has the feeling that "something is really wrong." Based on the results of the evaluation, the patient is deemed competent to make decisions about his care. As a result, a meeting is set up with the oncologist, the patient, and the patient's partner and nephew to discuss diagnosis and prognosis.

In this case, it became clear that the patient's nephew's request not to disclose diagnosis did not reflect the patient's wishes and preferences and was perhaps motivated by other agendas. In addition, because of the patient's current capacity, the previously designated health-care proxy is not operative. Maintaining a focus on the patient allowed the team to operate outside the complex family conflict and take steps to understand the patient's needs.

In some cases, patients who are competent to make decisions may choose to defer to family members. The care team should assess whether this represents an expression of autonomy or is the result of coercion.

CASE VIGNETTE 8.2

Alvaro Rosado is an 81-year-old Latino, admitted to the hospital with recurrent gastric cancer with metastases to liver and omentum, weight loss, nausea, vomiting, and pain in his throat. He lives with his wife and has three adult daughters who all live within two miles from the parents' home. They take turns visiting their parents ensuring that someone will be with them for a few hours every day. They all report being extremely close. The patient's first language is Spanish, and he only speaks a few words of English. Alvaro immigrated to the United States from Mexico when he was 40 years old, with his wife. He has full code status and does not have advance directives, but he has appointed the wife as his health-care proxy agent.

The oncologist believes that given the extent of the disease and the patient's current performance status, further disease-modifying treatment would not be tolerated and is unlikely to add any benefit. His prognosis is considered to be in the order of months. The oncologist would like to share this information directly with the patient and also discuss his decision to be full code. However, the family strongly disagrees with this approach. An adversarial relationship develops between the oncologist and the family, with each party strongly polarized. At this point, the oncologist requests a palliative care consult to help communicating with the family. The palliative care team organizes a family meeting with the oncologist and the patient's family to explore the concerns.

The patient's wife is adamant that the patient should not be told about the cancer recurrence even though he has been feeling increasingly ill, nor should he be told about his prognosis. She reported that when he was initially diagnosed, five years prior, he immediately became extremely depressed and developed suicidal ideation with a plan to walk into traffic. His wife explained that it was extremely difficult to convince him to receive treatment for depression as well as chemotherapy. He accepted an antidepressant from his primary care physician, whom he trusted, and he received regular visits from his priest. The suicidal ideation and mood improved, but the family described that time as extremely challenging.

According to the wife, if the patient was told directly about the cancer recurrence he would "just give up and die." She insists that the patient would not be able to "emotionally handle" the news and that he should just be told that he has some medical problems that required him to be hospitalized but that these are being taken care of. His wife insists they should respect her wishes, given that she knows him best and she has his best interests at heart. She adds that on some level her husband is aware that he will not get better, but he cannot be told anything directly because that would make it "more real" and, therefore, unbearable. The daughters agree with their mothers' perception and literally beg the team not to speak directly with their father. They are convinced that the patient's quality of life would be irreparably damaged if he knew that he only has a limited amount of time left.

The patient's wife and daughters also share with the palliative care team that they felt guilty for telling the patient he had stomach cancer when he was first diagnosed. One of the daughters felt especially guilty because she had pushed her mother to disclose the diagnosis. She thought knowing that it was cancer would give her father something to fight. Because her father had worked hard to overcome different challenges in his life, she thought he would fight like he had at other times in his life—for example, after losing jobs. However, she admits that when health was concerned he always deferred to his wife and wanted her to make decisions for him.

They also share that in their culture patients are never told that they are going to die; it is up to the family to protect them and take care of them until they die by making sure they remain hopeful and optimistic. They add that they have the right to protect their father from what they believe would be unbearable stress and suffering.

The oncologist, however, thinks the patient should be made aware of the reality of his diagnosis so that he will be able to make decisions about goals of care. He states that the patient has a right to know that he has a limited time.

A palliative care clinician who was also a native Spanish speaker offered to meet with the patient and evaluate his current mood and understanding of his medical situation. The clinician assured the family that he would not disclose any information to the patient and the family would be welcome to be present during the interview. The family agreed and the interview took place in the patient's room.

CLINICIAN: Good morning Mr. Rosado. My name is Dr. Mendez. I have heard so much about you from your wife and your daughters, and I must say you have a really devoted family.

PATIENT: Oh, you speak Spanish! Where are you from?

The patient and the clinician spend a few minutes talking about life in Mexico, where the clinician and the patient are both originally from. The patient comments that it is very important to stay true to one's culture and values. After the clinician feels that some rapport and trust has been established, he focuses on the illness by taking an indirect approach.

CLINICIAN: So, I heard you are here at the hospital because you have had a lot of problems with your stomach?

PATIENT: Yes, but I am feeling better. They gave me good medication for nausea and pain and it helps.

CLINICIAN: I am glad to hear that. But I also heard from your wife that you went through a difficult time five years ago when you got sick. (The clinician uses indirect language, but it is clear that both patient and clinician are aware that they are talking about the diagnosis of cancer.)

PATIENT: I can't even talk about it, it was really bad. I felt like a stone had fallen on my head and I could not get up. I could not get out of bed in the morning and my wife was very worried about me. She was making good food and good soups to give me energy, but nothing worked. I was like dead. Dead in my heart.

CLINICIAN: I am so sorry to hear it was so difficult.

PATIENT: Yes, I had no hope. I went to the doctor to do some tests because my stomach hurt. Then he called my wife and spoke to her. Then she spoke to our daughters and then they decided to speak to me. I think it was a mistake to tell me, because I could not be strong. My wife and my daughters can be very strong, but I don't like hospitals, and I don't like doctors, and I don't like being sick. I am a strong worker, I have been all my life, but I don't want to hear about illness.

CLINICIAN: Do you mean to say it would have been better for your wife and daughters to keep your illness a secret?

PATIENT: They could tell me that I had a stomach problem and that I needed some treatment, but they did not need to tell me it was cancer. Even the doctor who knows me well told my wife not to tell me it was cancer but just to say that it was a stomach problem. I went to his office for the treatment. The treatment made me very sick and very tired, so I did not have the energy to do anything. You can do something if you hear you are sick, but when you hear that you have cancer it's like being dead. I would just want to go home and be with my family and then die when it is my time.

CLINICIAN: Of course; and you have such a devoted family, and I heard you have grandchildren, correct?

PATIENT: Yes, five grandchildren.

CLINICIAN: I am going to leave very soon so you can be with your family, but could you just tell me what helped you feel better when you had the illness five years ago?

PATIENT: The doctor gave me some other medication saying that it would make me feel strong again in my mind, and I would be able to get out of bed and do things. So, one morning I got up and it smelled good in the kitchen and I was happy to see that my wife had made a good soup I like. That was the sign that I was feeling stronger again.

CLINICIAN: That is a great description; I bet your wife makes wonderful soups (both clinician and patient turn toward the patient's wife and everyone smiles). Now how are you feeling being here in the hospital?

PATIENT: I know that I have to be here because I have a stomach problem again, and I need some medication but I am very sick, I know.

CLINICIAN: Because it was so difficult when you got sick five years ago we want to make sure that we do things the right way that will help you this time. Would you like the doctors to talk to you about your stomach problem? Or would you like the doctors to talk to your wife and daughters?

PATIENT: No, no, I want them to talk to my wife and to my daughters. They can make all decisions. I don't want to talk to anybody about anything. I'm feeling better, and I don't want to feel like I did five years ago. My wife knows me, and she can talk to the doctors for me. She always talks to the doctors for me, even when I have a cold, or when I have the flu. So, she can talk to them now. I talk to you because you speak my language, but I don't like talking to doctors. So, please tell them.

CLINICIAN: I am so glad we had this conversation, so I will make sure to tell everyone that you want them to talk to your wife. And you said your wife knows you very well, right?

PATIENT: We have been married for 50 years. I hope I can go home soon, because I don't like hospitals. But I know I am very sick.

CLINICIAN: Thank you so much for talking with me and letting me know what's important to you. It was really good meeting you.

PATIENT: Yes, thank you. Please, talk to my wife. She knows.

From the interview, it is clear that the patient had significant difficulty coping with the initial diagnosis of gastric cancer. What the patient described as "a stone fell on my head" appeared to be a metaphor for depression. The patient has a strong opinion about how his initial diagnosis should have been handled. He is clear that he does not wish to be given any direct information by the doctors and that his wife and his daughters should be in charge of those communications. The patient is adamant that he wants to go home and be given some medication to make him feel better. His words to the clinician indicate that he has a sense that he's extremely ill and that his current illness may be related to the original illness. However, he is not willing to confront the situation directly and chooses an avoidant style to protect himself from emotional distress. Therefore, even though he is competent to make decisions, he has decided that he does not wish to make medical decisions, or to be involved in medical decisions. He has chosen to defer decisions to his wife and his daughters.

The palliative care clinician who interviewed the patient stated that the benefit of disclosing information should be weighed against the likely distress it would cause the patient. He commented that his decision to defer to his wife could be understood as an expression of his autonomy and decision-making ability. He recommended a referral to hospice to provide additional support to the patient and the family, allowing the patient to remain home. The wife asked that the word "hospice" not be used, to avoid creating distress for her husband. She was reassured that the word "hospice" did not need to be used and that the program could be described as special support services to receive better care in the home.

At this point, everyone appeared to be in agreement. The patient was referred to hospice, and a hospice admission was arranged for that afternoon. At the end of the day Alvaro was discharged home with hospice care. His wife and daughters were appreciative that his doctors had taken the time to "really understand him" and respect his culture and his values.

ABUSE AND NEGLECT IN SERIOUS ILLNESS AND AT END OF LIFE

Patients with serious illness represent a vulnerable population and may become the victim of abuse. Palliative psychologists have a role in recognizing possible signs and assessing patients and families accordingly. The goal in these complex and challenging situations is to develop an interdisciplinary plan that not only ensures the safety of the patient but also addresses the need for psychological support at a time when they are most vulnerable (Wygant, Bruera, & Hui, 2014).

While many family caregivers are extremely devoted to their loved one, the stresses of living with serious illness can have a disruptive impact on family dynamics. Drug or alcohol use or abuse on the part of a caregiver can increase risk for abusive behavior. In rural communities, where access to resources is limited, family caregivers may become especially isolated and overwhelmed by the task of caregiving.

Patients often become dependent on their spouse or significant other for financial as well as personal care. Therefore, they may be reluctant to report instances of abusive behavior for fear of retaliation, or fear of being sent to a nursing home if it is determined that the home is not safe. The patient may have become more isolated as a result of the abuse, and also from physical and functional deterioration and cognitive deterioration. As a result, they may not be able to access a support network.

The terms "domestic violence" and the more recent "intimate partner violence" (IPV) are often used interchangeably. Intimate partner violence reflects the intent to broaden the understanding of abuse, as possible in any type of intimate relationship. It has been described as "any behavior within an intimate relationship that causes physical, psychological, or sexual harm to those in the relationship" (World Health Organization, 2012, p. 1). It has also been defined as a "pattern of assaultive and coercive behaviors that may include but are not limited to physical injury, psychological abuse, sexual assault, progressive social isolation, economic control, stalking, deprivation, and intimidation, threats to do harm to the individual, their family members, and even their pets."

Victims do not easily report the abuse. Patients who are not specifically asked are not likely to report it (Nelson, Bougatsos, & Blazina, 2012). They may feel shame, self-blame, emotional distress, fear of retaliation, or fear of the stigma of being a victim of abuse. Some only think of physical violence as abuse and may not recognize emotional and verbal abuse.

CASE VIGNETTE 8.3

Brenda is a 63-year-old woman with advanced ovarian cancer. She is admitted to a palliative care unit for management of a recurrent bowel obstruction. The patient had been admitted twice in the past six months, but on those occasions the obstruction had resolved after a few days, and she had been discharged. She is married and has a teenage son. She lives in a rural area about an hour-and-a-half drive from the hospital. Diagnosed with cancer two years prior, she underwent chemotherapy. The oncologist and the nurse thought the patient was pleasant, her mood was optimistic, and her son and husband were supportive. The patient had been on time for all the medical follow-ups with the oncologist and rarely canceled an appointment. During this most recent admission, however, it is noticed that she never receives any visitors. When asked about her husband and her son, she states that her husband works all day with a local contractor and cannot drive the long distance to visit her at the hospital. Brenda states that at night he needs to stay home with their son, but he calls her on the phone every night. However, she appeared sad and withdrawn. The obstruction resolves, but the patient appears frail with some difficulty ambulating. The nurse and social worker are concerned that the patient may not have enough support at home and suggest a home health aide. She patient declines, saying her husband will care for her. When the nurse asks if it would be possible to speak on the phone with her husband, she starts crying and says he is working and they should not bother him. A palliative care consultation is requested, and the palliative care nurse and psychologist meet with the patient.

At the meeting, the patient appears weak, sad, and becomes easily tearful during the conversation. Although she has always been private and unwilling to talk about her husband and her son, she acknowledges that the situation at home is difficult. She shares that her husband lost his job and drives long distances every day just to fill in with different contractors in the area. When asked how her husband is coping emotionally with the stresses of work and her illness, she becomes tearful and says he is angry and stressed out. When the psychologist asks her directly if her husband had ever become abusive toward her or her son, she adamantly denies it and comments, "He doesn't abuse me. He cannot contain his anger, but he has never touched me. It is my role as a wife to help him when he's angry. I just don't have enough strength now."

The palliative psychologist gently explores the meaning of the patient's words. Though her husband has not been physically violent, he often yells at her, blames her illness for all of his difficulties, pounds his fist on the table in anger, and call her names. He often refuses to help her bathe but is unwilling to allow anyone else to help, including a neighbor's wife who has offered. He blames her for his sexual frustration, as they have not been able to have sexual relations since her illness due of her physical discomfort. When asked about the impact of this situation on her son, the patient says he spends most of the time in his room or with friends, and she is careful to not let him know about the marital problems. She explains that her husband and son are close and spend time together on weekends. When asked about any family or friends who could visit her and provide support, the patient shares she has a sister who lives about 20 miles away, but her husband does not like her and does not want her to visit. He also becomes upset if the patient speaks to her sister on the phone, because he is convinced they will criticize him for losing his job. At the end of the meeting the patient comments tearfully, "I know he is not a very good husband, but he is the only support I have." She is aware her disease is worsening and does not want to create more disruption by confronting her husband. The option of a transfer to a facility is explored and, to the team's surprise, the patient readily agrees that this seems to be the best option to "have some peace."

The interview evidenced that Brenda was experiencing verbal and emotional abuse. Additionally, her spouse's refusal to help her bathe or allow for help is a form of neglect. Her prognosis at this point was considered to be in the order of months, and it appeared that a home discharge, even with hospice, may not be the safest option. A report to Adult Protective Services was considered, as the patient was a vulnerable adult due to the advanced disease. However, it was also important not to create a situation that would cause even more distress for this patient, who was rapidly approaching end of life.

With the patient's consent, the palliative care team invited her husband to the hospital to discuss his wife's condition. Obviously upset, initially he demanded that his wife be discharged home. The team shared that unfortunately the disease had progressed, and his wife's prognosis was poor. They also gently approached the topic of caregiving and commented and acknowledged the difficulties he was facing being a primary caregiver for his wife and caring for his son.

It was tactfully mentioned that his wife would continue to deteriorate and that her physical needs would become more urgent and difficult to meet. He reluctantly acknowledged that he had difficulty managing his stress and that his precarious job situation, combined with his wife's illness, created an almost unbearable situation. He tearfully explained feeling that he was failing his family. The team described the option of a transfer to a facility 10 miles from their home, where his wife could receive the care needed. He and his son could visit daily and focus on spending quality time together. The husband agreed and the patient was transferred two days later.

In processing this complex and emotionally challenging case, after the patient's discharge, the clinicians involved in this patient's care expressed feeling relieved that she had not been discharged home but also expressed feelings of sadness about her situation.

Overall, the clinicans felt that everything had been done to honor the patient's wishes and not add to her suffering. They also admitted that the case triggered strong countertransference with wishes to "save" the patient and the son from the difficult home environment, and some expressed difficulty understanding how the patient would consider her husband a source of support.

Patients with advanced disease may have few options for living arrangements, especially if they do not have trusted family members or close friends nearby, or live in rural areas, or have few financial resources. For some patients, the only option to escape the abusive relationship is to leave the home and be transferred to a nursing facility where they may have to remain until their death. This situation may limit the possibility of having other family members visit. In many cases, it is not possible to find an optimal solution that does not involve additional losses for the patient. For this reason, every course of action taken by palliative care clinicians should be the result of careful consideration with identification of available sources of support to minimize patients' distress.

CONFLICT AMONG FAMILY CAREGIVERS AND HEALTH-CARE PROVIDERS

Health-care providers may develop the impression that a patient is being pressured by family members to change medical decisions previously made or to make decisions that are contrary to the patient's preferences. Blackler (2016) defined family pressure or coercion as "occurring when caregivers employ verbal threats, harassment, berating, intimidation, or other manipulative tactics designed to force vulnerable patients to change well-established beliefs or preferences" (p.184). She described a case in which a patient with advanced cancer who had voluntarily signed a DNR decided to rescind it based on pressure from his wife. After much discussion and several changes, the patient agreed to follow the family's wishes and was intubated and in the ICU for two weeks before his death. This case is described as creating moral distress for the ICU staff, who felt the patient's real wishes and preferences were not being honored by the wife.

This kind of scenario is always complex because the patient and family caregiver relationships are affected by many cultural factors and preexisting dynamics within a family—and these are factors often unknown to medical providers. Therefore, when ethical concerns are raised about patient autonomy, it is necessary to fully explore the issues involved and how they are affecting the patient's care and ability to have preferences respected.

If the patient lacks the capacity to make decisions for health care, and it is believed that the family is acting against the patient's best interest by requesting nonstandard medical interventions, ethical and legal steps can be taken to protect the patient. However, if the surrogate decision-maker is requesting lawful medical interventions that are accepted medical practice—which may be accepted by some health-care providers but discouraged by others—the situation can become more complex. The family caregiver charged with making decisions may face real challenges trying to exercise substituted judgment, especially when end-of-life preferences were never discussed (Patel & Ackermann, 2016). In this case, it is even more difficult for family caregivers to separate their personal preferences from those of the family member for whom they are making decisions.

When the patient has the capacity to make decisions, but appears to be placing a family caregiver's preferences ahead of her own, clinicians may feel alarm and anger toward the family. These feelings can create moral distress and a sense of futility in clinicians. Polarizations can occur, with a desire to "save" the patient from what is perceived as a disrespectful and disruptive family caregiver. Thus, the staff may begin relating to the family caregiver as uncompassionate, losing the opportunity to develop alliances and to provide much-needed support.

Palliative psychologists can play an important role in identifying the presence of undue pressure that is damaging the patient by providing in-depth psychological evaluations of complex family dynamics. They can also help clinicians experiencing distress recognize their countertransference.

CASE VIGNETTE 8.4

Paul was a 58-year-old African American man referred to palliative care for emotional support following a diagnosis of cancer of the pancreas metastatic to the liver. The patient had been experiencing weight loss and fatigue for about two months. His primary care physician performed an ultrasound of the abdomen in his office and referred the patient to a local cancer center, where a CT scan confirmed the diagnosis of cancer. Chemotherapy to slow progression of disease was initiated. The patient lived with his wife and two adult children. He also had a daughter from a previous marriage. The relationship between his daughter and his current family was tense and often a source of conflict. The nurses reported to the oncologist that during the first round of chemotherapy the patient cried incessantly and appeared distressed. His wife sat next to him and held his hand quietly. When the nurses approached the wife, she commented that she was worried about her husband and did not know how to help him.

This situation prompted the referral to palliative care, and the patient was referred to the psychologist of the cancer center, who also served as a consultant for the palliative care team. During the first session the patient admitted feeling overwhelmed and anxious about the diagnosis and limited prognosis. He mentioned he would like to learn techniques to relax and manage stress. He also wanted to learn to manage what he described as negative thoughts, which made him feel that there was no reason to pursue treatment. He was struggling with finding the motivation to continue treatment given the limited expected outcome but felt he "had to fight" for his wife and children.

The weekly therapy sessions offered the patient the opportunity to explore his ambivalence about treatment. He was benefiting from self-hypnosis techniques that helped him relax during the chemotherapy session and also at home. On one occasion he expressed the need to "be in control" and "back in charge" because he felt as if everyone else was trying to make decisions about what kind of medical care he should receive. He admitted feeling lost.

The therapist gently raised the issue of advance care planning by saying, "It is normal to feel lost in the medical system; there are so many things happening, so fast, and you are also dealing with the stress of illness and treatment. Some people feel that it is important to let everyone know how they would like to be treated by the doctors if they become so ill that they are unable to speak for themselves. Of course, we all hope that that will not happen to any of us for a very, very long time. However, planning ahead is something that makes some people feel that they can be in charge of what kind of medical procedures they are going to receive if they are so ill that they cannot make decisions."

The session focused on exploring the meaning of decision-making at the end of life, and the patient acknowledged he was worried about his wife and his children fighting over what kind of medical treatments he would receive. The psychologist stated that involving the patient's oncologist, whom he trusted, in this conversation could be beneficial and offered to invite her to one of the next therapy sessions. The patient was agreeable and commented that the doctor would be "coming to my territory," meaning the therapy session, and this made him feel more empowered. The oncologist and the patient's wife joined the following session.

The patient was active in the session, and after much discussion and information sharing with his physician he decided to appoint his wife as his health-care proxy agent. He also decided to sign an advance directive and a living will clarifying that he would not want to receive any life-prolonging treatments such as mechanical ventilation or intubation. He commented that he wanted to ensure that his children would not question his wife's decision and create additional distress for her. At the next therapy session the patient and the psychologist discussed ways that he could talk about his decisions with his children to prevent future problems and ensure everyone would be in agreement. It was decided that the children would be invited to the next therapy session; however, his daughter from a previous marriage refused to be in the same room with his other children. A separate session for the patient and his daughter was scheduled and the patient had the opportunity to discuss his wishes. The following two therapy sessions were focused on allowing the patient to discuss his decisions and his wishes with his children. The sessions were emotional with high levels of grief expressed by all. However, at the end of the session, the patient commented that for the first time since his diagnosis he felt he "could make things happen on my own terms" and also do all he could to minimize additional distress when he would be at the end of his life.

In the case just described, the psychologist took a gentle but active role in facilitating the patient's advance care planning. This process was framed as a way of gaining more sense of control at a time when the patient felt weakest in this regard. The several therapy sessions that followed allowed the patient to not only understand and express his goals and wishes but also experience a deep emotional connection with his children.

References

American Medical Association. (1947). Code of Ethics. In: Encyclopedia of Bioethics, 1995, Vol.5. New York, NY: Simon & Schuster.
American Psychological Association. (2010). *Ethical principles of psychologists and code of conduct*. http://www.apa.org/ethics/code/. Retrieved on January 20, 2017.
American Psychological Association (2013). Guidelines for psychological practice in health care delivery systems. *American Psychologist*, 68(1), 1–6.
Beauchamp, T. L., & Childress, J. F. (2001). *Principles of biomedical ethics* (5th ed.). New York: Oxford University Press.
Billings, J. A. (2011). Terminal extubation of the alert patient. *Journal of Palliative Medicine*, 14(7), 800–801.

Billings, J. A. (2012). Humane terminal extubation reconsidered: The role for preemptive analgesia and sedation. *Critical Care Medicine, 40*(2), 625–630.

Blackler, I. (2016). When families pressure patients to change their wishes. *Journal of Hospice and Palliative Nursing, 18*(4), 184–191.

California Board of Psychology Laws and Regulations. (2015). *California board of psychology*. Charlottesville, VA: LexisNexis.

Campbell, M. L. (2004). Terminal dyspnea and respiratory distress. *Critical Care Clinics, 20*, 403–417.

Ditto, P. H. (2006). Self-determination, substitutive judgment, and the psychology of advanced medical decision making. In J. L. Werth & D. Blevins (Eds.), *Psychosocial issues near the end of life: a resource for professional care providers*. Washington, DC: American Psychological Association.

Freyer, F. J. (2016). When you die, will your wishes be known? *Globe*, May 12, 2016. https://www.bostonglobe.com/metro/2016/05/11/wishes-for-end-life-care-often-ignored-survey-finds/Pna4jQN3V1MqxYKTJWLFaP/story.html. Retrieved on August 16, 2016.

Fritch, J., Petronio, S., Helft, P. R., & Torke, A. (2013). Making decisions for hospitalized older adults: Ethical factors considered by family surrogates. *Journal of Clinical Ethics, 24*(2), 125–134.

Nelson, H. D., Bougatsos, C., & Blazina, I. (2012). Screening women for intimate partner violence: A systematic review to update the US preventive services task force recommendation. *Annals of Internal Medicine, 156*(11), 796–808.

O'Mahoney, S., McHugh, M., Zallman, L., & Selwyn, P. (2003). Ventilator withdrawal: Procedures and outcomes. Report of a collaboration between a critical care division and a palliative care service. *Journal of Pain and Symtpoms Management, 26*, 954–961.

Patel, A. V., & Ackerman, R. J. (2016). Care of patients at the end of life: Surrogate decision making for incapacitated patients. *FP Essentials, 447*, 32–41.

Periyakoil, V. S., Kraemer, H., & Neri, E. (2016). Multi-ethnic attitudes toward physician-assisted death in California and Hawaii. *Journal of Palliative Medicine, 19*(10), 1060–1065.

Sharman, S. J., Garry, M., Jacobson, J. A., Loftus, E. F., & Ditto, P. H. (2008). False memories for end of life decisions. *Health Psychology, 27*(2), 291–296.

Teno, J. M., Gozalo, P. L., Bynum, J. P., Leland, N. E., Miller, S. C., Morden, N. E., ... Mor, V. (2013). Change in end-of-life care for medicare beneficiaries. *JAMA, 309*(5), 470–477.

Werth, J. L., & Kleespies, P. M. (2006). Ethical considerations in providing psychological services in end of life care. In J. L. Werth & D. Blevin (Eds.), *Psychosocial issues near the end of life: a resource for professional care providers*. Washington, DC: American Psychological Association.

World Health Organization. (2012). Intimate partner violence. http://www.apps.who.int/iris/bitstream/10665/77432/1/WHO_RHR_12.36_eng.pdf. Retrieved on October 20, 2016.

Wright, A. A., Keating, N. L., Ayanian, J. Z., Chrischilles, E. A., Kahn, K. L., Ritchie, C. S., ... Landrum, M. B. (2016). Family perspectives on aggressive cancer care near the end of life. *JAMA, 315*(3), 284–292.

Wygant, C., Bruera, E., & Hui, D. (2014). Intimate partner violence in an outpatient palliative care setting. *Journal of Pain and Symptom Management, 47*(4), 806–813.

Index

Page references for figures are indicated by *f*, for tables by *t*, and for boxes by *b*.

abuse, 259–262
Accelerated Recovery Program for Compassion Fatigue (ARP), 24
acute pain, 47, 48*t*
advance care planning, 249–250
advanced disease, 37–43
    case vignette 2.1, 42–43
    constipation, 39
    dyspnea, 37–39
    pain, 39–41, 40*b*, 41*t*, 42*t*
advance directive, 250–251
alienation, 161
alliance, therapeutic, 74
amitriptyline, 54
Analgesic Ladder, WHO, 50, 51*b*
anger, 163
anorexia, 211
anticipatory grief, 84–85, 84*t*
anticonvulsants, 55
antidepressants
    for depression, 95
    for pain, 54
anxiety, 96–102
    case vignette 3.4, 100–102
    clinical presentation, 96–97, 97*t*
    diagnostic considerations, 98–99
    medical causes, 97
    pharmacological treatment, 99–100
    psychological and integrative medicine approaches, 100
    psychosocial and spiritual factors, 98
    spiritual components, 162
APA ethics code, 240
APA *Guidelines for Psychological Practice in Health Care Delivery Systems*, 239
APA multicultural guidelines, 176, 177*t*
assessment
    palliative care, 16–17
    palliative psychology, 68

    areas covered, 70*t*
    characteristics, 69*t*
    depression, 90
    spiritual, 146, 151–152, 154
assessment, family caregivers, 114–117
    culture, 183–185
    family system, 114–115, 116*t*
    needs, 114, 115*t*
    sensitive issues and abusive behaviors, 117
assessment, psychological pain, 43–50, 45*b*
    classification, 47–50
        inferred pathophysiology, 48–49, 49*t*
        onset and duration, 47–48, 48*t*
        pattern, 49–50
    comorbid medical conditions, 44
    comorbid psychiatric conditions, 44
    consequences and impact, 46–47
    intensity, self-report, 44
    meaning attributed to pain, 46
    pathophysiology, inferred, 48–49, 49*t*
    patient distress as clinical target, 44–45
    physical *vs.* psychological pain, 44
    prognosis, 43–44
    psychological factors and psychotherapy interventions, 45–46
atheists, 156–157
attitudes
    competency, 2*b*
    protective, 25, 27*b*
autonomy, patient, 238, 249
    advance directive, 250–251

Baranowsky, A. B., 22
barbiturates, for palliative sedation, 233
barriers to care
    cultural, 180–181, 186–188
    pain management, 40–41, 41*t*
    treatment adherence, 78

268 Index

baseline pain, 49
beneficence, 240–242, 249
benzodiazepines
  for anxiety, 99–100
  for palliative sedation, 233
bereavement
  definition, 84t
  understanding and conceptualization, 124
bereavement care, for family caregivers, 124–130
  clinical features and outcome, 124–125
  complications
    bereavement-related depression, 126–128, 127t
    complicated grief, 125–126
    risk and protective factors, 128–129, 130b
bereavement-related depression, 126–128, 127t
bereavement support, for family caregivers, 130–137
  case vignette 4.2, 134–136
  case vignette 4.3, 136–137
  hospice, 130–131, 131t
  palliative care services, 131, 131t
  plan of care, 131–134
    co-morbid medical and psychiatric conditions, 133
    meeting caregivers where they are, 132–133
    needs and personal grieving style, 134
    protective factors and sources of strength, 133–134
    reassurance, 131–132
Blackler, I., 262
boundaries, psychotherapy, 75–76
breakthrough pain, 49–50
breathing, end-of-life, 224
burnout, professional, 19–20, 242
  therapies for, 23

cachexia, 211
cancer pain, 48
caregiving
  cultural aspects, 183–185
  styles, 111–112
carrier caregiver, 111
Cheyne-Stokes breathing, 224–225
chronic pain, 48, 48t
clinical interview, psychology, 17
codeine, 52
cognitive-behavioral therapy (CBT), 13–14, 60
  for anxiety, 96
  for burnout and compassion fatigue, 23
  for caregivers, 118
  culture and, 194
  for depression, 95
  for pain and distress, 37, 38–39, 45, 57, xxxi
  in psychological care, 67, 68, 81, 100
  in spiritual or religious care, 150–151

collectivist cultures, 178
Comas-Diaz, L., 195
communication
  culturally appropriate, 174, 180, 182t
  language, 241–242
community-based palliative care, 5
comorbidities, medical and psychiatric, 44
compassionate care, 144
  self-compassion practice, 30
compassion fatigue, 21–22, 22b, 24
competence, 244–245
competencies, palliative psychologists, 2
  APA multicultural guidelines, 176, 177t
  cultural aspects of care, 176–181, 177t, 179b
  end-of-life care, 207–208, 208b–209b
  legal and ethical aspects of care, 239–240, 241b
  palliative care, xii
  physical aspects of care, 36–37, 38b
  psychological and psychiatric aspects of care, 66–67, 67b–68b
  social aspects of care, 106–107, 108b
  spiritual, religious, and existential aspects of care, 146–147, 148b
  structure and process of care, 2b
complicated grief, 84t, 125–126
complicated grief therapy, 126
confidentiality, 245–246
conflict, family caregivers and health-care providers, 262–263
  case vignette 8.4, 263–264
consent, end-of-life care, 238–239, 247
constipation, advanced disease, 39
coordination of care, adequate, 8
corticosteroids, 53–54
cost-effectiveness, 7–8
countertransference, 75
cultural aspects of care, 173–201, xxxv
  assessment, 178
  barriers to care, 180–181
  caregiving, 183–185
  case vignette 6.1, 188–190
  case vignette 6.2, 199–201
  collectivist cultures, 178
  communication, 174, 180, 182t
  competencies, 176–181, 177t, 179b
  cultural dimensions of serious illness, 181, 182t
  culture-bound values, medicine and psychology, 190–194, 192t–193t
  decision-making style, 185
  fundamentals, 173–174
  language, 241–242
  medical culture relationship, 182, 184t
  palliative and end-of-life care
    barriers, 186–188
    cultural aggressions, 196–199
  palliative psychotherapy, 194–196, 195t
  prognosis, limited, awareness of, 185–186

self-awareness, psychologists', 180, 180t–181t
social justice issues, 178
sociopolitical context, 181–182, 183t
terminology, 174–176, 174t
cultural competence, 174t, 175
cultural humility, 174t, 176, 195
cultural sensitivity, 174t, 175
culture, 174t, 175
curiosity, 29–30

death, imminent, 221–228. *see also* end-of-life care
case vignette 7.3, 221–222
case vignette 7.4, 222–223
support, patient and family, 223–228, 227b
death rattle, 224–225
decision-making, medical, 248–259
advance care planning, 249–250
advance directive, 250–251
complex scenarios, addressing, 252, 253t–254t
health-care proxy, 251–252
less aggressive care, 248
medical ethics, 248–249
surrogate, 251
decision-making style, cultural, 185
delirium, end-of-life, 228–231
case vignette 7.5, 228–229
diagnosis, 229, 230
etiology, 230–231
hyperactive, 229
hypoactive, 230
management, 230, 231
delivery, palliative care, 3–6
community-based, 5
home-based, 5–6
hospice, 3–4
institution-based, 4–5
demoralization, 146
dependence, physical, opioids, 55–56
depression
advanced illness, 87–96
barriers to diagnosis and treatment, 88–89
clinical presentation, 87–88
diagnostic considerations, 90–93
grief reactions *vs.*, 91, 91t
on patient, family, and caregiver, 88
pharmacological treatment, 94–95
prevalence, by disease, 88
risk factors, 89–90, 89b
suicidal ideation, 93–94, 94b
on trust in physician, 87
bereavement-related, 126–128, 127t
vs. grief, 127, 127t
spiritual components, 162
depth of engagement, 25
desipramine, 54
dexamethasone, 53–54

dignity, patient
meaning and, 72
respect for, 243–244
distress
existential, 145
patient, 44–45
spiritual, religious, and existential, 158–163
alienation, 161
anger, 163
anxiety and depression, 162
case vignette 5.2, 158–161
guilt, 162–163
loss of faith or spiritual beliefs, 161
diversity, 174t, 175
domestic violence, 260
do not resuscitate (DNR) orders, 262
duloxetine, 54
dyspnea, advanced disease, 37–39

economic drivers, 7–8
eighth domain. *see* legal and ethical aspects of care
emotional demands, 24
emotional safety, 112
empathy, 28–29, 77
empowerment, 195, 195t
end-of-life care, 206–235, xxxv
APA on, xxix
competencies, 207–208, 208b–209b
cultural aggressions, 196–197
cultural barriers, 186–190
delirium, 228–231
case vignette 7.5, 228–229
diagnosis, 229, 230
etiology, 230–231
hyperactive, 229
hypoactive, 230
management, 230, 231
family caregiver satisfaction, 113–114
historical perspective, 206
medical context, 213–217
chronic progressive diseases, 213–215
medical–psychological factors interplay, 213, 214t
prognostication, psychological impact, 215–217
patient and family adjustment to, 206–207
psychophysical changes, expected, 209–213
hope for improvement, 210
physical changes, 209t, 210–212
psychological and cognitive changes, 209t, 212–213
refractory symptoms, 233–234, 233b
sedation, palliative, 232–235, 233b
signs of death, 207
transitions and communication, 217–218
case vignette 7.1, 218–220

end-of-life care (cont.)
    case vignette 7.2, 220–221
    when death is imminent, 221–228
        case vignette 7.3, 221–222
        case vignette 7.4, 222–223
        support, patient and family, 223–228, 227b
end of therapy, 76
ethical aspects of care. *see* legal and ethical aspects of care
ethical standards, 244–247
    competence, 244–245
    privacy and confidentiality, 245–246
    record-keeping, 246–247
    therapy, 247
    Universal Declaration of Ethical Principles, 178
ethical standards, psychology, 240–244
    APA ethics code, 240
    beneficence and non-maleficence, 240–242, 249
    fidelity and responsibility, 242–243
    justice, 243, 249
    rights and dignity, respect for, 243–244
ethics code, APA, 240
European Association for Palliative Care (EAPC), xxix
euthanasia, 232
evolution, palliative care models, 9–16
    after cessation of disease-modifying treatments, 9–10, 9f
    case vignette 1.1, 10–13, 12f
    case vignette 1.2, 13–15
    case vignette 1.3, 15–16
existential concepts, 145–146
existential distress, 145
existential psychology, 145
existential psychotherapy, 145–146

faith, loss of, 161
familism, 183
family caregivers, 105–137
    assessment, 114–117
        culture, 183–185
        family system, 114–115, 116t
        needs, 114, 115t
        sensitive issues and abusive behaviors, 117
    bereavement care, 124–130 (*see also* bereavement care, for family caregivers)
    identifying individuals, 105–106
    interventions supporting, 117–124
        case vignette 4.1, 123–124
        family meeting, 118–124 (*see also* family meeting)
        range, 117
        systematic review, 118
    risk and protective factors, 108–114, 109t
        caregiving styles, 111–112
        disease, patient's type, 112
        meaning attributed, 109
        needs assessment, 114–117, 115t
        negative impacts, 110–111
        perceived preparedness, 113–114
        personality traits, 111
        physical, emotional, and social, 111
        positive impacts, 109–110
        prevalence, 108
        roles, 108–109, 109t
        satisfaction with end-of-life care, 113–114
        stress, nursing tasks, 112–113
        symptom control, 113
        training and preparation, 112
family meeting, 118–122, 119t, 120t
    case vignette 4.1, 123–124
    functions and aspects, 118–119, 119t
    goals, 118
    setting, 118
    structure, 120–122, 120t
fentanyl, 52–53
Ferrell, B., 153–154
FICA spiritual tool, 154
fidelity, 242–243
fifth domain. *see* spiritual, religious, and existential aspects of care
Figley, C. R., 21, 22
financial sustainability, 7–8
first domain. *see* structure and process of care
forgiveness, 162, 163
fourth domain. *see* social aspects of care
Frankl, Victor, 31, 148–149

generalist palliative care, xv, xvib
generalist palliative psychology, xxi–xxiii, xxiit
Gentry, J. E., 22
global meaning, 147
goals
    palliative care, xiii
    palliative psychotherapy treatment, 75
God Concept, 155
God Image, 155
God Image Inventory, 155
grief
    anticipatory, 84–85, 84t
    complicated, 84t, 125–126
    definition, 84t
    vs. depression, 127, 127t
    preparatory, 84–85, 84t
grief reactions
    before death, 82–87
        case vignette 3.3, 86–87
        patients and family caregivers, 83
        supporting grieving process, 83, 85–86
        terminology, 83–85, 84t
    in professionals, 30
grieving process, supporting, 85–86

Guidelines for Psychological Practice in Health Care Delivery Systems (APA), 239
guilt, 162–163

half-life, 50–51
health-care proxy, 251–252
history, spiritual, 146, 153–154
home-based palliative care, 5–6
HOPE spiritual history tool, 154
hospice
 bereavement support, 130–131, 131*t*
 palliative care, 3–4
hospitalization, preventing, 6
humility, cultural, 174*t*, 176, 195
hydrocodone, 52
hydromorphone, 52
hyperactive delirium, 229
hypnosis, clinical, 57–59
hypoactive delirium, end-of-life, 230

inquiry, personal, 30
institution-based palliative care, 4–5
interdisciplinary teamwork, 1–2, 17
intimate partner violence, 260

justice
 ethical standards, 243, 249
 social justice, 178

Kent, E. E., 114
Kübler-Ross, Elisabeth, 31, 84

legal and ethical aspects of care, 238–264, xxxv
 abuse and neglect, 259–262
 autonomy, preserving patient, 238, 249
 competencies, 239–240, 241*b*
 conflict, family caregivers and health-care providers, 262–264
 consent, obtaining, 238–239, 247
 ethical standards, 244–247
  competence, 244–245
  privacy and confidentiality, 245–246
  record-keeping, 246–247
  therapy, 247
 ethical standards, psychology, 240–244
  APA ethics code, 240
  beneficence and non-maleficence, 240–242, 249
  fidelity and responsibility, 242–243
  justice, 243, 249
  rights and dignity, 243–244
 medical decision-making, 248–259

advance care planning, 249–250
advance directive, 250–251
 case vignette 8.1, 254–256
 case vignette 8.2, 256–259
 complex scenarios, 252, 253*t*–254*t*
 health-care proxy, 251–252
 less aggressive care, 248
 medical ethics, 248–249
 prognostic disclosures, family requests to withhold, 252–254
 surrogate decision-making, 251
Universal Declaration of Ethical Principles, 178
lone caregiver, 111

manager caregiver, 111
meaning
 attributions, 46, 109
 global, 147
 of the moment, 148
 in palliative psychotherapy, 72
 in psychospiritual care, 147–149
 situational, 147–148
 ultimate, 148
meaning-making, in psychotherapy, 164
Meaning-Making model, 147
medical culture, Western, 190–192
methadone, 53
microaggressions, 196
microassaults, 196
microinsults, 197
microinvalidations, 197
midazolam, for palliative sedation, 233
Mindfulness-Based Stress Reduction, 23
mixed pain syndromes, 49
morphine, 52
mourning, 84*t*
multicultural focus, 74, 174*t*, 175
multiculturalism, 174*t*, 175

nausea and vomiting
 from opioids, 56
 refractory, palliative sedation, 233
needs assessment, family caregiver, 114–117, 115*t*
neglect, 259–262
neuropathic pain, 48–49, 49*t*
nociceptive pain, 48, 49*t*
non-maleficence, 240–242, 249
nortriptyline, 54

OPEN-INVITE tool, 154
openness, 29–30
opiates, 51
opioids, 51–53
 adverse effects, 55–57

opioids (cont.)
  nausea and vomiting, 56
  patient and family concerns, 55
  physical dependence, 55–56
  psychoeducation, 55
  respiratory depression, 56
  sedation, 56–57
  tolerance, 55
 drug class, 51–52
 fentanyl, 52–53
 hydrocodone and codeine, 52
 hydromorphone, 52
 methadone, 53
 morphine, 52
 opium, 51
 oxycodone and oxymorphone, 52
 strong, 50
 weak, 50
opium, 51
opportunities, palliative psychology, 17–18
outcomes, palliative care, 6–8
oxycodone, 52
oxymorphone, 52

pagans, 157–158
pain. *see also specific topics*
 advanced disease, 39–41, 40b, 41t, 42t
 consequences and impact, 46–47
 intensity, self-report, 44
 meaning attributed, 46
 physical *vs.* psychological, 44
 psychological and existential, 45–46
 psychotherapy interventions, 45–46
 Total Pain, 4
pain classification, 47–50
 acute, 47, 48t
 breakthrough, 49–50
 cancer, 48
 chronic, 48, 48t
 inferred pathophysiology, 48–49, 49t
 mixed pain syndromes, 49
 neuropathic, 48–49, 49t
 nociceptive, 48, 49t
 onset and duration, 47–48, 48t
 pattern, 49–50
  baseline, 49
  breakthrough, 49–50
pain management
 barriers
  health-care-provider-related, 40–41, 41t
  patient-related, 40, 41t
  social and cultural, 41, 41t
 case vignette 2.2, 59–61
 case vignette 2.3, 61–63
 clinical hypnosis, 57–59
 Joint Commission standards, 39

 psychological assessment, scenarios requiring, 41, 42t
  case vignette, 42–43
 undertreated, consequences, 40, 40b
pain management, pharmacological, 50–63. *see also specific agents*
 adjuvant medication, 53–55
 anticonvulsants, 55
 antidepressants
  selective serotonin reuptake inhibitors, 54
  serotonin-norepinephrine reuptake inhibitors, 54
  tricyclic, 54
 corticosteroids, 53–54
 non-opioids, 50
 opioids, 50, 51–53, 55–57
 pharmacodynamics, 50
 pharmacokinetics, 50–51
 WHO Analgesic Ladder, 50, 51b
palliative care
 bereavement support, 131, 131t
 care delivery systems, xiii–xiv
 competencies, xii
 consultation model, xiii
 core principles, xiv
 definition, xi–xiv
 domains, xii, xiiib
 generalist, xv, xvib
 goal, xiii
 historical perspective, xi
 interdisciplinary model, xiii
 pediatrics, xiv
 philosophy, xii–xiii
 quality of life, xiii
 scope, 4
 specialist, xv–xvi, xvib
 stresses, of living with illness, xvi–xviii
palliative psychology. *see also specific topics*
 contributions, xxx–xxxi, xxxiit
 definition, xx
 domains, as specialist-level competency framework, xxxi–xxxiii
 generalist level, xxi–xxv, xxiit
 research fellowships, xxviii
 specialist, xxv–xxvi, xxviit–xxviiit
 as specialty, case for, xviii–xxi
 training, xxvi–xxx
palliative sedation, 232–235, 233b
partner caregiver, 111–112
Patient Self-Determination Act of 1991, 249
periodic breathing, 224
Persistent Complex Bereavement Disorder (PCBD), 84t, 125–126
personal inquiry, 30
pharmacodynamics, 50
pharmacokinetics, 50–51
pharmacological therapy

pain, 50–63 (*see also* pain management, pharmacological)
psychological (*see* psychopharmacology)
physical aspects of care, 35–63, xxxiv. *see also specific topics*
　advanced disease, 37–43
　　case vignette 2.1, 42–43
　　constipation, 39
　　dyspnea, 37–39
　　pain, 39–41, 40b, 41t, 42t
　assessment, psychological pain, 43–50, 45b
　fundamentals, 35–36
　pain management, pharmacological, 50–63
　symptom clusters, 36
physical dependence, opioids, 55–56
physical safety, 112
physician assisted dying (suicide), 232
pluralism, 195–196, 195t
positive mental and emotional states, conscious, 29
post-traumatic stress disorder symptoms, professional caregiver, 20, 21–22
preparation, family caregiver, 112
preparatory grief, 84–85, 84t
presence, therapeutic, 25
present-focused orientation, 30
privacy, 245–246
Professional Quality of Life Test (Pro-QOL), 24
professional self-care. *see* self-care, professional
prognosis, 43–44
　disclosures, family requests to withhold, 252–254
　prognostication, psychological impact, 215–217
prolonged grief disorder, 84t, 125–126
protective attitudes, 25, 27b
psychological and psychiatric aspects of care, 65–102, xxxiv. *see also specific topics*
　anxiety, 96–102
　assessment, 68, 69t, 70t
　competencies, 66–67, 67b–68b
　depression, 87–96
　grief reactions, before death, 82–87, 84t
　psychopharmacology, 77–82
　psychotherapy, palliative, 68–77
　　fundamentals, 68–73, 71t–72t
　　process and content, 73–77
psychology
　culture, Western, 190–194, 192t–193t
　etymology, 163
psychopharmacology
　anxiety, 99–100
　depression, 94–95
　role, palliative psychologist, 77–82
　　barriers to treatment adherence, 78
　　integrative care plan, 79–80
　　level1 (generalist), 78, 79t
　　level2 (specialist), 78–79, 79t
　　level3 (licensed psychologist), 78

psychospiritual care, patient and family, 147–151
　case vignette 5.1, 149–151
　historical perspective, 147
　meaning in, 147–149
psychostimulants, 95
psychotherapy. *see also specific types*
　boundaries, 75–76
　etymology, 163
　existential, 145–146
　Western culture, 190–194, 192t–193t
psychotherapy, palliative, 68–77
　culturally appropriate and relevant, 194–196, 195t
　dignity and meaning, 72
　fundamentals, 68–73, 71t–72t
　meaning and purpose, 72
　patient and family needs and therapy, 72–73
　principles, 68–69, 71t–72t
　process and content, 74–77
　　boundaries, 75–76
　　countertransference, 75
　　end of therapy, 76
　　multicultural focus, 74
　　ruptures, 75
　　single-session and short-term psychotherapy, 77
　　therapeutic alliance, 74
　　therapeutic setting, 74
　　treatment goals, negotiating, 75
　psychological factors and, 45–46
Puchalski, C. M., 153–154

quality of life, 4, 6, 7, 9, 36, 37, 40, xiii. *see also specific domains*

record-keeping, ethical, 246–247
reflection, ongoing, 31
reflexivity, 195, 195t
refractory symptoms, palliative sedation, 233–234, 233b
religion
　on cancer symptoms, 144
　definition, 145
　importance, 144
　patient *vs.* family views of, 144
respiratory depression, opioids, 56
responsibility, 242–243
rights, 243–244
role, palliative psychologist, 77–82
　case vignette 3.1, 80–81
　case vignette 3.2, 81–82
ruptures, 75

Saunders, Cecily, 4
screening, spiritual, 146, 152–153

second domain. *see* physical aspects of care
sedation
  opioids, 56–57
  palliative, 232–235, 233*b*
selective serotonin reuptake inhibitors (SSRIs)
  for depression, 95
  for pain, 54
self-awareness, 30
self-care, professional, 19–31
  burnout, 19–20, 23, 242
  compassion fatigue, 21–22, 22*b*, 24
  ethical imperative, 19–22
  interventions, 23–24
  post-traumatic stress disorder, 20
  risk and protective factors, 24–31, 26*t*–27*t*
    clinical complexity and system-related limitations, 26*t*
    complex cases, pressure to fix or resolve, 26*t*, 28
    curiosity and openness, 29–30
    demonstrating added value, pressure, 26*t*, 28
    depth of engagement, 25
    emotional demands, 24
    empathy, 28–29
    intensity of pace, family dynamics, and preexisting conditions, 25
    interdisciplinary team dynamics, 26*t*, 28
    length of treatment, 25
    ongoing reflection, 31
    positive mental and emotional states, conscious, 29
    present-focused orientation, 30
    protective attitudes, 25, 27*b*
    self-awareness and personal inquiry, 30
    self-compassion practice, 30
    self-empathy, 29
    self-knowledge, 29
    staff psychological support, 26*t*, 28
    therapeutic presence, 25
    therapeutic relationship, 24–25
self-compassion practice, 30
self-empathy, 29
self-knowledge, 29
serotonin-norepinephrine reuptake inhibitors (SNRIs)
  for depression, 95
  for pain, 54
setting, therapeutic, 74
seventh domain. *see* end-of-life care
situational meaning, 147–148
Smith-Stoner, M., 158
social aspects of care, 105–137, xxxiv. *see also specific topics*
  competencies, 106–107, 108*b*
  family caregivers, 105–137 (*see also* family caregivers)
    bereavement care, 124–130

    bereavement support, 130–137
    identifying, 105–106
    interventions supporting, 117–124
    risk and protective factors, 108–117, 109*t*
  palliative care team approach, 106
social justice issues, 178
social safety, 112
specialist palliative care, xv–xvi, xvi*b*
specialist palliative psychology, xxv–xxvi, xxvii*t*–xxviii*t*
specialized support, xiii
spiritual, religious, and existential aspects of care, 143–169, xxxiv–xxxv
  in atheists, 156–157
  clinical considerations, 154–156
  competencies, 146–147, 148*b*
  definitions, 145
  distress manifestations, 158–163
    alienation, 161
    anger, 163
    anxiety and depression, 162
    case vignette 5.2, 158–161
    guilt, 162–163
    loss of faith or spiritual beliefs, 161
  duration, 143
  fundamentals, 143–146
  in pagans and Wiccans, 157–158
  palliative psychology session, spirituality in, 163–169
    case vignette 5.3, 165–168
    case vignette 5.4, 168–169
    meaning-making, 164
    patient autonomy, 238, 249
    screening and history, 164
    therapeutic space, 163–164
  psychospiritual care, patient and family, 147–151
    case vignette 5.1, 149–151
    historical perspective, 147
    meaning in, 147–149
  spiritual assessment, 146, 151–152, 154
  spiritual history, 146, 153–154
  spiritual screening, 146, 152–153
spiritual beliefs, loss of, 161
spirituality
  on cancer symptoms, 144
  definition, 145
  importance, 144
  patient *vs.* family views of, 144
spiritual suffering, 144
staff psychological support, 26*t*, 28
stimulants, 95
stress
  caregiver, xvii–xviii
  caregiver nursing tasks, 112–113
  living with illness, xvi–xviii
structure and process of care, 1–31, xxxiii
  assessment, 16–17

competencies, 2b
delivery, U.S., 3–6
  community-based, 5
  home-based, 5–6
  hospice, 3–4
  institution-based, 4–5
evolution of palliative care models, 9–16
  after cessation of disease-modifying treatments, 9–10, 9f
  case vignette 1.1, 10–13, 12f
  case vignette 1.2, 13–15
  case vignette 1.3, 15–16
opportunities, 17–18
outcomes, 6–8
self-care, professional, 19–31
  ethical perspectives, 19–22
  interventions, 23–24
  risk and protective factors, 24–31, 26t–27t
teamwork, interdisciplinary, 1–2
Sue, D. W., 194
suffering
  factors, 35–36
  preventing, 35
  spiritual, 144
suicidal ideation, 93–94, 94b
symptom control, 113

teamwork, interdisciplinary, 1–2, 17
Temel, J. S., 6–7
Teno, J. M., 6
therapeutic alliance, 74
therapeutic presence, 25
therapeutic relationship, 24–25
therapeutic setting, 74
therapy. *see also* psychotherapy; *specific types*
  ethical standards, 247
third domain. *see* psychological and psychiatric aspects of care
tolerance, opioids, 55
Total Pain, 4
training
  family caregiver, 112
  palliative psychology, xxvi–xxx
traumatization, vicarious, 21–22, 22b
tricyclic antidepressants, 54

ultimate meaning, 148
Universal Declaration of Ethical Principles, 178

venlafaxine, 54
vicarious traumatization, 21–22, 22b

white privilege, 176
WHO Analgesic Ladder, 50, 51b
Wiccans, 157–158

Made in United States
Orlando, FL
12 December 2025